Frontiers in Cardiology for
The Eighties

Proceedings of an Advanced International Course on Selected Topics held at Punta Ala,
Italy, on 14th to 18th September, 1981

Frontiers in Cardiology for The Eighties

Edited by

L. DONATO and A. L'ABBATE

Institute of Patologia Medica,
University of Pisa and Institute of
Clinical Physiology, CNR, Pisa, Italy

ACADEMIC PRESS 1984

(Harcourt Brace Jovanovich, Publishers)

London Orlando San Diego San Francisco New York
Toronto Montreal Sydney Tokyo São Paulo

ACADEMIC PRESS INC. (LONDON) LTD.
24–28 OVAL ROAD
LONDON NW1

United States Edition published by
ACADEMIC PRESS INC.
(Harcourt Brace Jovanovich, Inc.)
Orlando, Florida 32887

British Library Cataloguing in Publication Data

Frontiers in cardiology for the eighties.
  1. Cardiology
  I. Donato, L. A.   II. L'Abbate, A.
  616.1'2   RC681
  ISBN 0-12-220680-0
  LCCCN 83-71683

Typeset by Oxford Verbatim Limited
Printed in Great Britain by Galliard (Printers) Ltd, Great Yarmouth

Contributors

R. ABBATE
Department of Internal Medicine, University of Florence, Viale Morgagni, 85, 50134 Florence, Italy

A. AGOSTONI
Clinica Medica VII, Ospedale "S. Paolo", University of Milan, Via di Rudini, 8, 20142 Milan, Italy

B. R. BARBER
Institute of Clinica Medica I, Padiglione Granelli, University of Milan, Via F. Sforza, 35, 20122 Milan, Italy

C. BARLASSINA
Institute of Clinica Medica I, Padiglione Granelli, University of Milan, Via F. Sforza, 35, 20122 Milan, Italy

G. BAROLDI
Institute of Clinical Physiology, CNR, Via Savi, 8, 56100 Pisa, Italy

A. BARTOLETTI
Department of Internal Medicine, University of Florence, Viale Morgagni, 85, 50134 Florence, Italy

A. BENASSI
Institute of Clinical Physiology, CNR, Via Savi, 8, 56100 Pisa, Italy

D. BEN-ISHAY
Internal Medicine Department, Hadassah Medical Organization, University Hospital, Mount Scopus, 91240 Jerusalem, Israel

H. H. BENTALL
Royal Postgraduate Medical School, University of London, Cardiothoracic Unit, Department of Surgery, Hammersmith Hospital, Ducane Road, London W12 OHS, UK

A. BIAGINI
Institute of Clinical Physiology, CNR, Via Savi, 8, 56100 Pisa, Italy

G. BIANCHI
Institute of Clinica Medica I, Padiglione Granelli, University of Milan, Via F. Sforza, 35, 20122 Milan, Italy

C. BRESCHI
Department of Internal Medicine, University of Florence, Viale Morgagni, 85, 50134 Florence, Italy

P. CAMICI
Institute of Patologia Medica, University of Pisa and Institute of Clinical Physiology, CNR, Via Savi, 8, 56100 Pisa, Italy

C. CARPEGGIANI
Institute of Clinical Physiology, CNR, Via Savi, 8, 56100 Pisa, Italy

CH.-H. CHALANT
Department of Cardiovascular Surgery, University Clinic St. Luc, UCL, 10 Hippocrate Avenue, 1200 Brussels, Belgium

S. CHIERCHIA
Cardiovascular Research Unit, Royal Postgraduate Medical School, Hammersmith Hospital, Ducane Road, London W12 OHS, UK

G. CROSS
Clinical Research Centre, Division of Bioengineering, Watford Road, Harrow, Middlesex HA1 3VJ, UK

D. CUSI
Institute of Clinica Medica I, Padiglione Granelli, University of Milan, Via F. Sforza, 35, 20122 Milan, Italy

P. DARIO
Centro "E. Piaggio", Faculty of Engineering and Institute of Clinical Physiology, CNR, Via Savi, 8, 56100 Pisa, Italy

D. DE ROSSI
Centro "E. Piaggio", Faculty of Engineering and Institute of Clinical Physiology, CNR, Via Savi, 8, 56100 Pisa, Italy

A. DISTANTE
Institute of Patologia Medica, University of Pisa and Institute of Clinical Physiology, CNR, Via Savi, 8, 56100 Pisa, Italy

C. T. DOLLERY
Royal Postgraduate Medical School, University of London, Department of Clinical Pharmacology, Hammersmith Hospital, Ducane Road, London W12 OHS, UK

L. DONATO
Institute of Patologia Medica, University of Pisa and Institute of Clinical Physiology, CNR, Via Savi, 8, 56100 Pisa, Italy

T. A. H. ENGLISH
Cardiac Surgical Unit, Papworth Hospital, Papworth Everard, Cambridge, CB3 8RE, UK

S. FAVILLA
Department of Internal Medicine, University of Florence, Viale Morgagni, 85, 50134 Florence, Italy

P. FERRARI
Institute of Clinica Medica 1, Padiglione Granelli, University of Milan, Via F. Sforza, 35, 20122 Milan, Italy

F. FRANCONI
Department of Pharmacology and Toxicology, University of Florence, Viale Morgagni, 65, 50134 Florence, Italy

L. GATTINONI
Institute of Anesthesia and Reanimation, Polyclinic Hospital, University of Milan, Via F. Sforza, 35, 20122 Milan, Italy

G. F. GENSINI
Department of Internal Medicine, University of Florence, Viale Morgagni, 85, 50134 Florence, Italy

S. GHIONE
Institute of Clinical Physiology, CNR, Via Savi, 8, 56100 Pisa, Italy

A. GIOTTI
Department of Pharmacology and Toxicology, University of Florence, Viale Morgagni, 65, 50134 Florence, Italy

S. GOLDSTEIN
Henry Ford Hospital, 2799 West Grand Boulevard, Detroit, Michigan 48202, USA

M. GUAZZI
Institute of Cardiology, University of Milan, Cardiovascular Research Centre CNR, Via Parea, 4, 20138 Milan, Italy

P. G. HUGENHOLTZ
Department of Cardiology, Thoraxcentre, University Hospital, Erasmus University, Postbox 1738, 3000 DR Rotterdam, The Netherlands

D. G. JULIAN
Department of Cardiology, Freeman Hospital, University of Newcastle upon Tyne, Newcastle upon Tyne NE7 7DN, UK

R. L. KINLOUGH-RATHBONE
Department of Pathology, McMaster University, 1200 Main Street West, Hamilton, Ontario, L8N 3Z5, Canada

M. B. KNUDSON
Cardiac Pacemakers Inc., 4100 North Hamline Avenue, PO Box 43079, St Paul, Minnesota 55164, USA

R. KREBS
Bayer AG, Pharma Research Centre, Department of Medicine, Aprater Weg. 5600, Wuppertal I, West Germany

A. L'ABBATE
Institute of Patologia Medica, University of Pisa and Institute of Clinical Physiology, CNR, Via Savi, 8, 56100 Pisa, Italy

L. LANDINI
Institute of Electronics, Faculty of Engineering, University of Pisa and Institute of Clinical Physiology, CNR, Via Savi, 8, 56100 Pisa, Italy

J. R. LANDIS
Henry Ford Hospital, 2799 West Grand Boulevard, Detroit, Michigan 48202, USA

A. LANTIS
Henry Ford Hospital, 2799 West Grand Boulevard, Detroit, Michigan 48202, USA

M. LAZZARI
Institute of Clinical Physiology, CNR, Via Savi, 8, 56100 Pisa, Italy

F. LEDDA
Department of Pharmacology and Toxicology, University of Florence, Viale Morgagni, 65, 50134 Florence, Italy

R. LEIGHTON
Henry Ford Hospital, 2799 West Grand Boulevard, Detroit, Michigan 48202, USA

D. LEVANTESI
Institute of Clinical Physiology, CNR, Via Savi, 8, 56100 Pisa, Italy

L. H. LIGHT
Clinical Research Centre, Division of Bioengineering, Watford Road, Harrow, Middlesex HA1 3VJ, UK

P. LUPI
Institute of Clinica Medica I, Padiglione Granelli, University of Milan, Via F. Sforza, 35, 20122 Milan, Italy

G. MANCIA
Institute of Clinica Medica IV, University of Milan and Centre of Clinical Physiology and Hypertension, Ospedale Maggiore, Via F. Sforza, 35, 20122 Milan, Italy

L. MANTELLI
Department of Pharmacology and Toxicology, University of Florence, Viale Morgagni, 65, 50134 Florence, Italy

C. MARCHESI
Institute of Clinical Physiology, CNR, Via Savi, 8, 56100 Pisa, Italy

M. MARZILLI
Institute of Patologia Medica, University of Pisa and Institute of Clinical Physiology, CNR, Via Savi, 8, 56100 Pisa, Italy

P. MARZULLO
Institute of Clinical Physiology, CNR, Via Savi, 8, 56100 Pisa, Italy

A. MASERI
Cardiovascular Research Unit, Royal Postgraduate Medical School, University of London, Hammersmith Hospital, Ducane Road, London W12 0HS, UK

G. MASOTTI
Department of Internal Medicine, University of Florence, Viale Morgagni, 85, 50134 Florence, Italy

M. G. MAZZEI
Institute of Clinical Physiology, CNR, Via Savi, 8, 56100 Pisa, Italy

A. MEARNS
Royal Infirmary, Bradford 9, UK

P. MEYER
INSERM U7/CNRS LA 318, Department of Nephrology, Hôpital Necker, 161 Rue de Sèvres, 75015 Paris, France

C. MICHELASSI
Institute of Clinical Physiology, CNR, Via Savi, 8, 56100 Pisa, Italy

J. G. MILLER
Laboratory for Ultrasonics, Department of Physics, Washington University, St Louis, Missouri 63130, USA

P. MONTORSI
Institute of Cardiology, University of Milan, Cardiovascular Research Centre, CNR, Via Parea, 4, 20138 Milan, Italy

M. A. MORALES
Institute of Clinical Physiology, CNR, Via Savi, 8, 56100 Pisa, Italy

E. MOSCARELLI
Institute of Clinical Physiology, CNR, Via Savi, 8, 56100 Pisa, Italy

A. MUGELLI
Department of Pharmacology and Toxicology, University of Florence, Viale Morgagni, 65, 50134 Florence, Italy

J. F. MUSTARD
Department of Pathology, McMaster University, 1200 Main Street West, Hamilton, Ontario, L8N 3Z5, Canada

G. G. NERI SERNERI
Department of Internal Medicine, University of Florence, Viale Morgagni, 85, 50134 Florence, Italy

E. O'BRIEN
Department of Clinical Pharmacology, Royal College of Surgeons in Ireland, St Stephen's Green, Dublin 2 and The Blood Pressure Clinic, The Charitable Infirmary, Jervis Street, Dublin I, Ireland

W. O'CALLAGAN
Department of Clinical Pharmacology, Royal College of Surgeons in Ireland, St Stephen's Green, Dublin 2 and The Blood Pressure Clinic, The Charitable Infirmary, Jervis Street, Dublin I, Ireland

K. O.'MALLEY
Department of Clinical Pharmacology, Royal College of Surgeons in Ireland, St Stephen's Green, Dublin 2 and The Blood Pressure Clinic, The Charitable Infirmary, Jervis Street, Dublin I, Ireland

M. A. PACKHAM
Department of Biochemistry, University of Toronto, Toronto, Ontario, Canada

C. Palombo
Institute of Clinical Physiology, CNR, Via Savi, 8, 56100 Pisa, Italy

A. Panetta
*Department of Internal Medicine, University of Florence, Viale Morgagni,
85, 50134 Florence, Italy*

M. Paoletti
Institute of Clinical Physiology, CNR, Via Savi, 8, 56100 Pisa, Italy

O. Parodi
Institute of Clinical Physiology, CNR, Via Savi, 8, 56100 Pisa, Italy

C. Patrono
*Department of Pharmacology, Catholic University, School of Medicine,
Via della Pineta Sacchetti 644, 00168 Rome, Italy*

G. Pelosi
Institute of Clinical Physiology, CNR, Via Savi, 8, 56100 Pisa, Italy

D. J. Phillips
*Department of Surgery, University of Washington, Seattle, Washington
98195, USA*

E. Picano
Institute of Clinical Physiology, CNR, Via Savi, 8, 56100 Pisa, Italy

L. Poggesi
*Department of Internal Medicine, University of Florence, Viale Morgagni,
85, 50134 Florence, Italy*

E. Polli
*Institute of Clinica Medica I, Padiglione Granelli, University of Milan, Via
F. Sforza, 35, 20122 Milan, Italy*

D. Prisco
*Department of Internal Medicine, University of Florence, Viale Morgagni,
85, 50134 Florence, Italy*

A. K. Ream
*Department of Anesthesia, Institute of Engineering Design in Medicine,
Stanford University Medical Center, Stanford, California 94305, USA*

G. Ritter
*Henry Ford Hospital, 2799 West Grand Boulevard, Detroit, Michigan
48202, USA*

D. Rovai
Institute of Clinical Physiology, CNR, Via Savi, 8, 56100 Pisa, Italy

F. Sabino
Institute of Clinical Physiology, CNR, Via Savi, 8, 56100 Pisa, Italy

R. Saracci
Section of Epidemiology and Biostatistics, Institute of Clinical Physiology, CNR, Pisa, Italy. Present address: International Agency for Research on Cancer, 150 Cours A. Thomas, 69008 Lyon, France

A. P. Selwyn
Royal Postgraduate Medical School, University of London, Cardiovascular Research Unit, MRC Cyclotron Unit, Hammersmith Hospital, Ducane Road, London W12 OHS, UK

R. Serokman
Henry Ford Hospital, 2799 West Grand Boulevard, Detroit, Michigan 48202, USA

S. Severi
Institute of Clinical Physiology, CNR, Via Savi, 8, 56100 Pisa, Italy

J. E. Shapland, II
Cardiac Pacemakers Inc., 4100 North Hamline Avenue, PO Box 43079, St Paul, Minnesota 55164, USA

I. Simonetti
Institute of Patologia Medica, University of Pisa and Institute of Clinical Physiology, CNR, Via Savi, 8, 56100 Pisa, Italy

G. Soots
Regional Hospital Center and University of Lille, Department of Cardiovascular Surgery A, Hospital of Cardiology, Boulevard du Professeur J. Leclercq, 59037 Lille Cedex, France

D. E. Strandness jr
Department of Surgery, University of Washington, Seattle, Washington 98195, USA

B. Taccardi
Institute of General Physiology and "Centro Simes", University of Parma, Via Gramsci, 4, 43100 Parma, Italy

R. Testa
Institute of Clinical Physiology, CNR, Via Savi, 8, 56100 Pisa, Italy

M. G. TRIVELLA
Institute of Clinical Physiology, CNR, Via Savi, 8, 56100 Pisa, Italy

F. UNGER
Surgical Clinic I, University of Innsbruck, Anichstrasse, 35, 6020 Innsbruck, Austria

C. M. VASU
Henry Ford Hospital, 2799 West Grand Boulevard, Detroit, Michigan 48202, USA

G. VALLI
Institute of Clinical Physiology, CNR, Via Savi 8, 56100 Pisa, Italy

G. VEZZOLI
Institute of Clinica Medica I, Padiglione Granelli, University of Milan, Via F. Sforza, 35, 20122 Milan, Italy

G. WEBER
Centre of Research on Atherosclerosis, Institute of Pathological Anatomy, University of Siena, Via Laterino, 8, 53100 Siena, Italy

D. R. R. WILLIAMS
University Department of Community Medicine, Addenbrooke's Hospital, Hills Road, Cambridge CB2 2QQ, UK

R. W. WISSLER
Department of Pathology and Specialized Center of Research in Athero-sclerosis, The University of Chicago, 950 East 59th Street, Chicago, Illinois 60637, USA

A. ZANCHETTI
Institute of Clinica Medica IV, University of Milan and Centre of Clinical Physiology and Hypertension, Ospedale Maggiore, Via F. Sforza, 35, 20122 Milan, Italy

Preface

When Bayer Italia expressed their idea of promoting a high level scientific initiative in the field of cardiology, we were initially rather sceptical.

We live in a time in which we have probably too many meetings and too many courses: these are not always scientifically or professionally rewarding.

However, thinking it over and discussing it with other people in our Institute, we gradually developed the idea on which this advanced course is based. The idea that the forefront of cardiology has been recently moving at such a fast pace, that even the most advanced groups in one field often lose track of what is happening next door, busy as they are following the progress of their subdiscipline. A classic example of this strabic attitude is the field of ischaemic heart disease with respect to that of hypertension. Different meetings, different societies, separate experts keep their own respective internal discussion going, despite the large overlap of the two diseases in epidemiological, pathophysiological and clinical terms. We thought therefore that it might be worth trying to identify a series of topics that usually live a separate life, but are *de facto* largely interdependent, and to have a range of experts discussing the new ideas, the new problems and the new perspectives in the common environment of the same meeting.

For their epidemiological dimensions and for the impact of changing concepts we chose arterial hypertension and ischaemic heart disease. Then, we thought it important to discuss new trends in the two types of intervention in cardiology: surgery and drugs. Finally it seemed important to devote a full day to discuss what can be expected from the technological revolution that is in progress today. It is not so common to have, in the same meeting, such a distinguished group of experts in the field of clinical and experimental cardiology, cardiac surgery, epidemiology, biophysics and bioengineering. For us, it was also one more way of testing the hypothesis on which our Institute in Pisa was built and operates, with its multilevel and multidisciplinary approach to cardiology.

We wish to thank our colleagues from the Royal Postgraduate Medical School and from the Division of Cardiovascular Medicine of the Henry Ford Hospital in Detroit for their help in preparing the programmes.

We wish to thank several people who worked for this programme, but particularly Mrs Hilda de Ruyter Biagini for her dedication and efficiency, both during the meeting and the preparation of the Proceedings, and Dr A. Biagini for his great help in the review of the galley proofs.

Finally of course we wish to thank particularly Bayer Italia for making all this possible with unrivalled generosity and for their true scientific intent, documented by the total freedom they gave us.

August 1983   *Luigi Donato*
                                                    Antonio L'Abbate

Contents

II. Advances in the Pathophysiology of Ischaemic Heart Disease

III. Progress in Clinical Pharmacology

IV. Perspectives in Heart Surgery and Extracorporeal Assistance

V. The Clinical Perspectives of
New Technologies

I. Advances in the Pathophysiology of Hypertension

Genetic Markers in Hypertension

P. MEYER

National Institute of Health and Medical
Research (INSERM), National Centre of
Scientific Research (CNRS),
Department of Nephrology, Hôpital
Necker, Paris, France

The genetic transmission of essential (or primary) hypertension primarily suggested by its familial aggregation, is now established by several clinical and animal studies. On the other hand, primary hypertension appears to result also from environmental factors, particularly from an excess of alimentary sodium. The disease appears thus to be a multifactorial process, a gene–environmental interaction.

Genetically hypertensive rats (SHR) have diffuse membrane changes which appear to be primary and involved in the mechanism of the disease as they result in an increased permeability to external Na^+. One of them is a deficiency in an outward Na^+,K^+-cotransport system which can easily be demonstrated in erythrocyte membranes.

A similar change affects red blood cell membranes in human essential hypertension. In our laboratory, Na^+ outward cotransport values were found to be 463 ± 126 and 200 ± 137 in 98 normotensives and 139 hypertensives respectively. This change appeared specific of essential hypertension and genetically determined, as it was observed in almost 50% of the children born of hypertensive parents. Most of them, aged less than 40 years, were normotensives. The low cotransport value, since it was found both in SHR and adult subjects with essential hypertension, may indicate a

Frontiers Cardiol. for the 80s.
0-12-220680-0

genetic propensity to develop hypertension with aging. It may thus have the characteristics of a biochemical marker allowing a selective prevention, salt restriction being recommanded to low cotransport patients.

Investigation of the Na^+ transport systems in erythrocyte membrane, which are genetically determined, has already been shown to be of interest in endogenous bipolar psychosis and in familial obesity. Essential hypertension represents an additional field for clinical investigation. A particular interest arises from the fact that the membrane alteration is probably involved in the pathogenesis of the disease.

Bibliography

Garay, R. P. and Meyer, P. (1979). *Lancet* **i**, 349.

Garay, R. P., De Mendonca, M., Elghozi, J. L., Devynck, M. A., Dagher, G., Pernollet, M. G., Grichois, M. L., Ben-Ishay, D. and Meyer, P. (1979). *Clin. Sci. mol. Med.* **57**, 329s.

Garay, R. P. and Meyer, P. (1979). *C. r. Acad. Sci. Paris* **288D**, 453.

Garay, R. P., Elghozi, J. L., Dagher, G. and Meyer, M. (1980). *New Engl. J. Med.* **302**, 769.

Garay, R. P., Dagher, G., Pernollet, M. G., Devynck, M. A. and Meyer, P. (1980). *Nature* **284**, 281.

De Mendonca, M., Grichois, M. L., Garay, R. P., Sassard, J., Ben-Ishay, D. and Meyer, P. (1980). *Proc. natn. Acad. Sci. USA* **77**, 4283.

Meyer, P., Garay, R. P., De Mendonca, M. and Guicheney, P. (1979). *Acta Endocrinol.* **225** (suppl.), 451.

Meyer, P. (1980). *Néphrologie* **1**, 133.

Dagher, G. and Garay, R. P. (1980). *Can. J. Biochem.* **58**, 1069.

Garay, R. P., Dagher, G. and Meyer, P. (1980). *Clin. Sci.* **59**, 1915.

Dagher, G. and Meyer, P. (1980). *Biomedicine* **32**, 111.

Le Quan-Bui, K. H., Devynck, M. A., Pernollet, M. G., Ben-Ishay, D. and Meyer, P. (1981). *Experientia* **37**, 169.

Montenay-Garestier, T., Aragon, I., Devynck, M. A. and Meyer, P. (1981). *Biochem. Biophys. Res. Com.* **100**, 660.

Meyer, P., Garay, R. P., Nazaret, C., Dagher, G., Bellet, M., Broyer, M. and Feingold, J. (1981). *Br. Med. J.* **282**, 1114.

Garay, R. P., Adragna, N., Canessa, M. and Tosteson, D. C. (1981). *J. Membr. Biol.* (in press).

Devynck, M. A., Pernollet, M. G., Nunez, A. M. and Meyer, P. (1981). *Hypertension* **3**, 397.

Elghozi, J. L., Dagher, G., Garay, R. P. and Meyer, P. (1981). *Biomedicine* (in press).

Cloix, J. F., Devynck, M. A., Pernollet, M. G. and Meyer, P. (1981). *Clin. Exp. Hypertension* (in press).

Susceptibility and Resistance to Hypertension in the Rat: Their Value in the Study of The Pathology of Hypertension

D. BEN-ISHAY

Department of Medicine and
Hypertension Research Laboratory,
Hadassah University Hospital,
Mt Scopus, Jerusalem, Israel

During the past two decades, hypertension research has made considerable progress through the development of several models of genetically hypertensive rats. The official nomenclature and origin of seven recognized hypertensive strains and their respective normotensive controls are listed in Table I.

These strains were found to be dissimilar in many ways, a fact which is not surprising, in view of the differences in their origin and the methods of selection. Dissimilarities have been observed with respect to age of onset and severity of hypertension, sensitivity to salt, behaviour patterns, and the participation of various pressor systems in blood pressure control.

The Japanese Spontaneously Hypertensive Rat (SHR) is the only strain that is commercially available, and has consequently been extensively studied. Hundreds of articles have been published on these rats, as evidenced by a recent report derived from questionnaires distributed among 980 re-

Frontiers Cardiol. for the 80s.
0-12-220680-0

Table 1 *Hypertensive rat strains and their respective normotensive controls*[a]

Nomenclature	Symbol	Source	City of breeding	Reference
1. Genetically Hypertensive Strain	(GH)	WISTAR	Dunedin (New Zealand)	Smirk and Hall, 1958
2. Dahl's Salt Sensitive Strain Dahl's Salt Resistant Strain	(DS) (DR)	Sprague-Dawley	Brookhaven (USA)	Dahl et al., 1962
3. Spontaneously Hypertensive Rat Strain Wistar Kyoto Strain	(SHR) (WKY)	WISTAR	Kyoto (Japan)	Okamoto and Aoki, 1963
4. Sabra Hypertensive Strain Sabra Normotensive Strain	(SBH) (SBN)	Sabra (WISTAR?)	Jerusalem (Israel)	Ben-Ishay et al., 1972
5. Lyon Hypertensive Strain Lyon Normotensive Strain Lyon Low Blood Pressure Strain	(LH) (LN) (LL)	Sprague-Dawley	Lyon (France)	Dupont et al., 1973
6. Milan Hypertensive Strain Milan Normotensive Strain	(MHS) (MNS)	WISTAR	Milan (Italy)	Bianchi et al., 1974
7. SHR-Stroke Prone Strain SHR-Stroke Resistant Strain	SHRSP SHRSR	SHR	Kyoto (Japan)	Okamoto et al., 1974

[a] *Clinical Science* **59** (Suppl. IV.), 487S.

searchers who had used the SHR model (Yamori, 1981). Yet, despite the extensive use of these animals, the validity of the spontaneously hypertensive rat as a model for human hypertension has been questioned.

This problem has been recently debated in the literature, and the reader is advised to consult the papers of Trippodo and Frohlich (1981) and McGiff and Quilley (1981) for a detailed review of the opposing views.

The proponents of the rat model have provided an impressive list of similarities between human essential hypertension and genetic hypertension in the rat (Trippodo, 1981).

The progressive haemodynamic alterations observed during the development of hypertension in SHR are quite similar to those occurring in man. Hypertension in adult rats, like in humans, is associated with normal cardiac output and increased total peripheral resistance (Pfeffer and Frohlich, 1973). The blood volume is usually normal or slightly decreased (Trippodo *et al.*, 1978), and the left ventricle gradually hypertrophies as an adaptive change to the increased vascular resistance (Frohlich, 1977). Renal haemodynamics in uncomplicated hypertension in SHR, like in humans, is characterized by normal GFR, normal or decreased renal plasma flow, increased filtration fraction, and increased renal vascular resistance (Beierwalters and Arendshorst, 1978). The participation of neural mechanisms in the elevated renal vasoconstriction could be documented in the rat by direct recording of renal sympathetic nerve activity (Judy *et al.*, 1976) and by renal denervation which could delay the onset of hypertension (Kline *et al.*, 1978). As in human hypertension, an increased vascular reactivity to various stimuli has been observed in SHR and in other genetically hypertensive strains, which was attributed, at least in part, to an enhanced sympathetic activity (de Champlain *et al.*, 1977). More recently, it has been suggested that an increased vascular smooth muscle reactivity could be caused by altered cellular membrane function (Blaustein, 1977; Haddy *et al.*, 1979). In support of this concept, abnormalities in sodium transport have been reported in red blood cells of both hypertensive humans and genetically hypertensive rats (De Mendonca *et al.*, 1981).

The major argument of the opponents of the hypertensive rat as an adequate model for human hypertension, is based on a fundamental physiological difference which exists between this species and other mammals, including man. It was shown that prostaglandins of the E series, and their precursors, exert a vasoconstrictor effect on renal vasculature, and tend to aggravate pre-existing hypertension in the rat, in sharp contrast to the vasodilator and antihypertensive action of these prostaglandins in other mammals (Malik and McGiff, 1975).

In addition, several other dissimilarities between human hypertension and genetic hypertension in rats have been pointed out: genetically hypertensive rats, unlike humans, are not prone to atherosclerosis, and the occurrence of myocardial infarction in rats is extremely rare. While hypertensive subjects are frequently overweight, SHR and GH rats tend to weigh less than their respective normotensive controls. Moreover, the usual antihypertensive measures, including salt restriction, diuretics and propranolol have been found to be inconsistently effective in SHR.

Methodological problems have also been encountered, due to dissimilarities between various SHR colonies obtained from commercial breeders. Differences have been observed with regard to age of onset and severity of hypertension (McGiff and Quilley, 1981), renal function (Mullins and Banks, 1976) and certain physiological responses (Sinaiko and Mirkin, 1978). It seems, therefore, that substrain breeding may induce unexpected deviations in the characteristics of the original strain, which should be kept in mind when comparing data on rats obtained from different sources. Another cause of concern has been the adequacy of the available normotensive controls, since SHR are genetically different from the Wistar Kyoto (WKY) strain from which it was originally derived. Consequently, observed differences between SHR and WKY may sometimes reflect genetic variations, rather than fundamental alterations relevant to hypertensive mechanisms.

It is beyond the purpose of this paper to present a comprehensive comparative analysis of the various strains of genetically hypertensive rats. However, two other rat models deserve special consideration, since they present certain distinct differences from SHR. Dahl's DS and DR rats and the Hebrew University Sabra, SBH and SBN rats have two important common features:

(a) DS and SBH rats do not develop frank spontaneous hypertension. Both strains are hypertension-prone, i.e., predisposed to becoming hypertensive following chronic excess salt intake, or other experimental manipulation. These animals can therefore be studied at well defined stages to obtain information on the pre- and early-hypertensive state.

(b) The normotensive controls, DR and SBN, are hypertension-resistant rats, developed simultaneously and from the same stock from which the hypertension-prone strains were originally selected.

In Dahl's rats, both renal (Dahl and Heine, 1975) and neurogenic mechanisms (Saavedra et al., 1980) seem to participate in the pathogenesis of hypertension. Kidneys of DS rats when compared to DR rats have a reduced natriuretic capacity leading to sodium retention (Tobian et al., 1977). Cross transplantation of kidneys between DS and DR animals have caused lowering of blood pressure in the DS and induced hypertension in the DR rats (Dahl and Heine, 1975). Identical results were also obtained by cross transplantation in the Milan rat (Bianchi and Baer, 1976), which strongly support the concept that the kidney plays an important role in the pathogenesis of hypertension in these strains.

In the Sabra, SBH substrain, the available evidence suggests that proneness to hypertension is associated with preference for salt (Ben-Ishay et al., 1976), a tendency of the kidney to retain sodium (Ben-Ishay, 1978) and alterations in erythrocyte Na^+ transport (De Mendonca et al., 1980).

In our view, the intriguing element of the Sabra model is the hypertension resistant SBN rat, with its amazing ability to maintain normal blood pressure, under experimental conditions that would ordinarily induce hypertension in a regular rat. In an attempt to elucidate the physiological basis of its resistance to hypertension, central and peripheral noradrenergic mechanisms have been compared in the two substrains. The results of these studies, summarized in Table 2, revealed significant differences in several parameters.

Table 2   *Comparison of central and peripheral noradrenergic activity in SBN and SBH rats*

SBN rats are characterized by:

1. Higher NA concentration in the medulla oblongata (Zamir *et al.*, 1978)
2. Decreased tyrosine hydroxylase in the medulla oblongata (Feuerstein *et al.*, 1979)
3. Decreased sensitivity of the NA dependent, cAMP generating system in the medulla oblongata (Kobrin *et al.*, 1981)
4. Elevated atrial NA, unaffected by Doca-salt (Le Quan-Bui *et al.*, 1981)
5. Lower plasma NA levels in response to stress (De Mendonca *et al.*, 1981)

On the basis of these findings, it was postulated that the increased noradrenaline (NA) content found in the brain stem of SBN rats, might exert a prolonged central hypotensive action, that could lead to a decrease in sympathetic activity. Indirect evidence for decreased cardiac sympathetic activity in SBN rats was recently provided by a study of cardiac NA in Doca-treated rats (Le Quan-Bui *et al.*, 1981). In that study, the NA concentration in atria of SBN rats was found to be significantly higher than in SBH or the paternal SB strain. Doca treatment caused hypertension, and a significant decrease in atrial NA in SBH and SB, while in SBN both the blood pressure and the atrial NA concentration remained virtually unchanged. The decrease in atrial NA in SBH and SB corroborates the findings of previous workers (de Champlain *et al.*, 1977) and presumably reflects increased release of neurotransmitter induced by cardiac sympathetic overactivity. On the other hand, the high atrial NA concentration in untreated and in Doca treated SBN is compatible with a decreased activity of cardiac adrenergic nerve endings. These results were recently confirmed in Dahl's rats (Saavedra *et al.*, 1981). When fed a high salt diet, the heart NA content decreased in the hypertension prone DS rat, but was unaffected in the hypertension resistant DR. These findings illustrate the value of the hypertension resistant rat as a more adequate control for the genetic hypertensive rat. They also emphasize the usefulness of the hypertension resistant rat as a model for the study of mechanisms that protect against the development of hypertension.

In conclusion, the genetically hypertensive rat has been extensively used as a model for the study of mechanisms of hypertension. As pointed out by

McGiff and Quilley in their recent review (1981), comparison of patho-genetic mechanisms between human and rat hypertension is of limited value, since little can be learned by comparing two unknowns.

On the other hand, the use of the genetically hypertensive rats offers several advantages over other animal models:

(1) The small size, rapid reproduction and relatively low cost renders the rat model available to most laboratories.
(2) Its short life span enables one to study the natural course and the complications of hypertension in the rat.
(3) There is a definite hereditary component in this type of hypertension, which renders this model most suitable for investigation by geneticists.

Future avenues of research in genetically hypertensive rats should prob-ably include:

(1) Systematic studies of the pre- and early hypertensive state, making use primarily of hypertension prone animals such as DS and SBH rats.
(2) Elucidation of mechanisms that protect against hypertension, using the unique hypertension resistant DR and SBN rats.
(3) Studies of membrane abnormalities, particularly in isolated elements of contractile and nervous tissue, and
(4) Attempts to identify the abnormal proteins that might constitute the genetic markers of hypertension in the various rat strains.

Acknowledgement

Supported in part by the Elefant Research Fund.

References

Beierwalters, W. H. and Arendshorst, W. J. (1978). *Circ. Res.* **42**, 721–726.
Ben-Ishay, D. (1978). *Jap. Heart J.* Suppl. **1**, 147–149.
Ben-Ishay, D., Saliternick, R. and Welner, A. (1972). *Experientia* **28**, 1321–1322.
Ben-Ishay, D., Dikstein, S. and Shalita, B. (1976). *Pflügers Arch.* **361**, 153–157.
Bianchi, G. and Baer, P. G. (1976). *Clin exp. Pharmacol. Physiol.* Suppl **3**, 15–20
Bianchi, G., Fox, U. and Imbasciati, E. (1974). *Life Sci.* **14**, 339–347.
Blaustein, M. P. (1977). *Am. J. Physiol.* **232**, c165–173.
Dahl, L. K. and Heine, M. (1975). *Circ. Res.* **36**, 692–696.
Dahl, L. K., Heine, M. and Tasinari, L. (1962). *Nature* **194**, 480–482.
de Champlain, J., Von Ameringen, M. R., Cousineau, D., Marc-Aurele, J. and Yamaguchi, N. (1977). *Postgrad. Med. J.* **53**, suppl. 15–30.

De Mendonca, M., Grichois, M. L., Garay, R. P., Sassard, J., Ben-Ishay, D. and Meyer, P. (1980). *Proc. natn. Acad. Sci.* **77**, 4283–4286.
De Mendonca, M., Guichency, P., Grichois, M. L., Ben-Ishay, D. and Meyer, P. (1981). *Experientia* **37**; 1087–1088.
Dupont, J., Dupont, J. C., Froment, A., Milton, H. and Vincent, M. (1973). *Biomedicine* **19**, 34–41.
Feuerstein, G., Zamir, N., Ben-Ishay, D. and Gutman, Y. (1979). *J. Neurochem.* **33**, 393–395.
Frohlich, E. D. (1977). *In* "Hypertension Physiopathology and Treatment" (J. Genest, E. Koiw and O. Kuchel, Eds), pp. 15–49. McGraw-Hill, New York.
Haddy, F. J., Pamnani, M. B. and Clough, D. L. (1979). *Life Sci.* **24**, 2105–2118.
Judy, W. V., Watanabe, A. M., Henry, D. P., Besch, H. R. Jr, Murphy, W. R. and Hockel, G. J. (1976). *Circ. Res.* **38** (Suppl. II), 21–29.
Kline, R. L., Kelton, P. M. and Mercer, P. F. (1978). *Can. J. Physiol. Pharmacol.* **56**, 818–822.
Kobrin, I., Ebstein, R., Belmaker, R. and Ben-Ishay, D. (1981). *J. Neurochem.* **36**, 1285–1287.
Le Quan-Bui, K. H., Devynck, M. A., Pernollet, M. D., Ben-Ishay, D. and Meyer, P. (1981). *Experientia* **37**, 169–170.
Malik, K. V. and McGiff, J. C. (1975). *Circ. Res.* **36**, 599–609.
McGiff, J. C. and Quilley, C. P. (1981). *Circ. Res.* **48**, 455–463.
Mullins, M. M. and Banks, R. O. (1976). *Am. J. Physiol.* **231**, 1365–1369.
Okamoto, K. and Aoki, K. (1963). *Jap. Circ. J.* **27**, 282–293.
Okamoto, K., Yamori, Y. and Nagaoka, A., (1974). *Circ. Res.* **34/35** (suppl. 1), 143–153.
Pfeffer, M. A. and Frohlich, E. D. (1973). *Circ. Res.* **32/33** (suppl. 1), 28–38.
Saavedra, J. M., Correa, F. M. and Iwai, J. (1980). *Brain Res.* **193**, 299–303.
Saavedra, J. M., McCarty, R., Fernandez-Pardal, J., Guicheney, P., Weise, V. and Iwai, J. (1981). 4th Intl. Symp. on SHR and related studies. Heidelberg.
Sinaiko, A. R. and Mirkin, B. L. (1978). *Circ. Res.* **42**, 381–385.
Smirk, F. H. and Hall, W. H. (1958). *Nature* **182**, 727–728.
Tobian, L., Lange, J., Azar, S., Iwai, J., Koop, D. and Coffee, K. (1977). *Trans. Ass. Am. Physns* **90**, 401–406.
Trippodo, N. C., Walsh, G. M. and Frohlich, E. D. (1978). *Am. J. Physiol.* **235**, H52–H55.
Trippodo, N. C. and Frohlich, E. D. (1981). *Circ. Res.* **48**, 309–319.
Yamori, Y. (1981). 4th Intl. Symp. on SHR and related studies. Heidelberg.
Zamir, N., Gutman, Y. and Ben-Ishay, D. (1978). *Clin. Sci mol. Med.* **55** Suppl. 4, 105–107s.

Renal Mechanisms in the Pathogenesis of Essential Hypertension

G. BIANCHI, D. CUSI, P. FERRARI,
C. BARLASSINA, B. R. BARBER,
G. VEZZOLI, P. LUPI and E. POLLI

Institute of Clinica Medica I, University
of Milan, Milan, Italy

Four types of renal dysfunction may theoretically be involved in the pathogenesis of essential hypertension: (1) an increase in vascular resistance, (2) a decrease in the glomerular ultrafiltration coefficient, (3) an increase in tubular ion reabsorption and (4) an alteration in the production of a substance such as renin, prostaglandin or kallikrein that affects systemic blood pressure. The difficulties to overcome in evaluating whether one or more of these kidney dysfunctions is involved in the pathogenesis of essential hypertension are: (a): the reciprocal effects of blood pressure and kidney function, which make it almost impossible to evaluate in an already hypertensive individual whether kidney dysfunction is primary or secondary to the hypertension; (b) the many factors extrinsic to the kidney that affect the relationship between kidney function and blood pressure; (c) the heterogeneity of the genetic and environmental possible pathogenetic factors which make the population of essential hypertensives probably inhomogenous (Bianchi, 1980a; Bianchi et al., 1980b).

For these reasons, we have carried out our studies in both humans with essential hypertension (Bianchi et al., 1979a, 1980, 1981; Bianchi, 1980a; Guidi et al., 1980) and rats (Bianchi et al., 1973, 1974, 1975a, b, 1979b; Baer and Bianchi, 1976; Fox and Bianchi, 1976) with genetic or "essential" hypertension during the prehypertensive and the developmental phase, trying to measure as many extrarenal factors as possible, in order to discriminate primary from secondary kidney dysfunctions. When young normotensive offspring of hypertensive parents were compared to young normotensive offspring of normotensive parents the following differences and similarities were found: in the former renal vascular resistance and plasma renin are lower while GFR and 24h-urinary output are higher. Other factors (cardiac index, plasma volume, plasma catecholamine, 24 h urinary excretion of aldosterone and electrolytes) are similar in the two groups (Bianchi *et al.*, 1979a). Studies carried out by others have indicated that 24 h urinary excretion of kallikrein is also lower in the first group. These results seem to rule out renal dysfunctions, (1), (2) and (4) and do indicate a primary alteration in tubular handling of Na and water probably due to a tubular cell membrane transport abnormality.

Rats of the Milan Hypertensive Strain (MHS) were compared with rats of the Milan Normotensive Strain (MNS) at three ages: before, during and after the development of hypertension in the MHS. In the prehypertensive stage, MHS have greater 24 h water intake, urinary outputs and the fraction of the cardiac output that goes to the kidney, while the plasma and urine osmolalities, ratio of the kidney weight to body weight, urine kallikrein and plasma renin are lower (Bianchi *et al.*, 1975b). At this age GFR tends to be higher in MHS (Baer and Bianchi, 1976; Bianchi *et al.*, 1979b). During the development of hypertension, renal sodium retention develops and in adult hypertensive MHS most of the differences from controls tend to disappear. Kidney cross-transplantation experiments between MHS and MNS showed that hypertension follows the kidney (Bianchi *et al.*, 1973, 1974; Fox and Bianchi, 1976). These findings are consistent with the hypothesis that increased tubular reabsorption may be the primary abnormality that causes the differences in kidney function and blood pressure between MNS and MHS.

In order to see whether or not cell membrane transport abnormality is involved in the development of hypertension, we have studied red cell membrane transport to establish: (1) whether the abnormalities in red cell membrane transport are consistent with other red cell abnormalities, present while physiological conditions are still preserved and with kidney function abnormalities that very likely are the direct cause of hypertension (De Mendoca *et al.*, 1980; Bianchi *et al.*, 1982; Cusi *et al.*, 1981a,b); (2) whether the red cell membrane abnormality and the level of blood pressure segregate together or independently in the hybrid generations of back-cross experiments (Stewart, 1972, Festing, 1979). As compared to MNS rats, the red cells of young MHS rats have faster Na–K cotransport through the cell membrane ($44 \cdot 19 \pm 6 \cdot 55$; $24 \cdot 20 \pm 4 \cdot 1$ rate constant h 10^{-3}; $P < 0 \cdot 01$), lower intracellular Na content ($2 \cdot 34 \pm 0 \cdot 23$; $2 \cdot 65 \pm 0 \cdot 08$ mmol 1^{-1} RBC; $P < 0 \cdot 001$) and smaller cell volume ($44 \cdot 3 \pm 0 \cdot 54$; $50 \cdot 2 \pm 0 \cdot 6\,\mu^3$; $P < 0 \cdot 001$) (Ferrari *et al.*, 1982). All these findings are consistent with accelerated outward cell membrane transport of Na in the MHS, with a resetting of the volume and the Na content of the cells to a relatively lower level than in MNS. These findings are also consistent with the lower kidney weight and kidney water content, expressed both as a total and as a percentage of wet kidney weight, in the MHS, as compared to the MNS in the presence of an equal number of nephrons, and with an accelerated transtubular ion transport in the MHS.

Assuming that the differences in red blood cell volume and kidney weight between MNS and MHS are in some way linked to the differences in cell membrane transport, we measured these two parameters and the blood pressure in the second generation hybrids obtained by the "back-cross" of the first (FI) generation of hybrids with the two original parental strains: MHS and MNS. There was a significant inverse correlation ($P < 0.01$) between red cell volume in the prehypertensive stage and the blood pressure level that developed in the same animal when adult. An inverse correlation ($P < 0.025$) was also found between kidney weight and blood pressure, measured simultaneously in adults. Moreover, calculation of the number of loci responsible for the blood pressure difference yielded an estimate of two loci. These results strongly support the hypothesis that the differences in the three traits (red cell volume, kidney weight and blood pressure) between the two strains are genetically linked and may be caused by the same two pairs of alleles.

Regarding a line of research that may give more fruitful results in the future, in our opinion the multidisciplinary approach: genetic, biochemical and physiological, in animal models, that we have just summarized may offer an opportunity to discover new types of genetically determined pathogenetic mechanisms, that may be responsible for hypertension in discrete subgroups of patients, through subtle modifications of kidney function. In fact, once such a mechanism has been elucidated in the animal model, it may be possible to find markers for the same mechanism in humans. Probably the best known example of this type of interaction between animal models and humans hypertension is that of the Goldblatt experiment. After the demonstration that constriction of the renal artery can raise blood pressure clinicians were stimulated to search for an analogous condition in humans and found a discrete group of patients with hypertension due to renal artery stenosis.

References

Baer, P. G. and Bianchi, G. (1976). *Clin. exp. Pharm. Physiol.* Suppl. **3**, 41.
Bianchi, G. (1980a). *In* "Frontiers in Hypertension Research", New York, May 19–21, (Ed. J. H. Laragh).
Bianchi G. (1980b). Int. Symposium on New Trends in arterial Hypertension Cellular Pharm. and Physiol. Deauville, 30 October to 1st November.

Bianchi, G., Fox., U., Di Francesco, G. F., Bardi, U. and Radice, M. (1973). *Clin. Sci. mol. Med.* **45**, 135s.

Bianchi, G., Fox, U., Di Francesco, G. F., Giovannetti, A. M. and Pagetti D. (1974). *Clin. Sci. mol. Med.* **47**, 435.

Bianchi, G., Fox, U., Pagetti, D., Caravaggi, A. M., Baer, P. G. and Baldoli, E. (1975a). *Kidney Inter.* **8**, S165.

Bianchi, G., Baer, P. G., Fox, U., Duzzi, L., Pagetti, D. and Giovannetti A. M. (1975b). *Circ. Res.* **36**, and **37**, suppl., I–153.

Bianchi, G., Cusi, D., Gatti, M., Lupi, G. P., Ferrari, P., Barlassina, C., Picotti, G. B., Bracchi, G., Colombo, G., Gori, D., Velis, O. and Mazzei D. (1979a). *Lancet* **i**, p. 173.

Bianchi, G., Baer, P. G., Fox, U., Duzzi, L., Caravaggi, A. M. and Möhring, (1979b). *Jap. Heart J.* **20** (suppl. I), 173.

Bianchi, G., Cusi, D., Barlassina, C., Duzzi, L., Caravaggi, A. M., Lupi, G. P., Gatti, M., Velis, O., Como, G. and Salvioli, G. (1980c). *La Ric. Clin. Lab.* **10**, 163.

Bianchi, G., Caravaggi, A. M., Cusi, D., Barlassina, C., Lupi, G. P., Duzzi, L., Gatti, M., Ferrari, P. and Velis, O. (1981). *In* "Hypertension in Children and Adolescents" (Eds, G. Giovanelli *et al.*). Raven Press, New York.

Bianchi, G., Cusi, D., Ferrari, P., Barlassina, C., Ferrandi, M. and Guidi, E. (1982). *In* "Nephrology" (G. M. Berlyne, S. Giovanetti, S. Thomas, Eds), Vol. 30, p.192. S. Karger, Basel.

Cusi, D., Barlassina, C., Ferrandi, M., Lupi, G. P., Ferrari, P. and Bianchi, G. (1981a). *J. Exp. Clin. Hypertension 1981* **3**, 871.

Cusi, D., Barlassina, C., Ferrandi, M., Palazzi, P., Celega, E. and Bianchi, G. (1981b). *Clin. Sci.* **61**, 335.

De Mendoca, M., Grichois, M. L., Garay, R. P., Ben-Ishay, D., Sassard, J., Bianchi, G., Caravaggi, A. M. and Meyer, P. (1980). *In* "Int. Symposium on Intracellular Electrolytes and Arterial Hypertension". Univ. Press, Munster, Germany, G. Thieme.

Ferrari, P., Cusi, D., Barber, B., Barlassina, C., Vezzoli, G., Duzzi, L., Minotti, E. and Bianchi, G. (1982). *Clin. Sci.* **63**, 619.

Festing, M. F. W. (1979). *In* "Notes on Genetic Analysis. Inbred Strain in Biomedical Research", p. 81. Macmillan, London.

Fox, U. and Bianchi, G. (1976). *Exp. Phar. Physiol.* Suppl. **3**, 71.

Guidi, E., Bianchi, G., Dallosta, V., Cantaluppi, A., Vallino, F. and Polli, E. (1980). 7th Scientific Meeting of the Inter. Society of Hypertension, New Orleans, Louisiana, USA, May 11–14, 1980.

Stewart, J. (1972). Genetic variation in membrane transport of water and electrolytes. Role of Membrane in Secretory Processes, p. 127. North Holland Publishing Company, Amsterdam.

Neural and Psychological Factors in Hypertension

G. MANCIA and A. ZANCHETTI

Institute of Clinica Medica IV,
University of Milan and Centre of
Clinical Physiology and Hypertension,
Ospedale Maggiore, Milan, Italy

Since the discovery that the autonomic nervous system represents a mechanism of primary importance in regulation of circulation, the idea that hypertension might depend on a derangement in neural cardiovascular control has been a leading one in the investigation of this condition. This presentation will deal with four points that are currently thought to be key ones in this topic, a summary of which will be given in this report.

Is there evidence that nervous factors may produce a condition of high blood pressure, i.e. that they may have an intiating role in this disease? There is no doubt that such evidence is available thanks to a number of studies that have produced prolonged hypertension in animals through neuropsychological manipulation. The following are a few examples: (1) a prolonged elevation in blood pressure has been obtained in the monkey by operant conditioning, a stressful procedure which teaches the animal to perform in such a way as to avoid a painful stimulus (Herd *et al.*, 1969; Forsyth and Harris, 1970); (2) hypertension has been found to occur in male mice which behave as dominant within their colony, in clear contrast to the lower blood pressure values of other mice whose behaviour can be defined as subordinate or indifferent (Henry *et al.*, 1975); (3) a neurally-initiated hypertension may also be that of the spontaneously hypertensive rats, as in these animals the pressor and tachycardic responses to a stressful stimulus are much greater than in the normotensive comparisons even before hypertension has developed. Furthermore such development is slowed or pre-

Frontiers Cardiol. for the 80s.
0-12-220680-0

vented by drastically reducing the natural stimuli that occur in a rat's life (Folkow, 1975). Thus in this instance environmental factors may interact with an inherent hyper-reactivity of the defence mechanisms and the more powerful pressure rises that result may contribute to the development of what appears to be a "spontaneous" hypertensive state; (4) in contrast the time-honoured procedure of denervating arterial baroreceptors does not seem anymore a satisfactory model of neurogenic hypertension (Heymans, 1938). In this model prolonged blood pressure recording made in un-anaesthetized, undisturbed animals have shown that under this condition blood pressure is merely characterized by a pronounced lability (i.e. high but also low values) with an average only slightly different from that of the intact animals. This is so not only when arterial baroreceptors are dener-vated (Cowley, 1973), but also when denervation is extended to vagal receptors in the cardiopulmonary region, thus depriving the animal of all its negative feedback blood pressure controls (Mancia, 1981).

Is there evidence that neural influences, besides playing an initiating role, are important as secondary factors, i.e. they represent a mechanism that maintains blood pressure high in non-neurally initiated hypertensions? Such evidence is also available because destruction of sympathetic nerve terminals either at a peripheral or a central site is accompanied by a large reduction in blood pressure in neurally-induced hypertensions (destruction of nucleus tractus solitarii, SHR, etc.) and in DOCA and renovascular hypertension aswell (De Champlain, 1977). Furthermore, the development of renovascular hypertension in rats can be slowed or prevented not only by diffuse central or peripheral destruction of vasomotor structures but also by lesion of a tiny area in the anterior hypothalamus (Brody *et al.*, 1978). Finally, in reno-vascular hypertensive cats with the sino-aortic nerves cut, the elevated blood pressure shows a return to normotensive and even hypotensive values whenever the sympathetic vasoconstrictor tone is spontaneously turned off during REM sleep (Mancia and Zanchetti, 1980). Why under these circum-stances sympathetic circulatory control is activated is unknown, although current hypotheses are focused on the relationship between sodium and norepinephrine stores and release in the nerve terminals (De Champlain, 1977) as well as on the stimulating properties of angiotensin II at various central and peripheral sympathetic sites (Zimmermann *et al.*, 1968; Ferrario *et al.*, 1979).

What is the importance of neural factors in human, and particularly in essential hypertension? In this regard difficulties arise from the fact that (1) in man the disease is commonly seen at a variably advanced stage from its inception, primary vs secondary factors being usually indistinguishable and (2) all measures of sympathetic activity currently available (plasma cate-cholamines, direct recording of sympathetic traffic, estimation of vascular responses to sympathetic blockade) have important limitations. Neverthe-less, the results obtained largely suggest that in the majority of hypertensive subjects sympathetic activity is not substantially greater than that found in normotensive subjects. Other results extend this similarity to sympathetic circulatory control. For example our own studies with 24 h continuous and direct blood pressure recording in unrestrained conditions show that although absolute blood pressure variability increases progressively from normotensive subjects to subjects with moderate and severe essential hypertension, 24 h variation coefficient for blood pressure is similar in the three groups (Mancia *et al.*, 1980). Furthermore, the maximal hypotension induced by sleep has a similar magnitude in normotension, moderate and severe essential hypertension. Other similarities involve the pattern of the changes in blood pressure variability throughout the day and night, and the relationship of these changes with the concomitant heart rate alterations. These results suggest an undisturbed spontaneous neural modulation of circulation in essential hypertension.

Physiologically when blood pressure increases, baroreflexes reduce and even abolish sympathetic vasoconstrictor tone. An unchanged sympathetic activity in hypertension therefore suggests a *baroreflex abnormality in this condition*, which animal studies have shown to be a resetting of the reflex towards the higher blood pressure levels (McCubbin *et al.*, 1956). In man with essential or renovascular hypertension this phenomenon is particularly pronounced. For the carotid baroreceptor control of blood pressure (studied by the neck chamber technique) the set-point of the reflex is closer to the reflex threshold in hypertensive than in normotensive subjects (Mancia *et al.*, 1978, 1979). This feature implies that rather than being saturated, this antioscillatory mechanism for blood pressure is preserved in hypertension allowing sympathetic vasoconstrictor tone to be also preserved. This may account for the normal neural circulatory regulation that is found in this condition as well as for the effectiveness of antihypertensive treatment with sympatho-inhibitory drugs.

A further interesting feature that characterizes the baroreflex in hypertension is the selective impairment of its heart rate control. In our hypertensive subjects the ability of the carotid baroreceptors to modulate blood pressure, though reset towards the higher blood pressure values, was similar to that of normotensive subjects (Mancia *et al.*, 1978, 1979). On the other hand there is conclusive evidence that the baroreceptor–heart rate reflex, besides being reset, is markedly reduced in hypertension (Mancia *et al.*, 1978; Sleight, 1979). This may result from anatomical alterations (increased stiffness, atherosclerosis, etc.) of the aorta and the major intrathoracic arteries where aortic baroreceptors are located, as in man these receptors seem to play a major role in heart rate control (Mancia *et al.*, 1977). It may also be due, however, to central factors. In animals diencephalic influences during emotion and exercise can depress the baroreceptor ability to modulate the vagus while leaving the sympathetic efferent component of the reflex unaltered (Mancia and Zanchetti, 1980). These influences can act in a similar manner in man (Mancia *et al.*, 1982). Thus the selective impairment of the baroreceptor–heart rate reflex in hypertension suggests that upper brain centres are involved in some of the cardiovascular phenomena that characterize this disease.

References

Brody, M. J., Fink, G. D., Bruggy, J., Haywood, J. R., Gordon, F. J. and Johnson, A. K. (1978). *Circ. Res.* **43**, (suppl. 1), 1.

Cowley, A. W. (1973). *Circ. Res.* **32**, 564.

De Champlain, J. (1977). *In* "Hypertension" (J. Genest *et al.*, Eds), p. 76. McGraw-Hill, New York.

Ferrario, C., Barnes, K. L., Szilagyi, S. E. and Brosnian, K. B. (1979). *Hypertension* **1**, 205.

Folkow, B. (1975). *Clin. Sci. mol. Med.* **84** (suppl. 2), 205.

Forsyth, R. P. and Harris, R. E. (1970). *Circ. Res.* **26** (suppl. 1), 13.

Herd, J. A., Morse, W. H., Kelleher, R. T. and Jones, L. G. (1969). *Am. J. Physiol.* **217**, 24.

Henry, J. P., Stephns, P. M. and Santisteban, G. A. (1975). *Circ. Res.* **36**, 156.

Heymans, C. (1938). *N. Engl. J. Med.* **219**, 154.

Mancia, G. (1981). Atti 82°- Congr. Med. Interna, 462.

Mancia, G. and Zanchetti, A. (1980a). *In* "Physiology during Sleep" (J. Orem, Ed.), p. 1. Academic Press, London and New York.

Mancia, G. and Zanchetti, A. (1980b). *In* "Handbook of Hypothalamus" (J. Panksepp and P. A. Morgane, Eds), Vol. III, Part 13, p. 147. M. Dekker, New York.

Mancia, G., Ferrari, A., Gregorini, L., Valentini, R., Ludbrook, J. and Zanchetti, A. (1977). *Circ. Res.* **41**, 309.

Mancia, G., Ludbrook, J., Ferrari, A., Gregorini, L. and Zanchetti, A. (1978). *Circ. Res.* **43**, 170.

Mancia, G., Ferrari, A., Gregorini, L., Parati, G., Ferrari, M. C., Pomidossi, G. and Zanchetti, A. (1979). *Am. J. Cardiol.* **44**, 895.

Mancia, G., Ferrari, A., Gregorini, L., Parati, G., Pomidossi, G., Bertinieri, G., Grassi, G. and Zanchetti, A. (1980). *Clin. Sci.* **59**, 4013.

Mancia, G. *et al.* (1983). "Hypertension" (in press).

McCubbin, J. W., Green, J. H. and Page, I. H. (1956). *Circ. Res.* **4**, 205.

Sleight, P. (1979). *Am. J. Cardiol.* **44**, 889.

Zimmermann, B. G. and Gisslen, J. (1968). *J. Pharmacol. exp. Therap.* **163**, 320.

Salt and Dietary Factors in the Aetiology, Pathophysiology and the Treatment of Hypertension

D. R. R. WILLIAMS

University Department of
Community Medicine, Addenbrooke's
Hospital, Cambridge, UK

Introduction

At least two questions are raised by the title of this paper:

(1) Is exposure to dietary salt (and the usual focus of attention is dietary sodium) an important cause of essential hypertension?
(2) Is a reduction in salt intake an effective treatment in cases of established hypertension?

These questions are still the subject of much discussion and debate and it is the purpose of this paper to examine, particularly for the first question, the reasons for this continued controversy and to suggest some of the ways in which clarification may be achieved by future work in this field.

From the first of the above questions a third arises – the important public health debate about the effectiveness of a reduction in salt intake as a preventive measure in populations where hypertension and its sequelae are prevalent.

Frontiers Cardiol. for the 80s.
0-12-220680-0

A Failure to Distinguish between Questions of Therapy and Questions of Aetiology

It is important at the outset to distinguish between two debates – that concerning the role of salt in the aetiology of essential hypertension and that concerning the role of salt restriction in the treatment of the disease. The effectiveness (or otherwise) of salt restriction in the treatment of established hypertension does not necessarily relate to the question of whether exposure to salt is important in the aetiology of the disease. Similarly, because salt is (or is not) a cause of hypertension it should not be assumed that restriction of salt will (or will not) be effective in the treatment of hypertension. The mechanism or mechanisms by which the disease is brought about may be entirely different from the means by which the abnormality is maintained once established. Many of the debates in this and in other similar fields have often confused the questions of therapy with aetiology with a resulting lack of clarity.

In a similar fashion the debates on therapy and prevention are separate until proved otherwise. Evidence of the effectiveness of salt restriction in treating established hypertension does not necessarily have any bearing on the question of reduced salt intake as a public health measure for prevention.

Measurement Difficulties in Population Studies

The difficulties associated with the measurement of blood pressure in epidemiological studies will not be considered here. Equally formidable and equally important are the difficulties associated with the measurement of salt intake. Population studies relating salt intake to blood pressure (Donnison, 1929; Foster, 1930; Orr and Gilk, 1931; Shattuck, 1937; Kean, 1944; Takahashi et al., 1957; Kaminer and Lutz, 1960; Lowenstein, 1961; Shaper, 1962; Maddocks, 1967; Prior et al., 1968; Shaper et al., 1969; Oliver et al., 1975; Truswell, 1977; Ueshinia et al., 1981; Finn et al., 1981) have measured intake by a variety of methods, many of them unsatisfactory. The sodium content of foods as eaten is highly variable even for the same foods (mainly because of differences in cooking methods) and the analysis of duplicate portions has been recommended as the only satisfactory method of assessing sodium intake from diet data (McMance and Widdowson, 1978). In addition, only about 30% of ingested salt is added at the table (Bull and Buss, 1980) so that methods involving the estimation of table salt usage are of doubtful validity for the estimation of total salt intake.

The estimation of sodium excretion in urine has been widely used as a measure of sodium intake in population studies on the assumption that faecal and skin losses are negligible. Gleibermann (1973) comparing data on blood pressures and salt intakes from 27 population studies has demonstrated statistically significant positive linear correlations between both systolic and diastolic mean blood pressure values (expressed logarithmically) and mean salt intakes. Such inter-population comparisons have been held as supportive evidence of an aetiological role for salt in the aetiology of hypertension.

With few exceptions (e.g. Joossens, 1973; Pietinen *et al.*, 1979; Finn *et al.*, 1981) *intra* population comparisons have failed to demonstrate a convincing relationship between levels of blood pressure and salt (or sodium) intake for individuals. Failure to find such a relationship has been regarded as evidence favouring rejection of such a hypothesis.

The difficulties associated with the measurement of sodium excretion in individuals, however, are of a different magnitude to those associated with the measurement of means for groups because of the large day to day variation in individual intakes in populations with high or moderately high salt intakes. As discussed by Liu *et al.* (1979) a large number of 24 h urine collections are necessary in such populations to categorize individual sodium intake with acceptable accuracy and to ensure that any correlation that may exist between blood pressure and intake is not obscured by random measurement error. Hence a failure to demonstrate a relationship between blood pressure and sodium intake in intra-population studies is not necessarily indicative of a lack of relationship but is, in many cases, a reflection of lack of power of the studies performed.

Multiple Differences in Population Comparisons

Many of the population comparisons available in the literature have dealt with a small number of populations (sometimes two) with contrasting life styles and contrasting levels of blood pressure or prevalence rates of hypertension. Such studies give relatively weak support for the salt hypothesis since a difference in salt intake is often but one of the many differences in lifestyle reported between these populations. Other striking differences in dietary intakes and in levels of obesity, physical exercise etc. are often present. However, most such studies have shown that populations with high (or increasing) sodium intakes have high (or increasing) levels of mean blood pressure and those with lower (or decreasing) sodium intakes have lower (or decreasing) levels. The few studies that have failed to show this effect (e.g. Malhotra, 1970) are deficient on methodological grounds. Despite this, most available population studies must be regarded as unsatisfactory tests of the hypothesis that salt intake is a major causative factor in the aetiology of hypertension.

Other Causes, Competing and Interactive

Studies of human populations and animal experiments (Meneely *et al.*, 1957; Burstyn and Firth, 1975; Sriniuvasan *et al.*, 1980) have suggested that other dietary factors, e.g. sucrose, fat and potassium, may be important aetiological or protective factors in the development of hypertension. The influence of psychosocial factors in the aetiology of hypertension in man and in animals has also been considered (Henry and Cassal, 1969). The possibility that several exposures, either separately or acting synergistically may give rise to essential hypertension is a realistic one and there is some support from animal experiments to suggest that may be so in that the effect of psychological stress may enhance the hypertensive effect of sodium in genetically susceptible rats. The studies that allow such putative causal interactions to be examined in human hypertension are few.

Individual Differences in Susceptibility to Salt Intake

Individual differences, perhaps inherited, in susceptibility to salt and other dietary intakes are potential confounding factors in any experimental or epidemiological study of salt and hypertension. Inherited differences in susceptibility are well described in laboratory rats (Dahl *et al.*, 1974). Such differences in humans would contribute to a failure to demonstrate intra-population correlations between blood pressure and salt intake. The study of Pietinen *et al.* (1979) has demonstrated a statistically significant relationship in normotensive subjects with a family history of hypertension but no relationship in subjects without a family history. The presence or absence of a family history of hypertension is a crude indication of susceptibility but more refined indicators of susceptibility may be the individual differences in Na^+ and K^+ handling by cell membranes suggested by Garay and Meyer (1979) and described elsewhere in these proceedings.

Failure to Define the Correct Hypothesis

Alternative hypothesis for the mechanisms of essential hypertension have recently been discussed by Lever *et al.* (1981). In addition, they point out the important distinction between the testing of a hypothesis suggesting elevated blood pressure levels in all individuals exposed to a high salt intake and the hypothesis suggesting that such a response is seen in only some (perhaps genetically susceptible) individuals within the population. The studies required to test these hypotheses are of fundamentally different designs and at least some of the confusion in the debate has been the result of an inability to state precisely the hypothesis under scrutiny.

Present Intake vs Past Intake

The accuracy with which present salt intake reflects past salt intakes in individuals or in population groups is unknown. Also unknown is the critical period or periods, if any, during which exposure has an influence on the development of hypertension. If, in individuals, present intake is a poor reflection of past intakes then the case control method used successfully in other epidemiological investigations is of little value. Prospective studies offer the most useful means by which the salt hypertension hypothesis may be tested.

Conclusions

Despite these difficulties a number of conclusions may be drawn:

(1) Indirect evidence suggests that salt intakes are rising in some countries (the UK for example). This may be deduced from data on trends in the consumption of processed foods (which tend to be high in salt). The desirability of such an increase should be seriously questioned in the absence of any evidence suggesting that this level of salt consumption is safe.

(2) It is likely that exposure to dietary sodium is an important cause of hypertension in susceptible individuals though we cannot yet confidently predict the level to which the prevalence of hypertension would fall for any given reduction in mean population salt intake.

Salt and the Treatment of Hypertension

A number of observations can be made on this subject:

(1) Since the early discussions on salt restriction in the treatment of hypertension (Kempner, 1944) there has been a marked change in opinion from marked scepticism (*Lancet*, 1975) to a resurgence of interest (*Lancet*, 1978). The efficacy of severe salt restriction is not questioned but the evidence for modest salt restriction (to, say, 70–100 mmol of sodium/24 h, Morgan *et al.*, 1978) is more controversial.

(2) Part of the problem in demonstrating efficacy is that of adherence by the patient to the salt restricted diet and, in measuring this, the same problems of monitoring salt intake arise as were discussed above.

(3) Future studies must ensure sufficiently large sample sizes for the adequate statistical demonstration of a clinically important effect on blood pressure levels.

(4) The confounding effects of other changes induced by the dietary regime (intake of other electrolytes, changes in body weight etc.) must be adequately taken care of in the experimental design.

(5) The clinical heterogeneity of essential hypertension is probably of considerable importance with regard to treatment with salt restriction.

References

Bull, N. L. and Buss, D. H. (1980). *Proc. Nutr. Soc.* **39**, 30A.

Burstyn, P. G. and Firth, W. R. (1975). *Cardiovasc. Res.* **9**, 807.

Dahl, L. K., Heine, M. and Thompson, K. (1974). *Circ. Res.* **40**, 94.

Donnison, C. P. (1929). *Lancet* i, 6.

Finn, R., McConnochni, K., Box, D. E. D., Fennetry, A. G. and Green, J. R. (1981). *Lancet* i, 1097.

Foster, J. H. (1930). *N. Eng. J. Med.* **203**, 1073.

Friedman, R. and Iwai, J. (1977). *Proc. Soc. exp. Biol. Med.* **155**, 449.

Garay, R. P. and Meyer, P. (1979). *Lancet* i, 1066.

Gleibermann, L. (1973). *Ecol. Food Nutr.* **2**, 143.

Henry, J. P. and Cassal, J. C. (1969). *Am. J. Epidemiol.* **90**, 171.

Joossens, J. V. (1973). *Triangle* **12**, 9.

Kaminer, B. and Lutz, W. P. (1960). *Circulation* **22**, 289.

Kean, B. H. (1944). *Am. J. trop. Med.* **24**, 314.

Kempner W. (1944). *North Carolina Med. J.* **5**, 273.

Lancet leader. (1975). i, 1325.

Lancet leader. (1978). i, 1136.

Lever, A. F., Beretta-Piccoli, C., Brown, J. J., Davies, D. L., Fraser, R. and Robertson, J. I. S. (1981). *Br. Med. J.* **283**, 463.

Liu, K., Cooper, R., McKeever, J., McKeever, P., Byington, R., Soltero, I., Stamler, R., Gosch, F., Stevens, E. and Stamler, J. (1979). *Am. J. Epid.* **110**, 219.

Lowenstein, F. W. (1961). *Lancet* i, 389.

Maddocks, I. (1967). *Med. J. Aust.* **1**, 1123.

Malhotra, S. L. (1970). *A. J. Clin. Nutr.* **23**, 1353.

McMance, R. A. and Widdowson, E. M. (1978). "The Composition of Foods" 4th Edition, p. 10.

Meneely, G. R., Ball, C. O. T. and Youmans, J. B. (1957). *Ann. int. Med.* **47**, 263.

Morgan, T., Gillies, A., Morgan, G., Adam, W., Wilson, M. and Carney, S. (1978). *Lancet* i, 227.

Oliver, W. J., Cohen, E. L. and Neel, J. V. (1975). *Circulation* **52**, 146.

Orr, T. B. and Gilk, J. L. (1931). Special Rep. Series 155: "Studies of Nutrition", Medical Research Council.

Pietinen, P. I., Wong, O. and Alteschul, A. M. (1979). *Am. J. clin. Nutr.* **32**, 997.

Prior, A. M., Evans, J. G., Harvey, H. P. B., Davidson, F. and Lindsey, M. (1968). *N. Eng. J. Med.* **279**, 515.

Shaper, A. G. (1962). *Am. Heart. J.* **63**, 437.

Shaper, A. G., Leonard, P. J., Jones, K. W. and Jones, M. (1969). *E. Afr. med. J.* **46**, 262.

Shattuck, G. C. (1937). *Am. J. trop. Med.* **17**, 513.

Sriniuvasan, S. R., Berensen, G. S., Radhakrishnamurthy, B., Dalferes, E. R., Underwood, D. and Foster, T. A. (1980). *Am. J. clin. Nutr.* **33**, 561.

Takahashi, E., Sasaki, N., Taheda, J. and Ito, H. (1957). *Hum. Biol.* **29**, 139.

Truswell, A. S. (1977). "Diet and nutrition of hunter gatherers", *Ciba Foundation Symposium* **49** (New Series), 213.

Ueshinia, H., Tanigaki, M., Iida, M., Shimamoto, T., Konishi, M. and Komachi, Y. (1981). *Lancet* **i**, 505.

Preventing the Age Risk in Blood Pressure: Relevance, Feasability and Methods

K. O'MALLEY, W. O'CALLAGHAN and
E. O'BRIEN

Department of Clinical Pharmacology,
Royal College of Surgeons in Ireland
and The Blood Pressure Clinic, The
Charitable Infirmary, Dublin, Ireland

Serious consideration has been given to blood pressure levels in the elderly only in the last decade. There has been a slow but perceptible increase in interest in this important clinical problem dating from the late 1960s. Clearly the increased concern stems from the realization that raised blood pressure in the elderly is associated with significant morbidity and mortality. The mounting evidence provided by the ongoing Framingham Study on the inter-relationship of age, blood pressure and cardiovascular disease has been the main stimulus. While awareness of the problem has increased it must be stated that review papers on the subject probably greatly out-number important original reports. There is interest, but to date little information exists other than the epidemiological data which will allow us to make definitive statements. The poverty of data is illustrated by the observation of Koch-Weser (1978) that only 10% of the patients in 41 clinical studies of hypertension were over the age of 60 years. In this review we discuss the more important aspects of this problem, highlighting, where appropriate, gaps in our knowledge.

Frontiers Cardiol. for the 80s.
0-12-220680-0

High Blood Pressure: A Risk Factor in the Elderly

Both blood pressure and aging are continuous variables and therefore arbitrary cut-off points must be used if we are to classify people according to these parameters. In this paper we define elderly as those above 65 years and hypertension is defined as blood pressure in excess of 160/90 mmHg. Blood pressure both systolic and diastolic rise with age until about 50 years of age in both males and females. As age progresses diastolic pressure remains fairly constant in males but climbs further in females. In both sexes systolic pressure rises progressively into the ninth decade and thereafter falls slightly (Miall and Brennan, 1981). In quite a large number of people but particularly in those who become hypertensive the rise in systolic pressure dominates – disproportionate systolic hypertension (Koch-Weser, 1973). An extreme form of this is isolated systolic hypertension. Here the systolic blood pressure is greater than 160 mmHg and the accompanying diastolic is less than 95 mmHg (Kannel *et al.*, 1981). From the Framingham Study it is becoming increasingly obvious that the level of systolic blood pressure is a major risk factor for cardiovascular and cerebrovascular disease and this applies to isolated systolic hypertension as well as elevated systolic pressure combined with an increase of diastolic values (Table 1).

Stroke is two to four times more common in people with isolated systolic hypertension than in normotensive subjects. "While diastolic pressures related to stroke incidence, in the subjects with systolic hypertension the diastolic component adds little to risk assessment . . ." (Kannel *et al.*, 1981). In congestive heart failure and myocardial infarction blood pressure is also an important risk factor (O'Malley and O'Brien, 1980). In congestive heart

Table 1   *Risk of stroke according to systolic and diastolic blood pressure*

	2 year rate per 1000	
Systolic blood pressure mmHg[a]	Men	Women
< 140	5·0	3·3
140–159	9·4	8·0
⩾ 160	29·4	17·0
Diastolic blood pressure[b]		
< 90	29·4	17·0
90–94	12·0	14·9
⩾ 95	24·8	17·8

[a] DP < 95 mmHg; [b] SP < 160 mmHg; adapted from Kannel *et al.*, 1981.

failure systolic pressure also appears to be more important than diastolic. This is probably because cardiac work depends largely on systolic pressure (Tarazi and Gifford, 1978). In the elderly population the other risk factors for cardiovascular disease which operate in young people are of minor significance. Clearly blood pressure dominated as the major risk factor and systolic pressure has better predictive value than the diastolic pressure.

Measurement of Blood Pressure

The ability to measure blood pressure accurately is important but in the elderly there is some doubt as to whether we can do so. Spence *et al.* (1978) have published data which purport to show that cuff blood pressure measurement grossly overestimates diastolic blood pressure. In a selected group over the age of 60 years they found that cuff blood pressure exceeded the intra-arterial level by 10 mmHg or more in one-fifth of patients. Such findings, if confirmed, are important because they question ones whole approach to the detection and management of blood pressure in this age group.

Feasibility

We will consider feasibility under the headings – compliance, blood pressure reduction and benefit.

Compliance

The elderly have long been considered to be poor compliers with therapeutic regimens. We have not been able to find data to support this contention (O'Hanrahan and O'Malley, 1981). Clearly, patients who are confused or dementing cannot be relied upon to take medications but we suspect the average elderly hypertensive takes his medication as well if not better than any of his younger counterparts. Data from the Hypertension Detection and Follow Up Program study (HDFP, 1979) agrees with this view. Of patients who entered that study just as many patients in the age range 60–69 remained in follow-up for five years as did those in the 50–59 year age group. Both of these age groups were if anything better than the 30–49 year olds.

Blood Pressure Reduction

Is it possible to lower blood pressure in elderly hypertensives? The evidence from both the European Working Party on Hypertension in the Elderly

Group (EWPHE) Study (Amery *et al.*, 1981) and the HDFP study is that it is possible. In both studies the first drug employed was a thiazide diuretic. In the EWPHE Study the thiazide (plus methyldopa in a small percentage of cases) reduced sitting blood pressure by an average of 27/18 mmHg. In the HDFP study the elderly patients achieved goal blood pressure more often than did say the 30–49 year old group – 75% vs 49%. This indicates that not only do the elderly take their medication, but under the circumstances of these two studies blood pressure reduction occurs.

Reduction in Morbidity and Mortality

We do not know if treating mild to moderate hypertension in the elderly reduces mortality and morbidity. The mortality data from the HDFP study suggests that an aggressive approach to blood pressure management in the 60–69 year old range is worthwhile. The group thus managed showed an overall improvement in mortality, the stepped care group having a 16·4% lower mortality rate than did the referred group. This study does not compare active vs inactive drug regimens rather the mortality rates with two health care systems were compared. Hopefully the ongoing EWPHE study will give us a definite answer to this central question.

How to Lower Blood Pressure

As stated thiazide diuretics lower blood pressure in this age group. We do not have data on side-effects from the HDFP study but information from the EWPHE study shows that thiazide diuretics behave predictably. Thus there is an increase in fasting glucose of 12%. It is perhaps a little worrying that glucose intolerance which is itself a risk factor (at least in younger people) for ischaemic heart disease, should increase with thiazide treatment. Thus the balance between the increased risk invoked by the rise in blood glucose and the decrease likely with a reduction in blood pressure remains to be determined. Serum urate increased by 25% but there was no difficulty with clinical gout. Serum creatinine also increased. The rise in serum creatinine was presumably due either to a decrease in glomerular filtration rate commensurate with the fall in blood pressure or to an effect of the thiazide on renal secretory function. As triamterene is combined with the thiazide diuretic any change in potassium levels has been anticipated.

Beta Adrenoreceptor Blocking Drugs

In view of these side-effects with thiazides it is worth considering other antihypertensives as drugs of first choice in the management of hypertension in the elderly. There are many aspects of the pathophysiology of hypertension that are different in the young and the old. One of the most striking of these is the difference in the renin angiotensin aldosterone status. Low renin essential hypertension is a more common feature in the elderly. Weidmann *et al.* (1975) have shown that renin concentration, plasma renin activity and aldosterone concentrations are all lower in the elderly. Throughout life there tends to be an inverse relationship between serum renin levels and blood pressure and some authors (Niarchos and Laragh, 1980) hold that the decrease in renin in the elderly is merely a feedback inhibition induced by their higher arterial pressures. The low renin levels in the elderly would suggest that anti-renin agents such as beta adrenoceptor blocking drugs would be less effective in the treatment of hypertension than in the young. In a large study Buhler *et al.* (1975) found that older patients less often achieved goal blood pressure on long-term beta adrenoceptor blocking monotherapy (Table 2).

However various other studies do not confirm these findings (Birkenhager and de Leeuw, 1980). In studies that we have just completed (unpublished) we did not observe any case of failure of blood pressure to respond to atenolol, labetalol or nadolol. However, achievement of goal blood pressure levels is another matter and one that requires additional study.

Methyldopa

Methyldopa has been used in many studies including the EWPHE trial. In this study there does not appear to have been an excess of unwanted effects though in general we recommend caution in the use of centrally active drugs in the elderly.

Conclusions

High blood pressure is common in the elderly and it is a potent risk factor for cardiovascular disease and particularly stroke. Systolic pressure is an in-

Table 2 *Percentage of patients in whom diastolic blood pressure was normalized by beta adrenoceptor blocking drugs*

Age (years)	%
> 60	20
40–60	50
> 40	80

Buhler *et al.*, 1975.

dependent risk factor for stroke. It is feasible to lower blood pressure (systolic as well as diastolic) with thiazides but the pattern of response to beta blockers remains to be clarified. Many gaps in our knowledge need filling – not only those implied in the above statement but more information is required on the indications for treatment, drug of first choice, effects of treatment on mortality and morbidity, the pathophysiological significance of elevated systolic pressure and the best means of lowering systolic pressure.

References

Amery, A., De Schaepdryver, A. *et al.*, (1981). *In* "Hypertension in the young and old" (Eds, G. Onesti and K. E. Kim), 315–326. Grune & Stratton, New York.

Birkenhager, W. H. and de Leeuw, P. M. (1981). *In* "Hypertension in the young and the old" (Eds, G. Onesti and K. E. Kim), 309–313. Grune & Stratton, New York.

Buhler, F., Burkart, F., Lutold, B., Kung, M., Marbet, G. and Pfisterer, M. (1975). *Am. J. Cardiol.* **36**, 653–669.

Hypertension Detection and Follow Up Program Co-Operative Group. (1979). *JAMA* **242**, 2572–2577.

Kannel, W. B., Wolf, P. A., McGee, D. L., Dawber, T. R., McNamara, P. and Castelli, W. P., (1981). *JAMA* **245**, 1225–1229.

Koch-Weser, J. (1973). *Am. J. Cardiol.* **32**, 499–510.

Koch-Weser, J. (1978). **Herz 3**, 235–244.

Miall, W. E. and Brennan, P. J. (1981). *In* "Hypertension in the young and old" (Eds, G. Onesti and K. E. Kim), 277–283. Grune & Stratton, New York.

Niarchos, A. P. and Laragh, J. H. (1980). *Mod. Concepts cardiovasc. Dis.* **49**, 43–49.

O'Hanrahan, M. and O'Malley, K. (1981). *Br. Med. J.* **283**, 298–300.

O'Malley, K. and O'Brien, E. T. (1980). *N. Engl. J. Med.* **302**, 1397–1401.

Spence, J. D., Sibbald, W. J. and Cape, R. D. (1978). *Clin. Sci. mol. Med.* **55**, 399–4025.

Tarazi, R. C. and Gifford, R. W. Jr (1978). *In* "Hypertension: mechanisms, diagnosis and treatment" (Onesti, G. and Brest, A. N., Eds), 23–30. FA Davis, Philadelphia.

Weidmann, P., De Myttenaere-Burszteins, P., Maxwell, M. and De Lima, J. (1975). *Kidney Int.* **8**, 325–333.

Markers for Target Organ Damage?

S. GHIONE and L. DONATO

Institute of Clinical Physiology, CNR
and Institute of Patologia Medica,
University of Pisa, Pisa, Italy

Introduction

That high blood pressure (BP) is associated with increased risk of cardio-vascular (CV) disease and that lowering of even mildly elevated BP levels results in a significant fall of this risk are well-known concepts based on unequivocal evidence. They represent a major achievement of clinical research on arterial hypertension (HT) over the last decades and have gained wide acceptance in clinical practice, but probably, they also represent a somewhat reductive way of looking at the problem, which for several reasons does not leave one completely satisfied.

A major dilemma concerns *mild hypertension* (Mitchell Perry and McFate Smith, 1978). It affects the vast majority of people with elevated BP in a population, and, because of its high prevalence, a major part of the excess of mortality due to HT is associated with it. However, in mild HT the risk of the single individual and thus the benefit of treatment are very small: as suggested by the Australian Therapeutic Trial in Mild Hypertension for every 1000 mild hypertensives who regularly take treatment, in only seven will a major or minor morbid event be prevented every year (Editorial, *Lancet*, 1980). As Alderman and Madhavan (1981) recently synthesized the problem: "Is widescale therapy to help only a few justifiable?"

Moreover, in moving from epidemiological ground to the clinical approach to the individual patient (not necessarily with mild HT), we are faced with the problem of the *heterogeneity of the clinical history* of different subjects: some patients, despite a record of high blood pressure, never show cardiovascular complications, while others develop severe cardiovascular complications despite relatively low pressure levels or adequate response to the hypotensive treatment.

If we could sort out the complication-prone hypertensive subjects from the non-prone group, we would be in a position to guide our intervention more efficiently and the advantages in terms of cost/benefit would be self-evident.

The problem which thus arises is whether the risk is randomly distributed within a given range of BP levels and, if not, which other indicator(s) of increased risk could be identified that cooperate with BP levels in determining the occurrence and/or severity of cardiovascular complications.

The *ideal approach* would be that of the identification and effective measurement of the casual factor(s) which determine the susceptibility to CV injury: if such an approach were possible, obviously it would be feasible and practical to screen susceptible hypertensives by directly measuring the relevant factor(s).

An alternative, more *practical approach* resulting from the present lack of identification of the causal factors of CV injury may rely on our ability to prevent severe cardiovascular involvement essentially by picking up organ damage in the preclinical stages.

In the next section of this paper both approaches will be briefly discussed: the ideal one with the purpose of outlining some lines of reasoning that might help in the search for "the causal factor(s)"; the practical one, for pointing out the assumption and practical limitations of the current procedures, with the purpose of stressing the need for improved clinical methods.

In Search of "Causal" Markers for CV Injury

A "causal factor" determining the increased susceptibility to CV injury in hypertensives irrespective of the systolic and diastolic blood pressure readings, could operate at different levels. It could be that:

> some haemodynamic characteristics of the hypertensive state that escape current clinical observation, may vary in different individuals and may be relevant to the occurrence and/or the severity of the vascular changes;
> some factor related to the aetiology or to the pathogenesis of the hypertensive state may act with different intensity on the blood pressure level and on the vessels' wall;

some independent factor, either exogenous or endogenous, not directly related to the hypertensive state, may act as modulator of the severity of changes resulting from similar blood pressure levels.

Haemodynamic Characteristics of the Hypertensive State

Vascular changes occurring in the hypertensive state are currently referred to the exposure of the resistance vessels to supra-normal blood pressure levels. Although occasional BP measurements have been shown to be a good predictor of cardiovascular complication in epidemiological studies of adequate size, they may be inadequate to provide an estimate of the effective mechanical burden imposed on the peripheral vessels.

If we suppose that the peripheral damage resulting from high levels of arterial pressure is related to the integral amount of energy dissipated in the peripheral vascular structures, at least two possible alternatives should be considered in the attempt to explain individual differences.

Differences in the Short- and Long-term Time-profile of the Blood Pressure Between Measurements

The differences may originate from the variability in the response of BP to ordinary and exceptional events of life or, conversely, to different intensity of the emotional stress accompanying the measurement of BP. It may also reside in the chronobiological profile of BP.

Invasive monitoring of blood pressure is probably to be considered no more than a useful research tool. On the contrary, development of practical non-invasive methods might prove of real value in providing more representative estimates of the haemodynamic strain on the circulation.

If differences in the short-term profile of BP are difficult to evaluate, even more difficult is the assessment of differences in the long-term time-profile. On the other hand the importance of the time factor is suggested by the influence on cardiovascular complication of the different rates of rise of BP in Spontaneously Hypertensive Rats (SHR) (Okamoto *et al.*, 1974).

Differences in the Temporal Pattern of Energy Dissipation in Resistance Vessels

Differences in the aortic compliance result in differences in the amount of energy absorbed in systole and consequently affect the shape of the pulse pressure downstream, changing the concentration-in-time of the energy dissipation in resistance vessels. As aortic compliance decreases, pulse pressure increases, a sharper peak is present and energy dissipation is more concentrated in time.

The concentration-in-time of the impact of the pressure wave will tend to produce what we might call a "hammering effect" on the terminal vessels which is likely to induce intimal damage. To this effect, which is demonstrable in a hydraulic simulator of the circulation, might contribute high cardiac output, high heart rate, high ejection rate, low aortic compliance and high terminal resistance.

These considerations are in keeping with epidemiological evidence of the increased risk of CV sequelae for increasing systolic pressure in subjects with normal diastolic pressure as shown by recent analysis of the Framingham data (Kannel *et al.*, 1980).

It might be that, from this point of view, epidemiological studies relating incidence of CV disease to systolic and diastolic pressure might be pooling together different haemodynamic conditions that may be relevant in determining the clinical course of the individual patient. New methods based on Doppler velocimetry or other approaches may provide in the future better ways of characterizing these aspects.

Dissociation Between Vascular Damage and Hypertensive Effect

Although vascular damage is usually considered a consequence of the hypertensive state, some experimental and clinical evidence suggests that pathogenic factors may act directly on the vessels.

The search for endogenous humoral agents involved in the vascular and/or in the cardiac changes in HT has been intense in the last decade but yielded controversial results. It seems quite probable that the role of angiotensin, catecholamines, vasopressin and possibly other circulating factors will continue to represent an expanding field of interest in HT research in the eighties.

Salt has also been proposed to induce direct vascular damage: Limas *et al.* (1980) report that in a young, sodium fed SHR the aggravation of vascular changes actually precedes the onset of a steeper rise of BP. It is unclear whether these data reflect some vasculotoxic effect of sodium unrelated to BP or whether the vascular damage is secondary to some haemodynamic change (possibly even of BP) induced by sodium but undetectable by means of occasional BP measurements. Since the adverse effects of sodium on the vessels were not seen in non-hypertension-prone, control rats, these effects seem also to be related to genetic factors. Following up this line to reasoning it would be interesting to investigate about possible relationships between target organ damage and the recently proposed genetic cationic markers for HT (Meyer and Garay, 1981).

Independent Modulating Factors

In the last 30 years much effort has been devoted to the study of the so-called risk factors for CV disease. Up to 25 different risk factors have been described, ranging from age and sex, to blood constituents, to lifestyle, to exotic signs like diagonal ear-lobe crease (Davignon, 1977). The knowledge accumulated on the major risk factors (diet, smoking, exercise, hypertension) has already been converted into practice and substantial progress has been achieved in modification of risk factors in western populations. The decline in mortality rates in the last decade has been attributed to changes in these habits (Stamler, 1979).

Many questions however remain open and deserve extensive research in the future years. Among the most challenging questions are those concerning the role of *immunological* and *psychophysiological* factors in CV disease. The hypothetical model of how immunological factors (comprising autoantibodies, the complement system and HLA-antigens) might be interrelated in the development of vascular damage was proposed by Mathews *et al.* (1974) but, up to now, available data in this field, though suggestive, have provided only circumstantial evidence in favour of this hypothesis. The expanding knowledge on the mechanism on immunologically mediated tissue damage might however provide in the next future a better understanding on the pathogenesis of vascular damage in hypertension. On the other hand current developments in neurochemistry and neuropharmacology promise new insight in the mechanisms underlying CV regulation by the central nervous system (CNS). It is not unreasonable to hope that in the coming years a multidisciplinary approach involving the cardiovascular physiologist, the psychologist and the neuroscientist will restore the CNS to its primary integrating role of CV function and provide a substantial clarification of the pathogenesis of many CV diseases.

Picking up Preclinical Damage

The assumption that identification of cardiovascular injury in hypertensives at the preclinical stage might help in preventing severe organ damage rests on the following elements:

> that hypertensives with evidence of established CV abnormalities are both more likely to develop further damage and to benefit from hypotensive treatment, thus conferring a predictive and monitoring value to periodic functional assessment;
> that signs of preclinical involvement can be suitably identified and effectively quantified.

Predictive Value of CV Abnormalities

The VA intervention study has clearly shown that hypertensive subjects with detectable CV abnormalities have a higher probability of developing more severe injury, thus strongly suggesting that early preclinical signs could have a significant role in identifying subjects at risk (Veterans Administration Cooperative Study Group, 1972).

Reliability of Quantification of Early CV Injury

A procedure suitable for the detection of early cardiovascular changes should combine several different requirements:

from the point of view of the *information provided*, it should assess both the functional state of the heart and that of the small blood vessels;
from the point of view of the *quality of information*, it should provide consistent and reproducible results expressed in quantitative terms;
from the point of view of the *methodology*, it should combine simplicity and low cost (because of the large number of subjects to be evaluated), non-invasivity (because of the mildness of the condition) and sensitivity (because of the rather subtle changes which should be recognized).

The difficulty in matching the above requirements will be shown both for cardiac and microvascular evaluation in the following paragraphs.

Cardiac Evaluation by Echocardiography

Because of safety, absence of patient discomfort, ease of performance and quality of information, echocardiography (ECHO) would appear a method of choice for evaluation of cardiac involvement in HT. Its superiority with respect to other non-invasive methods (EKG, X-rays, etc.) appears to be without doubt. An indirect indication for that has been provided by our group, showing that out of several non-invasive parameters of cardiac hypertrophy the ECHO-determined left ventricular (LV) wall thickness correlates best with BP levels (Palombo et al., 1980). In a group of unselected and untreated HT patients a correlation coefficient of 0·67 was found between interventricular septal thickness (IVST) and BP, thus indicating that at least up to 50% of the variability of IVST can be "explained" on the basis of the concurrent BP levels.

However, ECHO evaluation of LV wall thickness is far from being satisfactory. In a group of 20 HT patients the reliability of an ECHO measurement by blind reading of different observers indicated that inter-observer variability was larger than inter-individual variability (Palombo et al., 1980). Similar results were reported by Felner et al. (1980) who, not unreasonably, conclude that this method is "semiquantitative at best". Thus there is an urgent need for further refinements and more reliable tools for the assessment of cardiac involvement in mild to moderate HT.

Reliability of Ocular Fundus Examination

As regards the assessment of vascular involvement, the examination of the ocular fundus (OF) still represents a cornerstone in clinical practice since it provides a unique insight on the functional state of the vascular district. However, the evaluation of the OF is affected by a disturbingly high degree of subjectiveness, as has been shown in diabetic patients (Sussman *et al.*, 1982). A recent study by our group tends to confirm the importance of this difficulty, at least in the presence of a moderate degree of HT. In this study (Ghione *et al.*, 1982) four different skilled observers examined the OF of 50 mild hypertensive patients randomly chosen out of those attending our outpatient clinic. As indicated in Fig. 1, the degree of agreement was rather

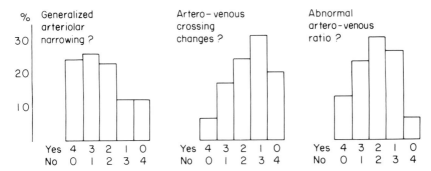

Figure 1. Agreement on subjective judgement on the presence of vascular signs in the fundus oculi of hypertensive patients. Fifty hypertensive patients randomly chosen out of those attending our outpatient clinic were evaluated by four independent observers (three ophthalmologists and one cardiologist). In the histograms the height of each bar represents the percentage of eyes for which a given combination of responses was obtained (e.g. for the question "Is generalized arterial narrowing present?" in 24 out of the 100 eyes examined all observers agreed on the response "yes", in 26% three observers gave a positive and one a negative answer etc.).

low and, for some parameters (particularly for those indicating the lowest degrees of vascular involvement) it approached that expected if the diagnosticians, instead of examining the patient, had given their response on the basis of pure guesswork.

   The collection of the image of OF on a "hard copy" (for instance a slide) for further evaluation, may represent a significant improvement and is already practicable today, while computer assisted analysis should be explored in view of a much more radical progress towards the standardization of these important data.

Conclusions

Hypertension is a "soft" indicator of risk for CV damage and the use of other indicators should greatly increase the effectiveness of treatment and prognosis. Some "needy" areas for future research in this field have been outlined and briefly discussed. A full evaluation of their role would certainly require highly expensive, carefully planned, widescale, long-term studies. However clinical and experimental studies on target organ damage are also required in the direction of improving the reliability of the existing methods for its assessment.

It is difficult to forsee if the "target organ damage" problem will represent one of the "hot" frontiers in cardiovascular research in the next decade. At present, in any case, it can be stated that it represents a "poorly manned" frontier (Table 1).

Table 1   *The "popularity" of the different fields of interest in hypertension research*

Fields of interest	% of abstracts
(1) Pathophysiological mechanisms in human and experimental hypertension known (or thought) to be involved:	
(a) in BP elevation	62
(b) in target organ involvement	15
(2) Diagnostic problems on aetiology in hypertension	7
(3) Evaluation of target organ involvement	8
(4) Hypotensive treatment, effect evaluated	
(a) on BP	39
(b) on target organ involvement	3

The varying degree of interest of researchers on arterial hypertension is estimated on the basis of the content of the abstracts submitted to the VIII Scientific Meeting of the International Society of Hypertension held in Milan (1981). The frequency of abstracts oriented on the different fields is reported. According to their content abstracts could be assigned to one or more topics. (The figures represent the evaluation of the authors.)

Finally, it may not be unjustified to remind ourselves that, when we treat a hypertensive patient, we do so not for the sake of the blood pressure *per se*, but in the belief that we will prevent further target organ damage.

References

Alderman, M. H. and Madhavan, S. (1981). *Hypertension* **3**, 192–197.
Davignon, J. (1977). *In* "Hypertension, Physiology and Treatment" (J. Genest, E. Koiw and O. Kuchel, Eds), pp. 961–989. McGraw Hill, New York.
Editorial (1980). *Lancet* **i**, 1283–1284.
Felner, J. M., Blumenstein, B. A., Schlant, R. C., Carter, A. D., Alimurung, B. N., Johnson, M. J., Sherman, S. W., Klicpera, M. W., Kutner, M. H. and Drucker, L. W. (1980). *Am. J. Cardiol.* **45**, 995–1004.
Ghione, S., Giaconi, S. and Fommei, E. (1982). Manuscript in preparation.
Kannel, W. B., Dawber, T. R. and McGee, D. L. (1980). *Circulation* **61**, 1178–1182.
Limas, C., Westrum, B., Limas, C. J. and Cohn, J. N. (1980). *Hypertension* **2**, 477–489.
Mathews, J. D., Whittingham, S. and MacKay, I. R. (1974). *Lancet* **ii**, 1423–1427.
Meyer, P. and Garay, R. P. (eds) (1981). *Clin. exp. Hypertension* **3**, 569–895.
Mitchell Perry, H. and McFate Smith, W. (eds) (1978). *An. NY Acad. Sci.* **304**.
Okamoto, K., Yamori, Y. and Nagaoka, A. (1974). *Circulation Res.* (Suppl. I) **34**, **35**, 143–153.
Palombo, C., Levorato, D., Rossi, G., Antonielli, E., Donato, L. and Ghione, S. (1980). Abstracts of the VIIth Scientific Meeting of the International Society of Hypertension, New Orleans, May 11–14.
Stamler, J. (1979). *Circulation* **60**, 1575–1587.
Sussman, E. J., Tsiaras, W. G. and Soper, K. A. (1982). *JAMA* **247**, 3231–3234.
Veterans Administration Cooperative Study Group on Antihypertensive Agents (1972). *Circulation* **45**, 991–1004.

Antihypertensive Drugs: Attack on Pathogenetic Mechanisms

M. GUAZZI
and P. MONTORSI

Institute of Cardiology,
University of Milan, Cardiovascular
Research Centre, CNR, Milan, Italy

Studies reported in this presentation should be regarded as an attempt to answer the following two questions: (a) whether or not renin, *per se* may have a role in the pathogenesis of hypertension in humans (Brown *et al.*, 1979), and antihypertensive drugs interfering with the renin system lower blood pressure through this mechanism (Ferguson *et al.*, 1980; Laragh, 1980); (b) whether or not the hypothesis of primary hypertension as a consequence of an excessive arteriolar tone due to enhanced intracellular calcium ion concentration (Blaustein, 1977) may be supported on clinical grounds.

The first topic was approached by a new method. In fact, we induced acute unilateral reduction of the renal perfusion pressure (RPP) (a sort of duplication in man of the experimental Goldblatt kidney) and investigated the renin and the haemodynamic responses to this type of stimulus. We also studied the effects that beta-blockade may have on these responses. The RPP was interfered with, at a time when patients were subjected to diagnostic renal arteriography, through insertion into a renal artery of a balloon-tipped catheter and through modulated inflation of the balloon. The method has been described in detail elsewhere (Fiorentini *et al.*, 1981). In seven normotensive and 17 untreated primary hypertensive individuals subjected to this procedure, we found that (Fig. 1): (a) reduction of the renal perfusion pressure by 30–50% of control was a stimulus strong enough to elicit the

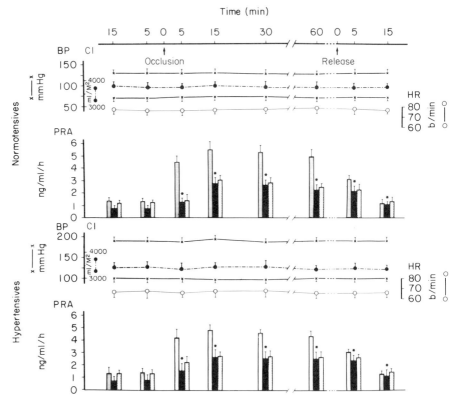

Figure 1. Means ± s.e. of systolic and diastolic blood pressure (BP), cardiac index (CI) and heart rate (HR) in a group of seven normotensive, and in a group of 17 primary untreated hypertensive subjects at various periods before, during and after 60-min unilateral reduction of the mean renal perfusion pressure by 50% of the baseline. Means ± s.e. of plasma renin activity (PRA) for the two groups in arterial (solid bars) and in the venous blood of the occluded kidney (dashed bars on the left) and of the contralateral side (dotted bars on the right) at the various periods, are also reported (*differences from the pre-occlusion period significant at P < 0·01) (Guazzi et al., 1981, by permission Cardiovasc. Res.)

maximal renin response obtainable by this method; (b) systemic (arterial) renin was already significantly augmented at 5 min after the beginning of arterial obstruction, reached a peak at from 15–30 min and then tended to decrease, although the mean values continued to be markedly higher than the baseline values until the obstruction was removed (60 min); (c) soon after the stimulus, venous renin and venous–arterial difference in renin activity in the occluded kidney became definitely elevated and remained elevated for the duration of the occlusion; (d) on the contralateral side, the venous–arterial difference in renin activity decreased progressively until 30 min after occlusion, when it was almost abolished, indicating that renin release from the nonoccluded kidney was suppressed; (e) the response was qualitatively and quantitatively similar in normotensive and hypertensive subjects; (f) despite the humoral reaction, in no case did systemic arterial pressure, heart rate and cardiac output change throughout the studies.

In nine untreated primary hypertensive patients subjected to the same degree of unilateral renal artery obstruction, for 30 min before and after i. v. infusion of propranolol (10 mg), we found that (Fig. 2), following the drug, the peak renin level in response to the mechanical stimulus was significantly lowered both in the systemic (arterial) and the venous blood from the occluded kidney, and the renin response was delayed, as compared to control. This proves that beta-blockade does interfere with the renal release of renin elicited with a mechanical stimulus. Baseline pressure, heart rate and cardiac output, however, were not affected by the occlusive procedure, both before and after propranolol.

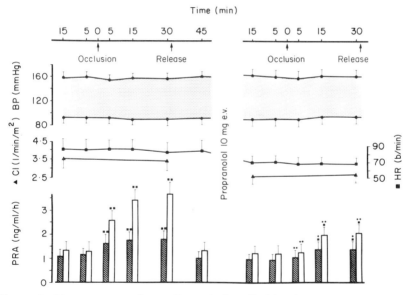

*Figure 2. Means ± s.e. of systolic and diastolic blood pressure (BP), cardiac index (CI) and heart rate (HR) in a group of nine primary hypertensives before, during and after 30 min unilateral reduction of the mean renal perfusion pressure by 50% of the baseline (left side). Means ± s.e. of the same variables at the same periods following 10 mg i. v. propranolol are also indicated (right side). Means ± s.e. of plasma renin activity (PRA) in the arterial and in the venous blood of the occluded kidney at the various periods are reported with dashed and open bars, respectively. (★★ differences from the pre-occlusion values significant at P < 0·01; ★ differences from the pre-occlusion values significant at P < 0·05; ** differences from the corresponding period before propranolol significant at P < 0·01; * differences from the corresponding period before propranolol significant at P < 0·05.)*

These data indicate that in man, either normotensive or hypertensive, unilateral RPP reduction duplicates the renin pattern of the Goldblatt kidney, but does not duplicate the hypertensive response. Although this evidence applies only to a short-lasting hyperreninaemia, it casts doubt on the possibility that enhanced renin availability, *per se*, can cause blood pressure elevation in humans, and that the pressure reduction following agents interfering with the renin system, such as blockers of the beta adrenergic receptors and of the converting enzyme, is the direct consequence of an effect on it.

As regards the second question, the hypothesis has recently been advanced that in primary hypertension a systemic dysregulation in sodium handling by the cell membrane exists involving the blood vessel smooth muscles, that leads to excessive intracellular calcium ion concentration, which, in turn, causes the vascular tone to increase and the blood pressure to rise (Blanstein,

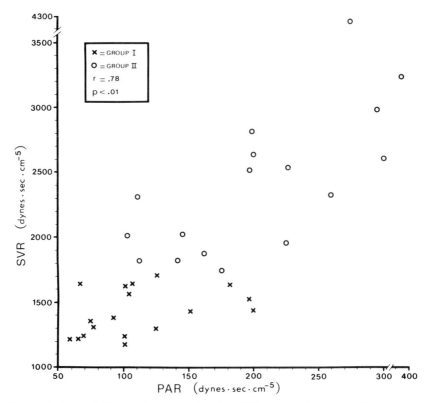

Figure 3. Correlation between systemic (SVR) and pulmonary (PAR) vascular resistance in 35 primary hypertensive subjects. Crosses identify patients with normal-sized left ventricle. Circles refer to subjects with left ventricular enlargement. (Guazzi et al., 1982, by permission.)

1977). In other words, intracellular calcium would have a primary role in the pathogenesis of essential hypertension. Clinical support for this speculation is lacking.

Starting from our previous observations that pressure in the pulmonary artery is higher than normal in systemic hypertension, and that this is due to elevated pulmonary vascular resistance (Olivari *et al.*, 1978), we decided to investigate further the haemodynamics of the lesser circulation in systemic hypertension, with the purpose of testing whether a common denominator may exist for the vasoconstriction that involves the two circuits, and whether intracellular calcium may have some responsibility.

We investigated systemic and pulmonary haemodynamics in 35 primary untreated hypertensive subjects before and after administration of nifedipine (10 mg), a calcium antagonistic agent (Guazzi *et al.*, 1977). We confirmed that in the baseline pulmonary arterial pressure and arteriolar resistance (PAR) are higher in hypertensive than in normotensive individuals of similar age. We also proved that: (a) elevation in PAR is not related to pulmonary blood flow and volume, pleural pressure, arterial PO_2, PCO_2 and pH, left ventricular filling pressure and function; (b) the level of systemic vascular resistance (SVR) significantly correlates with the level of

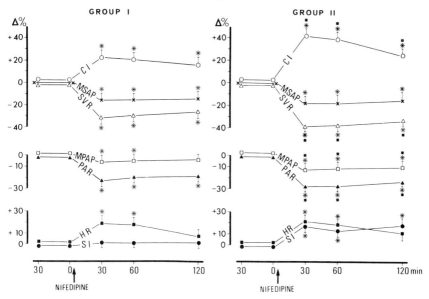

Figure 4. Average per cent variations from control, at various periods after nifedipine (10 mg), of mean systemic (MSAP) and pulmonary (MPAP) arterial pressure, systemic (SVR) and pulmonary (PAR) vascular resistance, cardiac index (CI), stroke index (SI) and heart rate (HR), in untreated primary hypertensive patients (Group I, 18 subjects with normal sized left ventricle; Group II, 17 subjects with left ventricular enlargement). * differences from baseline significant at P < 0·01.) (Guazzi et al., 1982, by permission.)

PAR (Fig. 3); (c) nifedipine helps one to reach normal pulmonary and systemic arterial pressures and significantly lowers both SVR and PAR; (d) per cent reduction in vascular resistance, following the drug, bears mutual relation with the baseline level of the same, both in the greater and lesser circulation (Fig. 4).

The failure to convincingly explain the increased pulmonary arteriolar resistance through the mechanisms that are currently indicated as responsible for pulmonary vasoconstriction, together with the correlation existing between SAR and PAR, consistently prospects the possibility that a common factor, whatever it is, produces vasoconstriction in the two circuits in hypertension. The qualitative and quantitative similarity in the response of pulmonary and systemic circulation to a calcium antagonistic agent, even though it is far from being a proof, does not contrast with the hypothesis that a widespread disorder in the intracellular calcium ion concentration may have a role in the pathogenesis of primary hypertension. If this were the case, calcium blockers might be regarded as a pathogenetic tool for treating primary hypertension.

References

Blaustein, M. P. (1977). *Am. J. Physiol.* **232**, c165.

Brown, J. J., Casals-Stenzel, J., Cumming, A. M. M., Davies, D. L., Fraser, R., Lever, A. F., Morton, J. J., Semple, P. F. and Robertson, J. I. S. (1979). *Hypertension* **1**, 159.

Ferguson, R. K., Vlasses, P. H., Koplin, J. R., Shirinian, A., Burke, J. F. Jr and Alexander, J. C. (1980). *Am. Heart J.* **99**, 579.

Fiorentini, C., Guazzi, M. D., Olivari, M. T., Bartorelli, A., Necchi, G. and Magrini, F. (1981). *Circulation* **63**, 973.

Guazzi, M., Olivari, M. T., Polese, A., Fiorentini, C. and Magrini, F. (1977). *Clin. Pharm. Ther.* **22**, 528.

Guazzi, M., Fiorentini, C., Olivari, M. T., Bartorelli, A., Magrini, F. and Bianciardi, C. (1981). *Cardiovasc. Res.* **15**, 637.

Guazzi, M. Polese, A., Bartorelli, A., Loaldi, A. and Fiorentini, C. (1982). *Circulation* **66**, 881.

Laragh, J. H. (1980). *In* "Topics in Hypertension" (Ed., Laragh, J. H.), 507–528. Yorke Medical Books, New York.

Olivari, M.T., Fiorentini, C., Polese, A. and Guazzi, M. (1978). *Circulation* **57**, 1185.

II. Advances in the Pathophysiology of Ischaemic Heart Disease

New Concepts in the Control of the Coronary Circulation

A. L'ABBATE, P. CAMICI,
M. G. TRIVELLA, G. PELOSI,
D. LEVANTESI and M. MARZILLI

Institute of Clinical Physiology, CNR
and Institute of Patologia Medica,
University of Pisa, Pisa, Italy

In the past decades, experimental research on coronary circulation has been focused mainly on the microcirculation. The effects of coronary stenosis and ventricular wall stress on coronary flow reserve, transmural flow distribution and regional ventricular function have been the object of extensive investigation for a long time.

Recently, clinical documentation of coronary vasospasm and the widespread acceptance of its fundamental role in the genesis of myocardial ischaemia is moving the interest in experimental research from the periphery to the proximal portion of the coronary circulation. Thus the large coronary arteries, which were previously either neglected or simply regarded as passive tubes, and the mechanisms underlying smooth muscle tone, will probably become the main object of extensive investigation in the eighties. Whether the peripheral coronary circulation will raise, in the future, less interest may now come into question.

The aim of this presentation is to illustrate some new aspects of the physiology of the peripheral coronary circulation which could stimulate new interest in this field.

Frontiers Cardiol. for the 80s.
0-12-220680-0

Assessment of Regional Vascular and
Extravascular Coronary Resistance

The availability of new methods, such as the radioactive microsphere technique, which can map the regional myocardial blood flow, has made it possible to apply the water-fall model, conceived by Permutt and Riley (1963) for the pulmonary circulation and applied to the total coronary vasculature by Downey and Kirk (1975), to the regional coronary circulation (L'Abbate *et al.*, 1979). The construction of regional pressure flow curves using regional flow values obtained at different coronary perfusion pressures, permits the separation of the vascular from the extravascular component of coronary resistance and the study of their distribution in different regions of the heart and in different layers of the ventricular wall.

By this method we were able to document, in the maximally dilated vascular bed, an opposite transmural gradient of vascular and extravascular resistance in the left ventricular wall (Fig. 1). In fact the pressure-flow curves of the outer and the inner third of the left ventricular wall differ in slope and intercept indicating lower vascular resistance and higher extravascular resistance in the subendocardium as compared to the subepicardium (L'Abbate *et al.*, 1980).

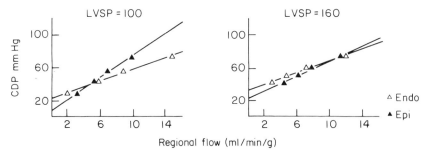

Figure 1. Regional pressure flow curves of the outer (EPI) and inner (ENDO) thirds of the left ventricular wall obtained during adenosine induced maximal vasodilation in two experiments with low (left) and high (right) left ventricular systolic pressure. Regional flow was obtained by radioactive microspheres technique. The difference in slope of the ENDO and EPI pressure-flow curves show the difference in intrinsic vascular resistance in the two layers, the resistance being lower in the ENDO. According to the waterfall model the higher intercept of the ENDO curves indicates higher extravascular pressure in this layer relative to the EPI. Because of the opposite behaviour of slopes and intercepts the two curves cross at a certain value of perfusion pressure. Above the cross-point, ENDO flow becomes higher than EPI flow, while the opposite occurs below the cross-point. This point, which corresponds to the value of coronary perfusion pressure at which perfusion is evenly distributed to the two layers, moves to the right when left ventricular systolic pressure increases.

This finding contrasts with the model of equally distributed intrinsic vascular resistance across the left ventricular wall proposed by Downey and Kirk (1975) on the basis of pressure–total flow curves. It explains why, in normal haemodynamic conditions, the subendocardial layer receives an equal or greater blood flow relative to the subepicardium even in the absence of autoregulation and in spite of a higher extravascular pressure; it also explains why it becomes selectively ischaemic in the presence of a low perfusion pressure such as that produced by a coronary stenosis.

In spite of the fact that this method does not allow us to obtain any information on phasic changes in resistance during the cardiac cycle, since microshere flow is an average flow, it appears to provide a unique opportunity for mapping intramyocardial vascularity and pressures and studying the relationship between endoventricular pressures, intramyocardial forces and coronary blood supply.

Increase in left ventricular preload proportionately affects the intercept of the pressure–flow curve indicating an increase in intramyocardial vascular compression (Ellis and Klocke, 1980). Preliminary results from our laboratory indicate that in the maximally dilated coronary bed the cross-point of the pressure–flow curves moves up or down according respectively to the increase or decrease in the afterload of the left ventricle (Trivella *et al.*, 1980) (Fig. 1). Thus for the same perfusion pressure and in absence of autoregulation, myocardial transmural distribution can be largely different depending on the values of ventricular pre- and after-load.

New Dimension and Availability of Coronary Flow Reserve

It is generally accepted that a brief period of ischaemia evokes the maximal coronary reserve and that peak flow during reactive hyperaemia is the maximal available flow at any given coronary perfusion pressure.

Recent data from our laboratory have documented that prolonged intracoronary infusion of adenosine produces: (1) an immediate, rapid (few seconds) vasodilation quantitatively similar to the one induced by transient ischaemia; (2) a slow, progressive, further vasodilation which in 20–40 min doubles the peak reactive flow value and remains constant up to 2 h infusion (L'Abbate *et al.*, 1981a). After the initial, rapid vasodilation, when peak hyperaemic flow is reached, transient ischaemia has no more effect on coronary flow. Thus an unexpected additional coronary reserve is elicited by a prolonged exposition of coronary vasculature to adenosine, suggesting a vasodilatory mechanism additive to transient ischaemia with a different time course.

Additional information derives from the analysis of the flow time-course and the effect of transient ischaemia following adenosine interruption. Flow decreases to control value in 10–20 min. Similarly to the increase of flow during adenosine infusion, the decrease is initially rapid and then slow.

However, during flow decrease, transient ischaemia produces at any time a reactive hyperaemic response, restoration of hyperaemia being immediate, when flow is still higher than control peak reactive flow (Fig. 2).

These observations are consistent with the hypothesis of two dilatory mechanisms:

(1) a fast one, that is quickly triggered by adenosine and transient ischaemia, and is quickly restored when adenosine infusion is discontinued;
(2) a slow one, that is slowly activated during prolonged adenosine infusion and is slowly reset following adenosine interruption.

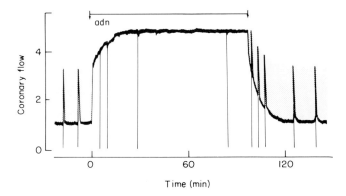

Figure 2.   Time course of coronary flow changes during prolonged intracoronary adenosine (ADN) infusion. Infusion starts at time 0. Before this time, reference value of peak reactive flow is obtained by two brief periods (30 s) of stop flow. Adenosine produces an immediate increase of flow which reaches the value of peak reactive hyperaemia in a few seconds. Thereafter flow continues to increase with a much slower rate reaching a plateau in about 20 min. Following the intial, rapid, vasodilation, transient ischaemia does not affect coronary flow. When adenosine infusion is stopped, flow immediately starts to decrease at a rapid and later at a slow rate. During flow decrease, reactive hyperaemia is immediately restored and transient ischaemia initially increases flow to values higher than reference post-ischaemic hyperemia. The dark area outlines the magnitude of hyperaemic response.

These findings raise new questions on the mechanism of coronary autoregulation and bring in the possibility that different portions of the coronary flow reserve could become available under acute or chronic dilating stimulation.

Even or Uneven Coronary Vasodilation in Response to Different Stimuli

Vasodilating coronary response to a maximal stimulus applied to the entire circulation is considered to be qualitatively and quantitatively uniform across the left ventricular wall, eliciting a parallel increase in flow in both subendocardium and subepicardium, on the condition that the stimulus does not affect at the same time the transmural distribution of coronary driving pressure. This is the case for hypoxia, transient ischaemia and for some vasodilating drugs such as adenosine and dypiridamole, which have been studied in respect of this question.

Recent reports from our laboratory, (L'Abbate *et al.*, 1981b), however, have shown that the transmural response of the coronary vasculature to a pharmacological vasodilating stimulus can be uneven. In fact, following carbochromen, while an increase in total flow quantitatively similar to, or slightly higher than the one induced by transient ischaemia is reached, (Fig. 3) a much higher vasodilatation in the subepicardium, as compared to the subendocardium, is recorded (Fig. 4). This uneven vasodilation causes a reduction of the ENDO/EPI flow ratio to approximately 50% of the control

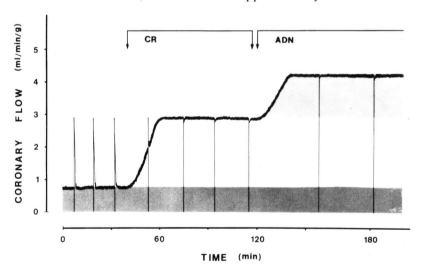

Figure 3. Time course of coronary flow increase during i.v. carbochromen and subsequent adenosine intracoronary infusion. Carbochromen produces an increase in flow similar to reference peak reactive values as determined during the control period. Substitution of carbochromen with adenosine produces a further increase in flow. During pharmacological vasodilation, once peak reactive flow value has been reached, brief periods of ischaemia do not produce reactive hyperaemia. The dark area outlines the control flow.

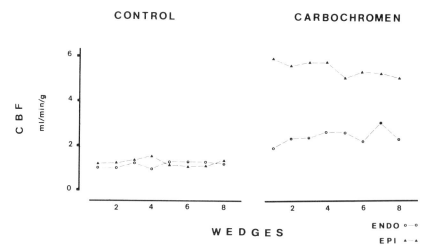

Figure 4.   Flow profile of subendocardium (ENDO) and subepicardium (EPI) of a transverse slice of the heart (unrolled and divided into eight wedges) during control (left) and carbochromen (right). During control flow is similar in the two layers. Carbochromen produces an increase in flow which is prominent in the subepicardium.

value. Subsequent infusion of adenosine increases total flow and moves the ratio back to the control by a prevalent increase in the subendocardial flow. These data, in addition to those reported by Domenech and MacLellan, (1980), who documented a dishomogenous vasodilating effect following beta$_2$ adrenergic receptors activation, in the same direction as we found for carbochromen, and those reported by Gross *et al.* (1981), who documented an uneven vasodilation in the opposite direction, following acetylcholine, lead to the hypothesis that different types of "receptors" are either evenly or unevenly distributed in the coronary vasculature.

Conclusion

The results of our studies on coronary microcirculation showed that the mechanisms regulating myocardial perfusion and coronary vasodilation are still far from being fully understood.

The finding of a coronary reserve much greater than previously thought, the hypothesis of different "receptors", with a different time course response and different intramyocardial distribution, challenge some of the traditional concepts on coronary autoregulation. They could represent the clue to a new direction for the future research on the physiology of coronary microcirculation.

References

Domenech, R. J. and MacLellan, P. R. (1980). *Circ. Res.* **46**, 29–36.

Downey, J. M. and Kirk, E. S. (1975). *Circ. Res.* **36**, 753–760.

Ellis, A. K. and Klocke, F. J. (1980). *Circ. Res.* **46**, 68–77.

Gross, G. J., Buck., J. D. and Warltier, D. C. (1981). *Am. J. Physiol.* **240**, H941–H946.

L'Abbate, A., Marzilli, M., Ballestra, A. M., Camici, P., Trivella, M. G. and Taddei, L. (1979). *G. ital. Cardiol.* **9**, 231–241.

L'Abbate, A., Marzilli, M., Ballestra, A. M., Camici, P., Trivella, M. G., Pelosi, G. and Klassen, G. A. (1980). *Cardiovasc. Res.* **14**, 21–29.

L'Abbate, A., Camici, P., Trivella, M. G., Pelosi, G., Davies, G. J., Ballestra, A. M. and Taddei, L. (1981a). *Cardiovasc. Res.* **15**, 282–286.

L'Abbate, A., Trivella, M. G., Camici, P., Pelosi, G., Levantesi, D., Taddei, L. and Marzilli, M. (1981b). *G. ital. Cardiol.* **11**, 663–670.

Permutt, S. and Riley, R. L. (1963). *J. Appl. Physiol.* **18**, 924–932.

Trivella, M. G., L'Abbate, A., Camici, P., Ballestra, A. M., Pelosi, G. and Taddei, L. (1980). VIII European Congress of Cardiology, Paris. p. 221. (abstract)

Angina Pectoris: Biorhythm, Myocardial Necrosis and Sudden Death

A. BIAGINI, C. CARPEGGIANI,
S. SEVERI, M. G. MAZZEI, R. TESTA,
C. MICHELASSI, P. MARZULLO,
A. MASERI[1] and A. L'ABBATE

Institute of Clinical Physiology, CNR and
Institute of Patologia Medica, University
of Pisa, Pisa, Italy; [1]Royal Postgraduate Medical
School, University of London, Cardiovascular
Research Unit, Hammersmith Hospital,
London, UK

In the seventies the deeply believed theory, that increased myocardial demand in the presence of critical coronary atherosclerotic stenosis was the only important cause of angina pectoris, was actually discredited by the objective documentation that coronary vasoconstriction, or other factors interfering with coronary blood supply, are usually responsible for angina at rest (Guazzi *et al.*, 1971; Maseri *et al.*, 1975, 1977). In addition it has been shown that "variant" angina is not the only electrocardiographic manifestation of coronary vasospasm, indeed S-T segment depression or T wave changes can be caused by coronary vasospasm as well (Maseri *et al.*, 1977,

Work partly supported by a grant of the CNR on Preventive Medicine – Atherosclerosis and by AR. Med., Medical Research Association, Pisa, Italy.

1977; Chierchia *et al.*, 1980; Parodi *et al.*, 1981). It was also objectively demonstrated that coronary vasopasm may occur in vessels with an extremely variable degree of coronary atherosclerosis and that in those patients with severe critical stenosis, angina at rest due to vasoconstriction may be associated with the traditional form of exertional angina (Maseri *et al.*, 1978).

Continuous electrocardiographic and haemodynamic monitoring of patients with angina at rest showed that pain is a late marker of ischaemia and that prolonged episodes of ischaemia with severe impairment of left ventricular function may be completely asymptomatic (Chierchia *et al.*, 1980). More recently continuous electrocardiographic ambulatory monitoring has shown that asymptomatic myocardial ischaemia may be quite frequent in some individuals (Golding *et al.*, 1973; Shang and Pepine 1977; Selwyn *et al.*, 1979) and electrocardiographic monitoring in CCU documented the high incidence of ischaemic attacks during the night (Maggini *et al.*, 1978; Biagini *et al.*, 1981a).

Furthermore the studies of patients with frequent anginal attacks at rest have shown that coronary vasospasm may cause myocardial cell damage even in absence of electrocardiographic sign of necrosis (Biagini *et al.*, 1981b), may cause sudden death (Maseri *et al.*, 1978; Maseri, 1979) and may be one of the causes of myocardial infarction (Maseri *et al.*, 1978).

In this paper we will discuss the results of our research in the last years in the field of biorhythms of vasospastic angina, myocardial cell damage and sudden death, three areas which will likely continue to be the object of our clinical research in the near future.

Biorhythms

The use of the Holter monitoring technique in patients with angina at rest allowed us to objectively document the frequency and distribution of ischaemic attacks during the day as well as during longer periods of time. In a preliminary study (Biagini *et al.*, 1981a) performed on a group of 10 consecutive patients with variant angina we have observed that ischaemic episodes with ST elevation have a particular distribution during 24 h periods with a preponderance during the first hours of the morning (Fig. 1). Out of these episodes the symptomatic ones (18% in this series) were equally distributed during 24 h; thus their incidence in respect of the total number of ischaemic episodes was minimal during the night and maximal during the day, probably because of a higher threshold to painful stimuli during the night time. This finding is in accordance with other reports in the literature (Golding *et al.*, 1973; Maseri *et al.*, 1978). On the contrary episodes characterized by ST segment depression do not show any particular distribution during the 24 h (Salerno *et al.*, 1981). It is also interesting to observe that medical treatment effective on the frequency of the ischaemic attacks does not abolish the daily distribution of episodes with ST elevation (Biagini *et al.*,

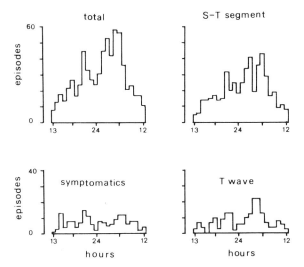

Figure 1. The daily distribution of the ischaemic episodes of 10 consecutive patients with angina at rest are presented in this picture. In panel A the total number of the ischaemic episodes recorded during a total of 48 days of continuous electrocardiographic monitoring by Holter technique are reported. The curve that represents the temporal distribution of the ischaemic episodes has a bell shaped contour with a peak at 5 a.m. The symptomatic episodes (panel B) don't have any particular pattern and their percentage in respect of the total episodes is minimal during the night and maximal during the day. In panel C and D the distributions of the episodes characterized by ST segment changes and T wave changes are presented. During the period of observation none of the patients was on drug administration but nitrates during the symptomatic episodes.

1981a). The "circadian" distribution seems not to be related to those hormones known to have a circadian rhythm (Biagini *et al.*, unpublished data).

Long periods of Holter monitoring also allowed us to recognize in most of the patients with variant angina the existence of rhythms of longer duration (Fig. 2). Although duration differed from patient to patient, it ranged in the majority of cases from 7 to 11 days.

In addition, the use of Holter monitoring has also shown in many patients with variant angina the existence of periodicity with much shorter duration, from a few minutes to 15–20 min. The results obtained in one patient during the night, from midnight to 6 a.m., during which he presented 28 ischaemic episodes, all asymptomatic, are shown in Fig. 3. It is interesting to note that this particular patient, as many others in our series, presented also a clear daily distribution with the described prevalence of the ischaemic episodes during the night in addition to a long-term periodicity of about 7 days.

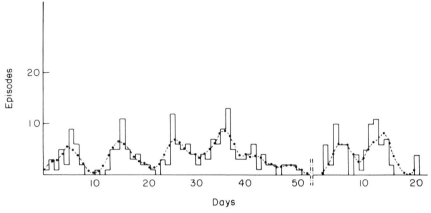

Figure 2. Histograms of the number of ischaemic episodes/day presented by one patient with angina at rest, obtained during a 52- and 20-day period of continuous electrocardiographic monitoring. The dotted line represents the best fit of the experimental data. The cyclic period in this particular patient was around 11 days, and was not correlated with the pharmacological therapy.

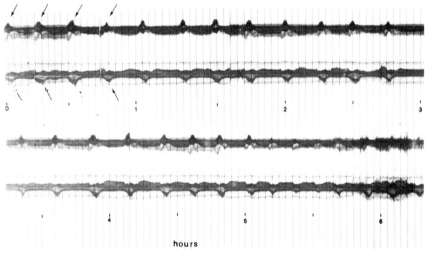

Figure 3. Analogic compact format of two electrocardiographic tracings obtained in one patient with angina at rest, monitored from midnight (time 0) to 6.30 a.m. by Holter technique. The first and third strips show the analogic compact format of an inferior lead while the second and the fourth strips show an anterior lead. The distance between two vertical lines is 3 min. In 6·5 h 28 ischaemic episodes (indicated by the arrows) characterized by ST segment elevation in the inferior lead and specular ST segment depression in the anterior lead are recognized. The distance between each episode is about 15–20 minutes. All the episodes were asymptomatic.

Thus in the same patient, irrespective of medical treatment, hourly, daily and day to day cyclic variation in the number of ischaemic episodes can be documented. This finding confirms the clinical knowledge of spontaneous worsening and waining of the disease. The documentation of these spontaneous variations strongly suggests the opportunity of long periods of monitoring in patients with variant angina, particularly when the evaluation of drugs in short- and medium-term clinical trials is requested.

Although the reasons for this complex ciclical manifestation of myocardial ischaemia are still obscure, the documentation of such biorhythms can address research on the pathophysiology of coronary vasospasm.

Myocardial Necrosis

The finding that the great majority of episodes of transient electrocardiographic changes are asymptomatic raises the question of their pathological significance. To answer this question, additional techniques capable of monitoring other parameters related to ischaemia are needed.

Angiographic (Biagini *et al.*, 1982a), scintigraphic (Parodi *et al.*, 1981), haemodynamic (Chierchia *et al.*, 1980) and echocardiographic (Distante *et al.*, 1979) studies tend to exclude that different mechanisms underline the two conditions. In a preliminary report (Biagini *et al.*, 1982b) we have observed, in the same patient that as compared to the symptomatic episodes, the asymptomatic ones are on the average of shorter duration and show less marked electrocardiographic alterations.

The detection of the actual number of ischaemic episodes has clinical and prognostic relevance as each episode can lead to a certain amount of cell damage, and frequent episodes can produce a progressive loss of myocardial tissue equivalent to a myocardial infarction (Biagini *et al.*, 1981b). For this reason we have conducted a study in 15 patients characterized by frequent ischaemic episodes, symptomatic and asymptomatic, in whom there was no clinical or electrocardiographic evidence of the occurrence of an acute myocardial infarction. The patients were characterized only by transient, completely reversible electrocardiographic changes indicative of myocardial ischaemia. In those patients serum enzymes of necrosis, such as myoglobin, creatine kinase MB form, and hydrossibutirric dehydrogenase were monitored and myocardial scans with ^{99m}Tc pyrophosphate performed. The serum time–activity curves had a crescendo–decrescendo pattern with a time course similar to that observed during myocardial infarction for both myoglobin and creatine kinase MB in seven patients, with a peak exceeding the normal upper limit in four cases. The ^{99m}Tc pyrophosphate myocardial scan was negative in one patient and positive in four while a diffuse but faint deposition of the tracer in the myocardial region was present in three patients. The results obtained in this series have shown that myocardial cell damage can follow episodes of acute transient myocardial ischaemia and that a strict connection can exist between ischaemic episodes, symptomatic or not, and loss of tissue.

Sudden Death

One point of particular clinical interest is the relationship between transient myocardial ischaemia and sudden death. The presence of coronary athero-sclerosis has been found a decisive factor in sudden death, however it does not explain *per se* the triggering mechanism of sudden death; in fact patients who die suddenly show at autopsy a remarkable variability in coronary involvement ranging from minimal to severely atherosclerotic vessels. Thus, the anatomic situation may *per se* favour or predispose, but not cause sudden death. In experimental animals acute ischaemia, as it occurs after ligation of a coronary artery, causes arrhythmias and sudden death. Similarly, in man, life-threatening arrhythmias were occasionally observed during ischaemic episodes caused by coronary vasospasm. To investigate the role of transient ischaemia at rest on the pathogenesis of sudden death we decided to perform a prospective study in patients with variant angina, the form of vasospastic ischaemia more frequently associated to potentially fatal arrhthymias (Fig. 4). Data are derived from a transversal and longitudinal observation of 187 patients with variant angina treated with medical therapy (Severi *et al.*, 1981). During hospitalization, 32 patients had serious arrhythmias asso-ciated with transient ischaemic episodes while 155 had no arrhythmias. Comparing the two groups we tried to answer the questions whether arrhythmias during ischaemic episodes (1) could be predicted by some clinical, ECGraphic or angiographic findings and (2) could be of prognostic

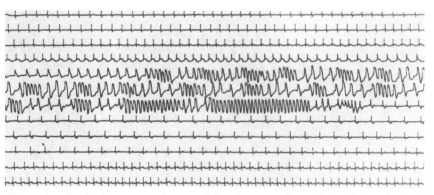

Figure 4. Analogic compact format of the electrocardiographic training obtained by Holter technique in one patient with angina at rest showing one ischaemic episode characterized by ST-segment elevation in the anterior lead and followed by runs of ventricular tachycardia.

value. We were unable to detect any significant difference between patients who developed arrhythmias and those who did not, regarding the incidence of previous myocardial infarction, of positive exercise stress test, of severity of coronary artery disease and of the abnormality of left ventricular function. In spite of these similar findings, early mortality in hospital was quite different, being 12% in the population with arrhythmias and 1·9% in the ones without arrhythmias. The mortality rate during the follow-up was very low in both groups, being on average 2·7% and 1·5% per year in patients with and without arrhythmias, respectively. Furthermore sudden death occurred in all cases but one, in patients who had had arrhythmias during ischaemic episodes while in the group of patients who had no arrhythmias only one-third of the causes of decease was sudden-death.

These data indicate that patients are at the greatest risk at the very onset of the symptoms or during the waxing phases of angina. The remarkably low incidence of sudden death as well as of other manifestations of ischaemic heart disease observed in the follow-up when patients received drugs known to prevent vasospasm suggests a new additional preventive approach to sudden death and to the clinical manifestations of heart disease.

The role of vasospastic ischaemia in triggering sudden death in the general population could be more important than suspected. In fact variant angina is only "an extreme of a continuous spectrum" of vasospastic ischaemia and less spectacular changes such as ST depression or T wave changes can underlie equally severe ischaemia. Furthermore because of the high frequency of asymptomatic episodes, sudden death can be the only clinical manifestation of ischaemic heart disease.

Acknowledgments

The authors greatly appreciate the secretarial assistance of Miss E. Campani, Miss D. Banti and Mrs H. Biagini de Ruyter.

References

Biagini, A., Carpeggiani, C., Mazzei, M. G., Testa, R., Michelassi, C., Antonelli, R., L'Abbate, A. and Maseri, A. (1981a). *G. ital. Cardiol.* **11**, 4.

Biagini, A., Mazzei, M. G., Carpeggiani, C., Buzzigoli, G., Zucchelli, G. C., Parodi, O., L'Abbate, A. and Maseri, A. (1981b). *Clin. Cardiol.* **4**, 301.

Biagini, A., Mazzei, M. G., Carpeggiani, C., Testa, R., Antonelli, R., Michelassi, C., L'Abbate, A. and Maseri, A. (1982a). *Am. Heart J.* **103**, 13.

Biagini, A., Testa, R., Carpeggiani, C., Mazzei, M. G., Emdin, M., Michelassi, C. and L'Abbate, A. (1982b). *In* "La Cardiopatia Ischemica Silente" (P. L. Prati, Ed.), p. 81. Lab. Schiapparelli, Roma.

Chierchia, S., Brunelli, C., Simonetti, I., Lazzari, M. and Maseri, A. (1980a). *Circulation* **61**, 759.

Chierchia, S., Lazzari, M., Simonetti, I. and Maseri, A. (1980b). *Herz* **5**, 189.

Distante, A., L'Abbate, A., Maseri, A., Landini, L. and Michelassi, C. (1979). *In* "Echocardiography" (Ed. Lancet, Ch. T.), p. 119. Martinus Nijhoff, The Hague.

Golding, B., Wolf, E., Tzivoni, D. and Stern, S. (1973). *Am. Heart J.* **86**, 501.

Guazzi, M., Polese, A., Fiorentini, C., Magrini, F., Olivari, M. T. and Bartorelli, C. (1971). *Br. Heart J.* **33**, 84.

Maggini, C., Guazzelli, M. Mauri, M., Chierchia, S., Cassano, G. B. and Maseri, A. (1978). *In* "Primary and Secondary angina pectoris" (Maseri, A., Klassen, G. A. and Lesch, M. Eds), p. 157. Grune and Stratton, New York.

Maseri, A. (1979). *Cardiovasc. Med.* **4**, 467.

Maseri, A., Mimmo, R., Chierchia, S., Marchesi, C., Pesola, A. and L'Abbate, A. (1975). *Chest* **68**, 625.

Maseri, A., L'Abbate, A., Pesola, A., Ballestra, A. M., Marzilli, M., Severi, S., Maltinti, G., De Nes, M., Parodi, O. and Biagini, A. (1977). *Lancet* **i**, 173.

Maseri, A., Severi, S., De Nes, M., L'Abbate, A., Chierchia, S., Marzilli, M., Ballestra, A. M., Parodi, O., Biagini, A. and Distante, A. (1978a). *Am. J. Cardiol.* **42**, 1019.

Maseri, A., L'Abbate, A., Baroldi, G., Chierchia, S., Marzilli, M., Ballestra, A. M., Severi, S., Parodi, O., Biagini, A., Distante, S. and Pesola, A. (1978b). *N. Engl. J. Med.* **299**, 1271.

Parodi, O., Uthurralt, N., Severi, S., Bencivelli, W., Michelassi, C., L'Abbate, A. and Maseri, A. (1981). *Circulation* **63**, 1238.

Salerno, J. A., De Marco, R., Medici, A., Previtali, M., Chimienti, M., Ray, M., De Servi, S., Tavazzi, L. and Bobba, L. (1981). In "Coronary Arterial Spasm" (Ed., Bertrand, M. E.), p. 126. Lab Dausse.

Selwyn, A. P., Fox, K. M., Oakley, D., Dargie, H. J. and Schillingford, J. P. (1979). *Br. med. J.* **2**, 1594.

Severi, S., Marzullo, P., Maseri, A. and L'Abbate, A. (1981). *Circulation* **64**, (Suppl. IV), 245.

Shang, S. J. Jr and Pepine, C. J. (1977). *Am. J. Cardiol.* **38**, 396.

Pathogenetic Mechanisms of Coronary Vasospasm

S. CHIERCHIA

Institute of Clinical Physiology, CNR, Pisa, Italy
and Royal Postgraduate Medical School,
University of London Cardiovascular Research
Unit, Hammersmith Hospital, London, UK

Although the importance of coronary vasospasm in the genesis of the different clinical manifestations of ischaemic heart disease is now well-established, the pathogenetic mechanisms responsible for it remain largely hypothetical. This is not surprising since large epicardial coronaries have been considered until recently only passive, rigid tubes and the interest of cardiac physiologists only recently directed towards their study.

This review will briefly summarize our own and others views on the pathophysiology of coronary vasospasm and report the experimental and clinical evidence supporting the different hypotheses.

Local Vascular Causes

Coronary vascular tone is likely to result from a dynamic equilibrium between vasoconstrictor and vasodilator stimuli acting on vascular smooth muscle. A critical reduction in coronary diameter could either result from an abnormal increase in vasoconstrictor tone in the presence of a reasonably preserved vasodilator reserve, or by the lack of vasodilatory forces able to counteract physiological vasoconstrictor stimuli.

This local equilibrium is obviously more likely to be altered by the presence of critical atherosclerotic lesions. On the one hand, the plaque

Frontiers Cardiol. for the 80s.
0-12-220680-0

itself can affect the homeostasis of vascular smooth muscle and produce a local hypersensitivity to vasoconstrictor stimuli; on the other hand, even minor changes in cross-sectional area due to vasoconstriction, can result in a complete occlusion of the vessel when the lumen is already severely reduced by the presence of a critical lesion.

McAlpin (1980) has recently suggested that a normal increase in vasomotor tone could be responsible for spasm superimposed on critical atherosclerotic lesions, while an "abnormal" increase should be postulated to explain spasm occurring on normal coronaries. However, should a normal increase in vasomotor tone be a common cause of spasm, it should be observed much more frequently in patients with severe coronary disease; moreover, the waxing and waning of symptoms, frequently observed in patients with vasospastic angina, suggests that factors other than atherosclerosis are likely to affect the threshold of excitability of coronary smooth muscle in response to vasoconstrictor stimuli. Vascular susceptibility to spasm could vary in relation to vessel wall alterations occurring in a particular phase of the atherosclerotic process and a variety of stimuli might then trigger vasoconstriction (Maseri et al., 1980), a circadian variation in sensitivity to spasm has also been described (Chierchia et al., 1978; Yasue et al., 1979), suggesting that humoral, nervous or neurohumoral factors, undergoing chronobiological variations, can also influence the occurrence of coronary vasospasm.

Possible Triggering Mechanisms

Autonomic Nervous System

The role of the autonomic nervous system in the genesis of coronary vasospasm has been repeatedly suggested. Stimulation of coronary alpha adrenergic receptors invariably results both in vivo and in vitro in contraction of large epicardial vessels of various animal species (Zuberbuhler and Bohr, 1965; Feigl, 1967; Drew and Levy, 1972). Pharmacological (Yasue et al., 1974) and reflex (Raizner et al., 1980) stimulation of the same receptors has been reported to precipitate coronary vasospasm in patients with variant angina. Administration of alpha adrenergic blocking agents occasionally prevents or reverses episodes of angina due to coronary vasospasm (Lewy et al., 1980; Yasue, 1980). Prolongation of the Q-T interval has been observed prior to episodes of variant angina and attributed to an increased sympathetic activity to the heart (Lewy, et al., 1980). The parasympathetic agent, metacholine, has also been reported to induce spasm (Endo et al., 1976; Stang et al., 1977) and the effect has been interpreted as consequent to a secondary release of noradrenaline by sympathetic nerve endings.

In our experience, alpha adrenergic stimulation only rarely precipitates coronary vasospasm in patients with variant angina (Chierchia *et al.*, in press). The "cold pressor" test appears ten times less powerful than ergonovine in provoking spasm and administration of phenylephrine, a pure alpha adrenergic agonist, is never effective. Continuous infusion of phento-lamine, an alpha-adrenolytic agent, failed to prevent the occurrence of episodes of vasospastic angina in five patients (Chierchia *et al.*, 1981). Prolongation of the Q-T interval prior to ischaemia was not confirmed in six patients with variant angina who recently came to our observation and were submitted to continuous Holter monitoring (Chierchia *et al.*, in press). In a systematic study, Robertson *et al.* (1979) failed to detect signs of generalized increase in sympathetic activity in a group of patients with vasospastic angina. More recently, the same authors reported a late increase in cardiac catecholamines levels during episodes of variant angina and suggested that increased sympathetic activity to the heart was probably a consequence rather than the cause of vasospastic myocardial ischaemia (Robertson *et al.*, 1981a).

Vasoactive Platelet Metabolites

The recent discovery of thromboxane A2 (TxA$_2$, Hamberg *et al.*, 1975), a potent vasoconstrictor released from aggregating platelets, and prostacyclin (PGI$_2$, Gryglewsky *et al.*, 1976), a powerful vasodilator with antiplatelet properties produced by vascular endothelial cells, opens a new field of research on the mechanisms locally controlling vascular tone. A local im-balance between TxA$_2$ and PGI$_2$ levels in the presence of endothelial lesions has been suggested as a possible mechanism of acute coronary vasoconstric-tion (Dusting *et al.*, 1979). Increased levels of TxB$_2$, the stable metabolite of TxA$_2$, have been found in both peripheral (Lewy *et al.*, 1979) and coronary sinus (Tada *et al.*, 1981) blood of patients with Prinzmetal's variant angina. However, administration of low dose aspirin (2mg/Kg/72 h), although reducing platelet thromboxane production to negligible levels, failed to prevent recurrence of ischaemic episodes due to coronary vasospasm (Robertson *et al.*, 1981b; Chierchia *et al.*, in press). Intravenous administra-tion of exogenous prostacyclin in six patients with variant angina induced obvious vasodilatation and markedly reduced *in vitro* platelet aggregation; repeated administration of the drug, alternated with equivalent periods of placebo, did not prevent the ischaemic episodes in five patients but con-sistently abolished the attacks in all four periods of infusion in one (Chierchia *et al.*, 1982). This observation suggests that, in some patients, a local or generalized decrease in prostacyclin could contribute to the genesis of coronary vasospasm.

During irreversible aggregation platelets also release serotonin, another powerful vasoconstrictor. The interest for serotonin in the pathogenesis of spasm has increased since the discovery that the vasoconstrictor effects of ergonovine, probably the most powerful agent used for the induction of coronary vasospasm, are mediated, *in vitro*, by serotonergic receptors (Henry and Yokoyama, 1980; Muller-Schweinitzer, 1980). Serotonin receptors could, therefore, represent a possible link between platelet aggregation and coronary vasoconstriction. As for many other hypotheses, this will also prove difficult to be checked in man, mainly because of the lack of specific and selective antagonists. Indeed, preliminary results seem to indicate that the coronary vasoconstrictor effects of ergonovine are not prevented by the administration of ketanserin, a relatively selective blocker of stubtype 2 serotonin receptors.

Other Possible Triggering Stimuli

After having shown the presence of a large number of subtype 1 histamine receptors on epicardial human coronaries, Ginsburg *et al.* (1980, 1981) have been recently able to precipitate coronary vasospasm by infusing histamine after H_2 receptor blockade with cimetidine. The patho-physiological relevance of this finding is not yet clear.

Prolonged hyperventilation with (Yasue *et al.*, 1978) or without (Pujadas *et al.*, 1981) Tris buffer infusion produces spasm in about 60% of patients with a positive ergonovine test. It is believed to induce coronary vasoconstriction by facilitating the entry of Ca^{2+} in coronary smooth muscle cells, resulting in activation of contractile proteins (Yasue *et al.*, 1978).

Conclusions

Despite the large number of clinical and experimental studies carried out in the last few years, the pathophysiological mechanisms underlying coronary vasospasm remain largely speculative. The few consistent observations obtained so far have ruled out some hypotheses but have not shed light on the actual triggering mechanisms of spasm.

The main difficulty in studying the problem is the fact that the genesis of spasm is probably multifactorial and the triggering mechanisms are likely to be different in different patients and, possibly, in the same patient at different times. The selection of patients, therefore, becomes crucial, since the same agonists or antagonists could produce different responses in different sub-sets of patients apparently presenting with the same clinical, angiographic and electrocardiographic characteristics.

Apparently, the only constant feature in patients with variant angina is the fact that coronary vasospasm is consistently precipitated by ergonovine and prevented by nitrates and calcium antagonists. Other powerful vasoconstrictors, such as phenylephrine and pitressin, or vasodilators, such as dipyridamole, phentolamine and prostacyclin, are generally not effective either in precipitating or preventing coronary vasospasm.

This observation suggests that vasospasm results from an interaction between the hypersensitive vascular smooth muscle and specific constrictor stimuli, rather than being the consequence of a non-specific vascular hypersensitivity to any vasoconstrictor stimulus. Similarly, reversal of spasm involves specific biochemical pathways activated by some drugs and not by others.

We believe that the study of the mechanism of action of drugs and other stimuli effective either in preventing or precipitating coronary vasospasm will provide many of the clues necessary for a better understanding of its pathophysiology.

References

Chierchia, S., Guazzelli, M., Maggini, C. and Maseri, A. (1978). *Circulation* **58**, 753.
Chierchia, S., Crea, F., Gasparetti, G., De Caterina, R. and Maseri, A. (1981). In "Les Alpha-bloquants, pharmacologie expérimentale et clinique", p. 203 Masson, Paris.
Chierchia, S., Patrono, C., Crea, F., Ciabatoni, G., De Caterina, R., Cinotti, G. A., Distante, A. and Maseri, A. (1982). *Circulation* **65**, 470.
Chierchia, S., Crea, F., Davies, G. Berkenboom, G. and Maseri, A. (in press). *Am. J. Cardiol.*
Chierchia, S., De Caterina, R., Crea, F., Patrono, C. and Maseri, A. (in press). *Circulation*.
Drew, G. M. and Levy, G. P. (1972). *Br. J. Pharmacol.* **46**, 348.
Dusting, G. J., Moncada, S. and Vane, J. R. (1979). *Prog. Cardiovasc. Dis.* **21**, 405.
Endo, M., Hirosawa, K., Kaneka, N., Hase, K., Inone, Y. and Komo, S. (1976). *N. Engl. J. Med.* **294**, 252.
Feigl, E. O. (1967). *Circ. Res.* **20**, 262.
Ginsburg, R., Bristow, M. E., Harrison, D. C. and Stinston, E. (1980). *Chest* **78** (suppl.) 180.
Ginsburg, R., Bristow, M., Kautrowitz, M. D., Bairn, D. S. and Harrison, D. (1981). *Am. Heart J.* **102**, 819.
Gryglewsky, R. S., Bunting, S., Moncada, S., Flower, R. J., and Vane, J. R. (1976). *Prostaglandins* **12**, 685.
Hamberg, M., Svennson, J. and Samuelson, B. (1975). *Proc. natn. Acad. Sci. U.S.A.* **72**, 2994.
Henry, P. D. and Yokoyama, M. (1980). *J. clin. Invest.* **66**, 306.
Lewy, R. I., Weiner, L., Smith, J. B., Walinsky, P., Silver, M. J. and Saia, J. (1979). *Clin. Cardiol.* **2**, 404.
Lewy, R. I., Wiener, L., Walinsky, P., Lefer, A. M., Silver, M. J. and Smith, J. B. (1980). *Circulation* **61**, 1165.
Maseri, A., Chierchia, S. and L'Abbate, A. (1980). *Circulation* **62** (suppl. V), 3.
McAlpin, R. W. (1980). *Am. J. Cardiol.* **46**, 143.
Muller-Schweinitzer, E. (1980). *J. cardiovasc. Pharmacol.* **2**, 645.
Pujadas, G., Tamashiro, A., Ruades, J. and Aldasoco, J. (1981). *Am. J. Cardiol.* **47**, 450, (abstr.).
Raizner, A. E., Chahine, R. A. and Ishimori, T. (1980). *Circulation* **62**, 925.

Robertson, D., Robertson, R. M., Nies, A. S., Oates, J. A. and Friesinger, G. C. (1979). *Am. J. Cardiol.* **43**, 1080.

Robertson, R. N., Bernard, Y. D. and Robertson, D. (1981a). *Circulation* **64** (suppl. IV) 245, (abstr).

Robertson, R. M., Robertson, D., Roberts, L. J., Maas, R. L., Fitzgerald, G. A. Friesinger, G. C. and Oates, J. A. *N. Engl. J. Med.* **304**, 998.

Stang, J., Kolibask, A. J. and Busk, C. (1977). *Am. J. Cardiol.* **39**, 326.

Tada, M., Kuzuya, T., Inone, M., Kodama, K., Mishima, M., Yanuda, M., Inui, M. and Abe, A. (1981). *Circulation* **64**, 1107.

Yasue, H. (1980). *Chest* **78** (Suppl.), 216.

Yasue, H., Touyama, M., Shimamota, M., Kato, H., Tanaka, S. and Akiyama, F. (1974). *Circulation* **50**, 534.

Yasue, H., Wagas, M., Omote, S., Takizawa, A., Miwa, K. and Tanaka, S. (1978). *Circulation* **58**, 56.

Yasue, H., Omote, S., Takizawa, A., Nagao, M., Miwa, K. and Tanaka, S. (1979). *Am. J. Cardiol.* **43**, 647.

Zuberbuhler, R. C. and Bohr, D. F. (1965). *Circ. Res.* **16**, 431.

Genesis of Atherosclerosis

G. WEBER

Centre of Research on Atherosclerosis,
Institute of Pathological Anatomy, University
of Siena, Siena, Italy

For atherogenesis, attention has been focused, for many years now, on the *hyperplastic smooth muscle cells reaction* to injuries mediated through endothelial lesions. The rôle of factors such as LDL or the platelet-derived-growth factor (PDGF) has been emphasized.

The presence and the rôle of *necrotic lesions* from the beginning of the natural history of the plaque (cf. Thomas *et al.*, 1977) have been rather neglected. We have been able (Weber, 1980; Weber *et al.*, 1980) to observe in transmission electron microscopy (TEM) that necrotic and necrobiotic smooth muscle cells are seldom to be found at all in the aorta of rabbits during early cholesterol atherogenesis, neither in the intima nor in the media. Those findings do not seem to simply depend on the necrogen effects of cholesterol auto-oxidation products; actually we have also observed quite similar lesions at TEM in rabbits subjected to immunological injuries (Weber *et al.*, 1980).

The importance of the aforementioned hyperplasiogen factors is certainly great but we feel that at least in a subsidiary way the hyperplasiogen effect of necrotic cells of the arterial wall should also be considered. Necrotic and necrobiotic lesions do not only take place at smooth muscle cell level but also at endothelial cell level (cf. Thomas *et al.*, 1977). As early as 7 days after the rabbits are given a 1% hypercholesterolic diet, large sheets or smaller groups of endothelial cells may be found at scanning electron microscope (SEM) examination to be detaching or to have detached from the aorta: some endothelial cell sheets have also been found by us circulating in the arterial blood (Weber *et al.*, 1978, 1979b). Morphometrically, the denuded

Frontiers Cardiol. for the 80s.
0-12-220680-0

areas represent 8% of the whole examined aortic surface (Weber and Toti, 1981).

Quite similar findings are still evident 15 days after the beginning of the hypercholesterolic diet: red blood cells and many platelets incorporated in a veil-like (maybe fibrin) deposition may at this period be seen adherent to parts of the denuded surface. Those data once more observed by us through the now disposable very sophisticated, highly reproducible, methodologies clearly confirm our previous observations (Weber *et al.*, 1970a, b; Weber and Toti, 1971a, b, c, d; Weber *et al.*, 1972a, b; 1973; 1974) so that those findings, far from being artificial, may have a real implication in the early phases of experimental atherogenesis.

The importance of *platelets* in promoting or helping the hyperplastic reaction of the smooth muscle cells cannot be undervalued. In effect, at freeze-etching examination, we have seen in the circulating platelets of rabbits on a short-term hypercholesterolic diet (Weber *et al.*, 1979a) and in human cases of familial type IIa hypercholesterolemia (Weber *et al.*, 1981a) a huge increase of the exocytotic processes taking place at the platelet membrane. The open canalicular system (OCS)-bound "protuberances" (cf. White and Clawson, 1980) are significantly increased and their increase has resulted biochemically linked with a huge increase of β-thromboglobulin secretion (preliminary results) which goes hand in hand, as is well known, with the secretion of factor IV and of PDGF (that promotes smooth muscle cell hyperplasia). Much work has to be done in the near future on platelets–wall relationships *in vivo* and *in vitro*.

As for the hyperplastic reaction of the arterial wall, here we must clearly remember that the early reactive phases of the arterial wall to atherogenic stimuli chiefly consist in a proliferation of smooth muscle cells, as was so clearly stressed at the Lindau Conference (Wolf, 1971). The presence of lipids and of macrophages (Wolman, 1974; Wissler, 1980; Stary, 1980) is verifiable only in a second moment, depending on the presence, the level and the nature of hypercholesterolemia. To avoid atherosclerosis not only should the accumulation of lipid be tentatively inhibited but also the hyperplastic reaction of the smooth muscle cells of the arterial wall. The number of smooth muscle cells in the arterial wall seems to be decidedly of relevance: in man, the most important atherosclerotic lesions are those of coronary arteries which are extremely rich in smooth muscle cells; atherosclerotic lesions develop much later for instance in the cerebral district not only at a clinical level (brain infarct usually appearing later in life than myocardial infarct) but also at autoptic gross inspection and even at histological examination of the arterial tree (Velican and Velican, 1981). The coronary arteries' lesions are much more precocious than those of the cerebral arteries. Also in animal models (rabbits, monkeys) under atherogenic stimuli lesions develop much later in cerebral arteries than in the aorta, coronary or carotid arteries.

In a collaborative work (now in progress) with the Wissler's SCOR Atherosclerosis Group of Chicago we have observed that 8–12 months after the beginning of the atherogenic diet the cerebral arteries are not affected by lesions while largely affected are not only the aorta but also the coronary and the carotid arteries. No endothelial nor smooth muscle cell lesions (or only really minimal) are appreciable at SEM and TEM examination of the cerebral arteries.

It must be noted here that in those arteries the endothelial cell lining does not lie directly over the internal elastic lamina but is separated from it by a thick basement membrane layer with sparse smooth muscle cells which are devoid of lipids. Does this thick basement membrane represent a morphological basis for hindering lipoprotein entrance into the cerebral arteries' wall or should other ultrastructural characters be looked for as well?

As in monkeys, also in rabbits submitted to an atherogenic diet, atherosclerosis of cerebral arteries does not appear at all or appears very late. But in the rabbit cerebral arteries there is no thick basement membrane layer underlying the endothelial cells. We have recently shown that in rabbits the concanavalin A (Con A) reactivity present in the aorta (Weber *et al.*, 1972a, 1973) as well as in the coronary, carotid and femoral arteries is extremely weak, almost completely absent at cerebral artery level (Weber *et al.*, 1981b), so that it might be inferred that a low amount or lack of lipoprotein–lipase activity (which after Dicorleto and Zilversmit, 1975; and Olivecrona *et al.*, 1976, has its site in the Con A reactive surface coat) could be a relevant factor in inhibiting or delaying the development of experimental atherosclerotic lesions of the cerebral arteries. We then extended similar research to the cerebral arteries of Cynomolgus monkeys (kindly provided by the *Istituto di Ricerche Biomediche*, Ivrea, Italy) kept on a normocholesterolic diet. We have tested the Con A reactivity at aortic and cerebral artery level: while the reaction was strongly positive at the aortic level it was negative in the cerebral arteries' endothelial cells (Weber *et al.*, 1981b).

These findings at cerebral artery level on which we have now been focusing your attention, throw light on and help explain the earlier involvement of the coronary arteries by atherosclerotic lesions vs the cerebral ones.

Comparative examination of endothelial cell cultures derived from different arterial districts may also help in future if their reaction and behaviour do keep being different to various stimuli. In conclusion, both human pathology observations and the study of animal models clearly show that important differences are revealed both at gross examination, light microscopic and ultrastructural level in different branches of the arterial tree so that a morphological basis for its different reactivities to atherosclerotic stimuli appears to exist.

References

Dicorleto, P. and Zilversmit, D. B. (1975). *Proc. Soc. exp. biol. Med.* **148**, 1101.
Gerrity, R. G. and Naito, H. K. (1980). *Artery* **8**, 208.
Olivecrona, T., Bengtsson, G., Hook, M. and Luidohl, U. (1976). *In* "Lipoprotein metabolism" (H. Greten, Ed.). Springer Verlag, Berlin.

Stary, H. C. (1980). *Artery* **8**, 205.

Thomas, W. A., Imai, H., Florentin, R. A., Reiner, J. M. and Scott, R. F. (1977). *Prog. Biochem. Pharmacol.* **13**, 234.

Velican, C. and Velican, D. (1981). *Atherosclerosis* **43**, 39.

Weber, G. (1980). *In* "Immunity and atherosclerosis" (P. Constantinides, F. Pratesi, C. Cavallero and T. Di Perri, Eds). Academic Press, London, New York, Toronto, Sydney and San Francisco.

Weber, G. and Tosi, p. (1971a). *Virchows Arch. a path. Anat. Physiol.* **353**, 325.

Weber, G. and Tosi, P. (1971b). Atti Simp. Internaz. Arteriosclerosi, Sanremo 29–30 May.

Weber, G. and Tosi, P. (1971c). *Path. Europ.* **6**, 386.

Weber, G. and Tosi, P. (1971d). VIII Congr. Naz. Soc. Ital. Micr. Elettronica, Milan 23–25 September.

Weber, G. and Toti, P. (1983). *Boll. Soc. ital. Biol. sper.* **57**, 2170.

Weber, G., Toti, P. and Cellesi, C. (1970a). *Arch. de Vecchi* **56**, 1.

Weber, G., Toti, P. and Cellesi, C. (1970b). *Arch. de Vecchi* **56**, 27.

Weber, G., Fabbrini, P., Barbaro, A. and Resi, L. (1972a). *Boll. Soc. ital. Biol. sper.* **48**, 1009.

Weber, G., Toti, P., Barbaro, A. and Resi, L. (1972b). *Boll. Soc. ital. Biol. sper.* **48**, 163.

Weber, G. Fabbrini, P. and Resi, L. (1973). *Virchows Arch. a Path. Anat. Physiol.* **359**, 299.

Weber, G., Fabbrini, P. and Resi, L. (1974). *Virchows Arch. a Path. Anat. Physiol.* **364**, 325.

Weber, G., Losi, M., Toti, P. and Vatti, R. (1978). *G. Arterioscl.* **3**, 203.

Weber, G., Bianciardi, G. and Pierli, C. (1979a). *Atherogenese* **4**, 33.

Weber, G., Losi, M., Toti, P. and Vatti, R. (1979b). *Artery* **5**, 29.

Weber, G., Orazioli, D., Fabbrini, P. and Resi, L. (1980). *G. Arterioscl.* **5**, 105.

Weber, G., Bianciardi, G., Toti, P., Widhalm, K. and Sinzinger, H. (1981a). 2nd Italian-Austrian Atherosclerosis Meeting, Igls 30 April–2 May, p. 41.

Weber, G., Fabbrini, P. and Resi, L. (1981b). *Boll. Soc. ital. Biol. sper.* **57**, 2176.

White, J. G. and Clawson, C. C. (1980). *Ultrastruct. Pathol.* **1**, 533.

Wissler, R. W. (1980). *In* "Atherosclerosis V" (A. M. Gotto, L. C. Smith and B. Allen, Eds). Springer Verlag, New York, Heidelberg and Berlin.

Wolf, S. (1971). The artery and the process of arteriosclerosis. Pathogenesis. Plenum Press, New York and London.

Wolman, M. (1974). *Atherosclerosis* **20**, 217.

The Elements of Regression of Advanced Atherosclerosis in Primates

R. W. WISSLER

Department of Pathology and Specialized
Center of Research in Atherosclerosis,
University of Chicago, Chicago, Illinois, USA

It is now clear that the major factor in atherogenesis in experimental animals as well as humans is cholesterol deposition in the intima and subintimal areas of the artery accompanied by smooth muscle cell proliferation.

While it is generally agreed that the deposition of stainable fat begins early in life, the contribution of these fatty streaks in lesion progression is controversial. There is little doubt, however, that most of the cholesterol and perhaps most of the lipid one can see and measure in both the fatty streak and the plaque comes from low density or very low density lipoprotein that makes its way through the endothelium and then becomes "bound" or "trapped" in the intima, partly by the proteoglycans and partly perhaps by means of the apo B receptors on the surface of the smooth muscle cells (Wissler, 1983).

Some of the most interesting recent findings regarding the lipid component of the lesion are related to the several forms of lipoproteins which may be atherogenic. It is now clear that cholesterol and saturated food fat feeding can result in an enlarged LDL particle with an enrichment of its cholesterol content, that LDL can circulate in several forms which Scanu and co-workers have labeled LDL-I, II, III, IV (Fless *et al.*, 1980) while work by Mahley (1980) indicates that some forms of VLDL in certain species may be particularly atherogenic (BVLDL in dogs) as may a particular type of HDL in some species (HDLc) which has a special component of arginine rich peptide and work by Getz and colleagues (Krishnaiah et al., 1980) in this Centre indicates that the apoprotein B of some LDL's and VLDL's may be made in the intestine as well as the liver following the feeding of a high cholesterol, high fat meal and may contain large quantities of an apo B peptide which is different from that which is usually made in the liver. It seems likely that LDL, rich in the intestinal type of apo B may, under some conditions, be a major contributor to atherogenesis.

A series of *in vitro* studies in our laboratory has demonstrated the importance of low density lipoproteins (LDL) from hyperlipemic serum in

(a) stimulating smooth muscle cell proliferation (Wissler et al., 1980a) and;

(b) permitting the intracellular assimilation of cholesterol esters in smooth muscle cells in much larger quantities than one would expect from the concentration in the serum (Wissler et al., 1981).

These and several other phenomena described recently constitute a part of an emerging cellular pathobiology (Wissler, 1979) and offer some of the elements of the potential for regression of the atherosclerotic plaque that are now evident (Wissler, 1978).

The direct data supporting the concept of regression have come from three kinds of studies:

(a) Extensive observations on human subjects both epidemiological and at the autopsy lesion level which have come from the consequences of warfare or experiments of nature in which large groups of wasting people were evaluated (Wissler, 1982).

(b) Numerous studies of regression of advanced experimental atherosclerosis in rhesus monkeys and swine (Daoud et al., 1976; Fritz et al., 1976; Wissler and Vesselinovitch, 1976; Wissler, 1982).

(c) Very recent studies of several series of small numbers of living human subjects studied by sequential arteriography both before and after vigorous therapy aimed at lowering serum lipid levels substantially (Barndt et al., 1977; Buchwald et al., 1978; Malinow, 1981).

We have now conducted ten studies of regression in the rhesus monkey, several of which have been reported (Vesselinovitch et al., 1976; Wissler and Vesselinovitch, 1976; Vesselinovitch and Wissler, 1978; Wissler, 1978, 1979, 1982). It is clear that substantial decrease in many plaque components can be quantitated in this species. Table 1 summarizes some of the gross evidence from three of these which indicates that the amount of the aortic surface covered by clearly evident lesions is much less after 12 months of therapy with any one of three types of therapeutic regimens. It is noteable, that not only does a low fat, low cholesterol ration favour regression but that an additive effect on regression can be demonstrated when cholestyramine therapy is added to dietary therapy and that substantial regression can be

Table 1 *Gross aortic lesions in three regression studies*

Groups	Atherogenesis and treatments		Gross aortic intimal lesions (Percentage of total)			
			RH XXVII (12 + 12 months)	RH XXXI (14 + 14 months)	RH XXXII (12 + 12 months)	Average
I	Coconut oil Butterfat Cholesterol	12·5% 12·5% 2·0%	62 ± 14·2	68 ± 9·5		66 ± 2·0
	Peanut oil Cholesterol	25·0% 2·0%			68 ± 3·9	
II	Coconut oil Butterfat Cholesterol	12·5% 12·5% 2·0%	84 ± 6·9	73 ± 4·8		82 ± 4·5
	Peanut oil Cholesterol	12·5% 2·0%			88 ± 4·3	
III	Low-fat, Low-cholesterol diet		23 ± 9·9			23 ±1·7
	Prudent diet: Corn oil Cholesterol	18·0% 0·05%		20 ± 8·4	26 ± 11·0	
IV	Low-fat, Low-cholesterol diet + Cholestyramine (2·5%)		10 ± 5·6			10 ± 1·5
	Prudent diet + Cholestyramine (2·5%)			7 ± 2·5	12 ± 3·4	
V	Coconut oil/Butterfat/ Cholesterol + Cholestyramine (2·5%)		31 ± 8·2	43 ± 12·0		32 ± 5·8
	Peanut oil/Cholesterol + Cholestyramine (2·5%)				23 ± 12·1	

produced when cholestryramine is simply added to the highly atherogenic diet.

Some of the lesion components have now been measured morphometrically in these animals, using both the point counting method (Vesselinovitch *et al.*, 1982) and the more recent, less laborious and more replicable computer-assisted digitizer that we have developed (Wissler *et al.*, 1980) with the help of Dr Gene Bond at Bowman Gray School of Medicine (Table 2). Furthermore, with Professor Giorgio Weber's collaboration, we have been able to document a strong component of healing of the endothelium over the severe atheromatous plaques (Weber *et al.*, 1977) and recently we have been able to confirm an important observation made earlier by Daoud and Fritz working with swine (Daoud *et al.*, 1976; Fritz *et al.*, 1976) indicating that cell mitotic activity in the plaque is markedly decreased during a regression regimen. Some of these characteristics of regression are reflected in the figure (Fig. 1).

While much remains to be done, it now appears to be firmly established that regression of advanced atherosclerosis is possible and that this will soon be an important area of study for human lesions.

We believe that the time is fast approaching when one of the best ways to test these results of therapy at the lesion level will be to utilize relatively small, carefully controlled groups of patients whose response to treatment will be documented quantitatively by means of autopsy-calibrated, computer-assisted, sequential, contrast-media angiography or by non-invasive ultrasound (echo) angiography. These should be much less complex and much more cost effective studies with less likelihood of flaws in design or execution as compared to the cumbersome, expensive, large-scale (mass clinical) trials (Wissler, 1982).

This should usher in a new era of prevention and regression, as well as aid in the development of approaches to atherosclerosis control where the

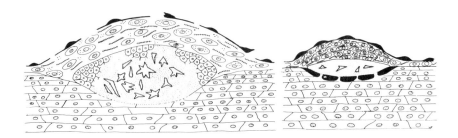

Figure 1. This is a diagrammatic representation of the major changes which seem to characterize regression of advanced atheromatous lesions in the rhesus monkey and in swine. Intracellular lipid virtually disappears and extracellular lipid decreases greatly. As endothelial damage heals, collagen and elastin condense and remodel. Reproduced from: R. W. Wissler, (1983).

Table 2 *RH XXXII Digitizer generated values for aortic lesion components*

Group	Dietary conditions		Total intimal lesion area (mm²)	Total lipid in lesion (%)	Intimal lesion thickness (mm)	Medial lesion (% of total media)
	First 12 months	Second 12 months				
I		Autopsied at 14 months (ref group)	0·40	50·6	0·19	4·5
II		Athero-diet continued	1·0	54·8	0·34	3·9
III	Atherogenic peanut oil diet with 2% cholesterol	Low fat, low cholesterol diet	0·47	20·5	0·18	2·2
IV		Low fat, low cholesterol and cholestyramine diet	0·23	9·7	0·11	0·5
V		Athero-diet and cholestyramine	0·54	9·9	0·20	1·5

effects of preventative and therapeutic measures will be documented in quantitative terms in living subjects at the lesion level.

References

Barndt, R., Blankenhorn, D. H., Crawford, D. M. and Brooks, S. H. (1977). *Ann. int. Med.* **86**, 139.

Buchwald, H., Auplatz, K., Knight, L. Guzman, I. and Varco, R. L. (1978). *In* "International Symposium State of Prevention and Therapy in Human Arteriosclerosis and in Animal Models" (W. H. Hauss, R. W. Wissler and R. Lehmann, Eds), p. 469. Westdeutscher-Verlag, Opladen, West Germany.

Daoud, A. S., Jarmolych, J., Augustyn, J. M., Fritz, K. E., Singh, J. K. and Lee, K. T. (1976). *Arch. Pathol. Lab. Med.* **100**, 372.

Fless, G. M., Kirchhausen, T., Fischer-Dzoga, K., Wissler, R. W. and Scanu, A. M. (1980). "Atherosclerosis V' (Proc. Vth Int. Symp.) (A. M. Gotto Jr, L. C. Smith and B. Allen, Eds), p. 607. Springer-Verlag, New York.

Fritz, K. E., Augustyn, J. M., Jarmolych, J., Daoud, A. S. and Lee, K. T. (1976). *Arch. Pathol. Lab. Med.* **100**, 380.

Krishnaiah, K. V., Walker, L. F., Borensztajn, J., Schonfeld, G. and Getz, G. S. (1980). *Proc. natn. Acad. Sci. USA* **77**, 3806.

Mahley, R. W. (1980). *In* "Atherosclerosis V" (Proc. Vth Int. Symp.) (A. M. Gotto Jr, L. C. Smith and B. Allen, Eds), p. 641. Springer-Verlag, New York.

Malinow, M. R. (1981). *Circulation* **64**, 1.

Vesselinovitch, D. and Wissler, R. W. (1978). *In* "International Symposium State of Prevention and Therapy in Human Arteriosclerosis and in Animal Models" (W. H. Hauss, R. W. Wissler and R. Lehmann, Eds), p. 127. Westdeutscher Verlag, Opladen, West Germany.

Vesselinovitch, D., Wissler, R. W., Hughes, R. and Borensztajn, J. (1976). *Atherosclerosis* **23**, 155.

Vesselinovitch, D., Wissler, R. W. and Schaffner, T. (1982). *In* "Nutrition and Heart Disease (H. Naito, Ed.), p. 121. S. P. Medical and Scientific Books, New York.

Weber, G., Fabbrini, P., Resi, L., Jones, R., Vesselinovitch, D. and Wissler, R. W. (1977). *Atherosclerosis* **26**, 535.

Wissler, R. W. (1978). *In* "Atherosclerosis Reviews", Vol 3 (R. Paoletti and A. M. Gotto Jr, Eds) p. 213. Raven Press, New York.

Wissler, R. W. (1979). *Artery* **5**, 398.

Wissler, R. W. (1982). *In* "Le Lipoproteine", (R. Paoletti and B. Lewis, Eds), p. 87. Gruppo Lepetit, Milan.

Wissler, R. W. (1983) *In* "Heart Disease: A Textbook of Cardiovascular Medicine", 2nd Edition (E. Braunwald, Ed.), 1221. W. B. Saunders Co., Philadelphia.

Wissler, R. W. and Vesselinovitch, D. (1976). *In* "Atherogenesis" (Proc. 1st Int. Symp.). *Ann. NY Acad. Sci.* **275**, 363.

Wissler, R. W., Fischer-Dzoga, K., Bates, S. R., Chen, R. M. and Eisele, B. (1980a). *Folia Angiologica* **28**, 32.

Wissler, R. W., Vesselinovitch, D., Schaffner, T. J. and Glagov, S. (1980b). *In* "Atherosclerosis V" (Proc. Vth Int. Symp.) (A. M. Gotto Jr, L. C. Smith and B. Allen, Eds), p. 757. Springer-Verlag, New York.

Wissler, R. W., Fischer-Dzoga, K., Bates, S. R. and Chen, R. M. (1981). *In* "Structure and Function of the Circulation" (C. J. Schwartz, N. T. Werthessen and S. Wolf, Eds), p. 427. Plenum Press, New York.

Mechanisms of Myocardial Damage and Its Reversibility

G. BAROLDI

Institute of Clinical Physiology, CNR, Pisa, Italy

The concept of a causal relationship between blood flow reduction and myocardial damage arose from the first post-mortem observations of obstructive lesions of the main coronary arteries. At present morphologic and functional changes at any level of the coronary system, as well as non-vascular conditions such as anaemia, cardiac hypertrophy, etc. suggesting a discrepancy between myocardial metabolic demand and nutrient supply, are thought to be the pathogenic background for the different clinical syndromes of "ischaemic heart disease" (IHD).

Little attention, however, has been paid to the various patterns of myocardial damage. The assumption is that all are consequent to ischaemia. In reality they are distinct morphologic entities each of which may have a specific pathogenic mechanism (Table 1). Each represents a different form of myocardial cell death which can be related to the three phases of its functional cycle: irreversible relaxation ("atonic death"), irreversible contraction, or better, hypercontraction ("tetanic death") and progressive loss of force of contraction and velocity of contraction and relaxation ("failing death").

In atonic death the myocardial cell is incapable of contraction and becomes passively stretched by the intraventricular pressure (systolic paradoxical bulging). Increased length of sarcomeres, elongation of the nuclei and thinning of myocardial cells are the earliest histologic signs reflecting this dysfunctional state. Within a few hours pathognomonic centripetal

Frontiers Cardiol. for the 80s.
0-12-220680-0

Table 1 Histologic pattern in different types of myocardial necrosis in CHD

Myocardium	Coagulation necrosis	Coagulative myocytolysis (Zenker necrosis)	Colliquative myocytolysis (myocytolysis)
Functional status	Irreversible relaxation (atonic death) + stretching by intraventricular pressure	Irreversible contraction (tetanic death)	Progressive loss of function (failing death)
Muscle fibre	Early thinning	Normal or swollen	Increasing oedema – vacuolization
Nucleus	Elongation – pycknosis progressive fading	Normal	Normal
Myofibrils	Elongated sarcomeres in normal registered order, even in late stage	Rhexis – Anomalous irregular cross band formations (coagulation of hypercontracted sarcomeres)	Progressive disappearance
Vessels	Secondary wall degeneration and thrombosis	Normal	Normal
Infiltration	Massive polymorphonuclear exudation	No early infiltrates. Possible late lymphocytes	No infiltrates
Extension – Location	In general unique massive focus of different size internal to transmural	Multiple (mono or pluricellular) disseminated or confluent foci of different size in any muscular layer	Focal subendocardial and peri-vascular, progressively spreading
Irreversible within	At least 20–60 min	Few minutes	?
Healing	In all the three different types: Removal by macrophages. Collagenization of empty sarcolemmal tubes		
Frequency in CHD: acute infarct	100%	100% external layer of infarct 77% in normal myocardium	43%
Sudden death	17% histologically demonstrated	72% unique demonstrable lesion 86% including cases with coagulation necrosis	8%

From: Baroldi, G., et al. (1979). Am. Heart J. 98, 20.

polymorphonuclear leukocytic infiltration occurs followed by vessel wall necrosis and fibrin thrombosis of the intramural vessels. The myofibrillar apparatus remains intact even within the last remnants of necrotic tissue undergoing organization. Improperly defined as "coagulation necrosis", this lesion is in general unifocal, being the specific structural change by which the histologic diagnosis of cardiac infarct is made.

The opposite pattern is shown in the tetanic death in which the myocardial cell is seen in extreme contraction. Hypercontraction with extreme shortening of the sarcomeres, myofibrillar rhexis and anomalous cross bands (coagulation of groups of hypercontracted sarcomeres) are the main structural characteristics. It is possible that this peculiar myofibrillar disruption is a consequence of the action of the normally contracting myocardium on the rigid, hypercontracted myocells. The lesion is multifocal with a tendency to become confluent. The number of cells involved in each focus may range from one to several to thousands. This type of damage, which is present in many human conditions, particularly in pheochromocytoma and experimentally reproduced by cathecolamine infusion, is always visible at the border of an acute infarct ("coagulation necrosis") and in most instances in the normal myocardium mainly in the region of the infarct (Silver *et al.*, 1980). In the majority of selected sudden coronary death cases, namely those with no history of IHD, no medical treatment or resuscitation attempts, this type of necrosis constitutes the unique acute demonstrable lesion (Baroldi *et al.*, 1979). The latter has been variously defined in the literature; miliary necrosis, catecholamine infarct or myocarditis, myofibrillar degeneration, contraction-band necrosis and coagulative myocytolysis. Due to its similarity to Zenker's necrosis of the skeletal muscle, perhaps Zenker's necrosis would be a preferable term.

The histologic hallmarks of the third type of damage, i.e. progressive intramyocellular oedema with vacuolization and disappearance of the myofibrils leading to "clear and empty" myocardial cells with an apparently normal nucleus, are indicative of a progressive functional reduction of contractility. Typically found in cardiomyopathies associated with low output syndrome, this lesion is seen in the subendocardial and perivascular layers of preserved myocardium in about half of the acute infarct cases and in 8% of sudden death cases, mainly those with extensive fibrosis. In the literature it is called vacuolar degeneration, sarcolysis, myofibrillolysis or myocytolysis. The latter term is the more popular one, but often indiscriminately used to indicate both this type of necrosis as well as Zenker's necrosis. To avoid confusion it is better to distinguish between coagulative myocytolysis or Zenker's necrosis ("tetanic" necrosis) and colliquative myocytolysis ("failing" necrosis) or myocytolysis *tout court*, if by this term we mean the latter lesion only.

The clear-cut morpho-functional pattern of each type of damage is evidence against the three types of structural change being different aspects of the same lesion and implies specific biochemical derangement and pathogenesis. This reasoning is consistent with the general rule that a specific pathogenic mechanism always induces the same type of damage. It is quite unlikely that different degrees of ischaemia may result in completely different morpho-functional patterns, or that one pattern may revert to another. In fact any infarct should be a mixture of the different lesions, since a transmural and chronological gradient of ischaemia exists because coagulation necrosis begins after a minimum of 20 min and is completely established only after one hour or more. On the other hand it is unlikely that a hypercontracted, fragmented myocell with rhexis of myofilaments and anomalous band formation would revert to a "relaxed" thin element with normal myofibrils or vice versa. Increasing intensity of a pathogenic cause results in a greater extension of the lesion but not in a different type.

At present we are investigating the correlation between biochemical and functional parameters and quantified extension of Zenker's necrosis by infusion of increasing doses of isoproterenol and noradrenaline in dogs. Increasing doses of these cathecolamines cause an increase in number and extension of Zenker necrotic foci, but do not produce coagulation necrosis or myocytolysis (Todd *et al.*, in press). Furthermore, from this study we found that at least three types of "contraction bands" can be distinguished. One, prominent at lower doses, is a transverse band which involves about 15 hypercontracted sarcomeres adjacent to the intercalated disc, the other portion of the myocell remaining normal. This "paradiscal" lesion is characterized by extreme shortening of sarcomeres showing thin, often fragmented transverse lines which seem to be remnants of the Z lines. The myofilaments maintain their longitudinal disposition, but without their normal sarcomeric structure. There is no rhexis or fragmentation of the myofibrils and the "band" does not show mitochondria. This type of contraction band may appear as a "clear band" (undetectable by the light microscope) or as a "dark band" (visible by the light microscope), or transitional patterns between these two can be observed.

A second type of "contraction band" is seen when the whole myocell is damaged. In this condition empty spaces or spaces filled by packed mitochondria alternate with total or partial transverse bands of hypercontracted sarcomeres with apparently thickened Z lines. The hypercontraction state of the latter as well as of the paradiscal lesion is deduced by the presence of folding of the sarcolemma, displacement of the mitochondria and by the frequent finding of waviness of the normal adjacent cells.

Finally at the site of biopsy samples a third type of "contraction band" limited to a zone of 0·2–0·5 mm in width along the cutting edge is detected. This lesion is probably due to the bioptic procedure per se and shows only hypercontracted sarcomeres in register, with thick Z lines, without rhexis or disruption of myofilaments.

With these findings two main questions arise. First what are the cause(s) and the pathogenic mechanism specific for each type of damage and, second, what does their presence together in the myocardium mean in IHD? We assume that IHD is an entity, even if not yet well defined which should not be confused with other, apparently similar, entities. For example infarct and/or sudden death may occur following involvement of a coronary artery by dissecting aneurysm or embolism. However these conditions are associated with diseases which are not part of the natural history of IHD. These examples as well as the experimental coronary occlusion demonstrate that a sudden reduction of the coronary blood flow is a mechanism capable of inducing infarct and/or sudden death. However, it must be recognized that the presence of longstanding disease, the presence of major complications of the IHD itself, the changes induced by medical interventions and resuscitation attempts, and the presence of other cardiac and non-cardiac disease can influence the clinical and pathological picture. Consequently it is important to separate these various categories in any study of the natural history of IHD. If only cases of IHD without any of these complicating conditions are studied, there is no conclusively documented direct cause–effect relationship between morphological and functional changes in the coronary arteries and the various clinical syndromes of IHD. It seems likely that coagulation necrosis found in IHD is caused by ischaemia. The mechanism(s) however, is (are) still controversial. Although it is not definitely proved, Zenker's necrosis and myocytolysis appear to be metabolic disorders of the myocardial cell without any relation to ischaemia. In support of this idea, Zenker's necrosis and myocytolysis occur in areas adjacent and near the infarct, where the nutrient flow should be adequate; otherwise extension of coagulation necrosis of earlier histologic age rather than other types of necroses, would be expected, a finding never observed in our cases (Baroldi *et al.*, 1974; Baroldi, 1983).

The causes and mechanisms of both Zenker's necrosis and myocytolysis are still a matter of speculation. The role of defects of the calcium and sodium pumps and the role of excess or depletion of cathecolamines is under investigation. As important a question is the meaning of these two types of damage when found in IHD, especially in relation to clinical course and mortality. Ventricular fibrillation and cardiac insufficiency are the main complications and causes of death. Zenker's necrosis and myocytolysis may represent the histologic hallmarks of a sympathetic or sympathetic-like disorder. Supporting this is the observation that both ventricular fibrillation and Zenker necrosis following acute coronary occlusion in dog can be prevented by beta-blocking agents (Baroldi *et al.*, 1977).

Considering these observations, several points can be raised. The first concerns the point of no return for each type of damage. Experimentally the irreversibility occurs in a few minutes for Zenker's necrosis, in about one hour for coagulation necrosis and the time limit is not yet determined for myocytolysis. This is too short for a possible therapeutical reversibility of the lesions. Therefore in patients with myocardial infarction it seems more appropriate and realistic to speak of prevention of metabolic damage of the normal non-ischaemic myocardium rather than reduction or limitation of the infarct size.

Another concern is to evaluate the various events which happen in the different patterns of IHD. During infarction, particularly when infarct is large, the sudden loss of contracting myocardium impairs the function of the cardiac pump as a whole. Data support the concept that the compensatory hyperfunction of the normal myocardium is mediated through the sympathetic nervous system. In people predisposed by congenital and acquired factors such as smoking, stress, pain, etc., a damaging sympathetic over-stimulation may occur particularly at the border of the infarct, where maximal mechanical tension should exist. In other words infarct *per se* may become the trigger mechanism leading to the above events resulting in ventricular fibrillation. On the other hand there is clinical evidence that most sudden coronary death cases, in one study 81% of patients resuscitated by defibrillation, do not show an infarct. In the latter condition congenital and/or acquired sympathicotonia *per se* may be responsible for the morpho-functional myocardial damage.

Last but not least, coronary spasm is the fashionable mechanism invoked to explain sudden events IHD. Spasm has been convincingly shown to be a fact and not an artifact. It occurs in angina and in acute infarct. It remains to be proved if the spasm is a primary or secondary phenomenon, and whether it plays a role in all clinical syndromes of IHD. Finally the cause of the spasm has yet to be established.

Experimental coronary occlusion is often associated with ventricular fibrillation in the first hour. It is possible to speculate that transient spasm may induce the same temporary loss of contraction as occurs in infarction, however, infarct is prevented because of early reflow. The spasm should last no more than 20 min. If occlusion lasts longer than 20 min and is followed by reflow, experimentally we see a type of myocardial damage which is associated with ventricular fibrillation and can be prevented by beta-blocking agents. This myocardial damage is a variant of Zenker's necrosis with rhexis of myofilaments and "contraction bands" associated with extensive haemorrhage and exudation; a pattern never seen in our cases of infarct and sudden death, and similar if not identical to the postsurgical haemorrhagic necrosis.

In conclusion IHD is still a field for speculation and working hypothesis, in which all the demonstrated facts should be considered and their significance and interrelation should be tested.

References

Baroldi, G. (1975). *Am. Heart J.* **89**, 742–752.

Baroldi, G. (1982). *In* "The Heart" (J. W. Hurst, Ed.), pp. 589–599. 5th Edition. McGraw-Hill Book Co., New York.

Baroldi, G. (1983). *In* "Cardiovascular Pathology" (Silver, M. D., Ed.), pp. 317–391. Churchill Livingstone Inc., New York. 1983.

Baroldi, G., Radice, F., Schmid, C. and Leone, A. (1974). *Am. Heart J.* **87**, 65–75.

Baroldi, G., Silver, M. D., Lixfeld, W. and McGregor, D. C. (1977). *J. molec. Cell. Cardiol.* **9**, 687–691.

Baroldi, G., Falzi, G. and Mariani, F. (1979). *Am. Heart J.* **98**, 20–31.

Silver, M. D., Baroldi, G. and Mariani, F. (1980). *Circulation* **61**, 219–227.
Todd, G. L., Baroldi, G., Pieper, G. M., Clayton, F. C. and Eliot, R. S., Experimental cathecolamine-induced myocardial necrosis. I Acute Morphologic patterns (in press).

The Genesis of Arrhythmias

D. G. JULIAN

Department of Cardiology, Freeman Hospital,
University of Newcastle upon Tyne, Newcastle
upon Tyne, UK

Arrhythmias, more specifically ventricular arrhythmias, remain the commonest mechanism of death in acute heart attacks, in spite of our success in treatment with drugs and electricity. Progress towards prevention is hampered by our inadequate knowledge of the mechanisms. Essentially, it has not been, as yet, possible to identify the precise cause of ventricular arrhythmias in man and we are dependent for our knowledge, first upon animal models of whose relevance we are uncertain and, second, upon the observation of certain phenomena in man which are associated with arrhythmias but which are not necessarily causal.

We must also remember that when arrhythmias occur during ischaemia or infarction, they may be due, not only to the direct effects upon the myocardium, but also to the generalized effects – the effects upon the CNS, upon sympathetic and parasympathetic activity, the changes in serum biochemistry and to local biochemical changes and, increasingly, to iatrogenic factors.

Let us first consider the animal models from an electrophysiological point of view. All arrhythmias may be regarded as being due either to enhanced automaticity or to re-entry, or both.

Perhaps the most popular animal model and that most relevant to myocardial infarction in the human is the dog model of Harris. In this model, ligation of a coronary artery leads to ventricular fibrillation within a few minutes in many animals. In those who survive, a period of some hours quiescence ensues before frequent and prolonged ventricular tachycardia develops. If reperfusion occurs during the quiescent period, ventricular fibrillation may occur.

Frontiers Cardiol. for the 80s.
0-12-220680-0

It has been found that ventricular fibrillation in the early phase is probably the result of re-entry within the ischaemic myocardium, which in turn results from slow depolarization, slow conduction and inhomogeneity. The ventricular tachycardia which occurs later is probably the result of enhanced automaticity of Purkinje fibres which become ischaemic but not infarcted. At a much later stage, ventricular arrhythmias may result from re-entry in territory adjacent to the infarcted area.

There is increased sympathetic activity following infarction with high levels of circulating catecholamines, whose effects are often adverse. It should be mentioned that in the cat model used by Sobel, alpha adrenergic stimulation appears to be an important arrhythmogenic factor. In many preparations, vagal activity protects against ventricular fibrillation, although bradycardia may, as is well-known, lead to ventricular arrhythmia in the human.

Other local and general biochemical factors must be emphasized. The interest in serum free fatty acids is waning but there is increasing concern that K depletion is a factor in arrhythmogenesis. We have undertaken a retrospective study which suggests that in a group of patients, none of whom have been on diuretics, ventricular fibrillation is more common in those whose K is between 3·0 and 3·5, than those with higher K levels.

It must also be emphasized that arrhythmias arise in very varying pathological conditions. Thus, when ventricular fibrillation causes instantaneous death, there is usually no thrombosis or infarction; the longer the time that elapses between the onset of the final episode and ventricular fibrillation, the more likely is thrombosis and infarction to be present. When ventricular fibrillation occurs several days after the onset, infarction is usually extensive.

We have been particularly interested in primary ventricular fibrillation – ventricular fibrillation occurring after infarction without pump failure. Our early CCU experience suggested a relationship between frequent and complex ventricular ectopic beats (especially R or T) and subsequent ventricular fibrillation. Later, Lown, on the basis of these observations and animal experiments, produced a classification of ventricular arrhythmia and he designated the more frequent and complex ventricular arrhythmia as "warning arrhythmias". Although for many years this concept was widely accepted and formed the basis for therapy, several workers, mostly Lie in Amsterdam and El-Sherif in Miami, have suggested that the so-called warning arrhythmias are as common in those who do not proceed to ventricular fibrillation as in those who do. Although we were impressed by these studies, we were concerned about certain aspects of them – notably the fact that some patients had received treatment before or during these studies, the changes in the frequency of the arrhythmias were not taken into account and the possibility that the significance of arrhythmia could change with time was not considered. Clinical experience also suggests close relationships between certain arrhythmic phenomena and ventricular fibrillation.

We therefore undertook a study that concerned patients within 3 h after the onset of infarction, none of whom had received anti-arrhythmic drugs, diuretics or beta-blockers in the preceding 72 h. Seventeen who developed ventricular fibrillation were compared with 21 apparently similar patients who did not.

Essentially, there was no difference in incidence of the various arrhythmias between the two groups within the first 12 h of the study. Of course, because ventricular fibrillation often occurred very early, non-VF patients were observed for a longer period. If this factor is taken into account R-on-T was more common in VF patients; other ventricular arrhythmias were not.

There was a striking difference between the prevalence of different ventricular arrhythmia at different times. Thus, ventricular fibrillation and R-on-T were most common in the first two or three hours, whereas ventricular arrhythmia, and especially ventricular tachycardia, persisted or even became more common towards 12 h. There was, furthermore, an increasing prevalence of R-on-T prior to ventricular fibrillation and ventricular fibrillation was initiated by R-on-T. The similarity of these findings those of the animal model of Harris is striking.

Late in-hospital ventricular fibrillation is different, being seen predominantly in those with antero-septal infarction with intraventricular conduction disorders. Post-hospital sudden death occurs especially in those with left ventricular dysfunction. Ventricular arrhythmias are statistically related, but probably are not causal. The best predictor may be exercise-induced ST changes soon after infarction. This observation must contain information about mechanisms.

Finally, we must remember the importance of drugs as arrhythmogenic agents; not only digitalis and diuretics, but anti-arrhythmic drugs. We must especially be concerned with drug interactions – such as quinidine and digitalis, amiodarone and digitalis, and, a new one – disopyramide and sotalol.

In summary, there are very numerous factors playing a role in the genesis of arrhythmias – anatomical, physiological, biochemical and pharmacological.

Characteristics of the Resuscitated Out-of-Hospital Cardiac Arrest Victim with Coronary Heart Disease

S. GOLDSTEIN, J. R. LANDIS,
R. LEIGHTON, G. RITTER,
C. M. VASU, A. LANTIS and
R. SEROKMAN

Henry Ford Hospital, Detroit, Michigan, USA

Most coronary heart disease deaths occur suddenly, outside the hospital. Many of these out-of-hospital cardiac arrest victims are being resuscitated because of well trained emergency medical squads (EMS). A study of these survivors may be able to increase our knowledge about the mechanisms of death in coronary heart disease (Baum *et al.*, 1974; Liberthson *et al.*, 1974a; Cobb *et al.*, 1975; Schaffer and Cobb, 1975). In this report, patients resuscitated outside the hospital after cardiac arrest due to coronary heart disease, will be discussed (Goldstein *et al.*, 1981). We will describe the clinical characteristics of these patients before their arrest, the event itself, and their immediate post-resuscitation course. We will correlate these observations with long-term survival of resuscitated patients.

* Supported by the National Heart, Lung and Blood Institute Grant N° H1 18800-07.

Methods

All emergency cardiac arrest runs occurring in three communities in Michigan and Ohio were collected between July 1, 1975 and June 15, 1979. All emergency cardiac runs were counted regardless of the status of the patient at arrival. Cardiac run was defined as the dispatch of an EMS for an event not related to trauma and associated with a cardiac arrest, either at arrival or during transit. A total of 1915 cardiac arrest events occurred before the arrival of the emergency unit and 250 occurred after the arrival of the unit for a total of 2171 events. Mean arrival time, calculated from the initial emergency call to the arrival of the EMS was 4·73 min. Of the 2171 patients, 81% were dead on arrival. Of the 417 patients who survived to reach the hospital, 27% died within the first day, 33% died before discharge and 40% were ultimately discharged alive. Of 166 patients successfully resuscitated, 142 were classified as having significant coronary heart disease. The 142 patients were classified into three groups using enzyme and electro-cardiographic information. Group 1 were acute myocardial infarctions (AMI) characterized by the development of new Q waves on serial electro-cardiographic tracings. Group 2 were ischaemic events (IE) that had evidence of myocardial ischaemia based on enzyme abnormalities and probably would be best characterized as subendocardial infarctions. They did not, however, develop a new transmural Q wave. Group 3 were patients with primary arrhythmic events (PAE) who did not develop any enzyme evidence of acute myocardial ischaemia following their events. Of the 142

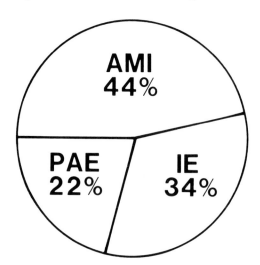

Figure 1.   Primary or precipitating event leading to sudden death in 142 victims with atherosclerotic heart disease studied by Goldstein and colleagues.

patients in whom a diagnosis of coronary heart disease was established, 62 (44%) were classified as acute myocardial infarction, 49 (34%) as ischaemic events, and 31 (22%) were considered to have a primary arrhythmic event (Fig. 1).

Results

The success of the out-of-hospital resuscitation is directly related to the arrival time of the EMS. If cardiac arrest was present upon arrival of the EMS, it was associated with a 6·5% (124 of 1913) success rate. If the arrest occurred after arrival, the success rate was 17·4% (45 of 258). The overall success rate was 7·8% for our entire population and was related to the duration of the arrival time of the EMS (Fig. 2). When the EMS arrived in less than 3 min, 10·2% (80 of 781) of the victims were resuscitated. The success rate fell precipitously as arrival time was prolonged. In those who had a cardiac arrest after arrival of the unit, either before or during transit, arrival time had little significance.

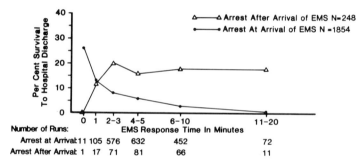

*Figure 2. Success of resuscitation related to emergency medical squad (EMS) response time. Total number in each group is less than in text because of incomplete response time data. (From Goldstein et al. (1981). Circulation **64**, 977; by permission of the American Heart Association, Inc.)*

Review of the clinical characteristics of the resuscitated victims prior to their arrest indicated that patients with a PAE were older than those with IE, who were, in turn, older than those with AMI. A history of angina was common in all three groups although the patients with AMI and IE were more often free of evidence of heart disease prior to their event. Cardiac arrest was the first cardiac event in 35% of the AMI patients. Most of the patients with PAE had a history of cardiovascular disease.

The survival experience for the patients classified according to the entry event subgroups is shown in Fig. 3, beginning from arrest event and for a maximum of 54 months of follow-up. The cumulative survival rates are significantly different ($P < 0.05$) among all three groups. The survival rate at

102   S. Goldstein et al.

Table 1   *Clinical characteristics of successfully resuscitated out-of-hospital cardiac arrest victims*

Entry event	Acute myocardial infarction (n = 62)	Ischaemic event (n = 49)	Primary arrhythmic event (n = 31)
Mean age (years)[a]	57·7	63·7	68·5
History			
Angina	53%(33)	53%(26)	61%(19)
Hypertension[b]	29%(18)	53%(26)	55%(17)
Digitalis therapy[c]	10%(6)	31%(15)	55%(17)
Myocardial infarction[c]	27%(17)	55%(27)	71%(22)
No history of the above[c]	35%(22)	16%(8)	6%(2)

Numbers in parentheses indicate number of patients. [a] Denotes all three pairwise differences significant at $\alpha < 0\cdot05$. [b]Denotes AMI significantly different from combined IE and PAE groups at $\alpha < 0\cdot05$. [c] Denotes PAE significantly different from combined AMI and IE groups at $\alpha < 0\cdot05$.

one year for the AMI patients was 89%, for IE 80%, and for the PAE 71%. This comparison is not adjusted for other relevant covariates, such as age, history of medications, or other signs and symptoms.

Using a Cox–Breslow life-table procedure (Cox, 1972; Breslow, 1975), covariate analysis model was constructed identifying the statistical importance characterizing survival experience of these 142 patients and classifying them into high- and low-risk groups. Based on the entry event, the high-risk

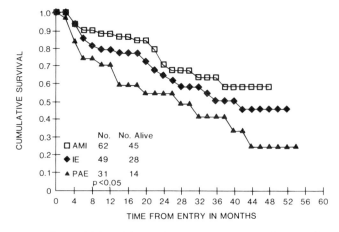

*Figure 3.   Unadjusted life-table analysis based on classification for all cardiac arrests. AMI = acute myocardial infarction; IE = ischaemic event; PAE = primary arrhythmic event. (From Goldstein et al. (1981). Circulation **64**, 977; by permission of the American Heart Association, Inc.)*

group was associated with the use of Digitalis before entry, highest BUN concentration during the acute event, pulmonary congestion on X-ray following the entry event, and classification of the event as PAE. Survival curves of the low-risk and high-risk groups are shown in Fig. 4. The low risk group includes 78% of the total survivors and the high risk makes up 22%. The one and two year survival rates for the low risk group were 85% and 69% and for the high risk group, 71% and 55% respectively ($P < 0.01$).

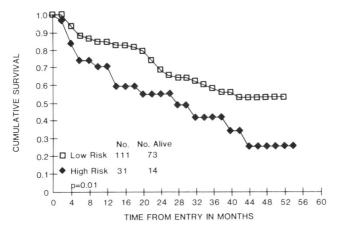

*Figure 4. Covariate-adjusted life-table analysis for high- and low-risk group for all deaths. (From Goldstein et al. (1981). Circulation **64**, 977; by permission of the American Heart Association, Inc.)*

Discussion

There is little question that the success rate of the out-of-hospital resuscitation by the EMS is in a large part related to the arrival time after the onset of the acute event, which is influenced by the topography and population density of the region served. Our units serve a large geographic area, encompassing rural, suburban and urban areas that are distinctly different from those described in other experiences limited primarily to highly urbanized areas. Thus, our mean arrival time of 4·73 min was relatively long compared with urban units (Cobb *et al.*, 1971).

Other studies (Gordon and Kannel, 1971; Baum *et al.*, 1974; Liberthson, 1974b; Cobb *et al.*, 1975) have noted that victims of cardiac arrest frequently have a history of cardiac disease, particularly of prior myocardial infarction. Death may be sudden, but it is usually not without some warning. Our study confirms these findings. The frequency and type of pre-existing heart disease, however, is different in the three groups. History of myocardial infarction was infrequent in patients with AMI. Cardiac arrest was the first cardiac

event in 35% of this group. However, the majority of cardiac arrest survivors have evidence of previous heart disease. In fact, 77% (110 of 142) of
the total group had a history of cardiac disease and 46% (66 of 142) had a
previous myocardial infarction. Prodromal symptoms were common in all
patients, but acute chest pain was more frequent as a prodromal symptom in
the AMI patients.

Liberthson *et al.* (1974b), in a combined clinical and pathologic study of
out-of-hospital cardiac arrest, observed that 39% of their patients experienced an AMI as an entry event, 34% had ischaemia without infarction, and
19% had no evidence of ischaemia or infarction. Our observations are
similar. In an autopsy study, Lovegrove and Thompson (1978) found that
20·5% of cardiac arrests were associated with acute infarction and 74·6%
were associated with a previous infarct. Post-mortem evidence of a recent
myocardial infarction (Rissanen *et al.*, 1978) was observed in 26% and early
infarction in 51% of witnessed deaths within 24 h. Approximately 10% of
these witnessed deaths occurred in patients who had large hearts, a history
of hypertension, congestive heart failure and no evidence of recent infarction. Baum *et al.* (1974) noted that only 19% of their resuscitated patients
after out-of-hospital arrest had electrocardiographic evidence of a transmural infarction. An additional 38% had ischaemia or necrosis without
infarction determined by elevation of the LDH isoenzyme, and 43% had
neither electrocardiographic or enzyme evidence of new infarction or
necrosis. We observed a greater frequency of transmural infarction and a
similar frequency of ischaemia using different enzyme criteria. Myerburg *et
al.* (1980), found evidence of an acute subendocardial or transmural myocardial infarction in 36% of out-of-hospital resuscitated cardiac arrests
based on electrocardiographic or enzymatic criteria, although the enzyme
criteria were not stated. Our own experience indicates that evidence of
myocardial infarction and myocardial ischaemia is a major associate of
out-of-hospital cardiac arrest and was found in over three-quarters of the
resuscitated victims.

Analysis of survival of the population resuscitated is important to our
understanding of the natural history and mechanism of death in patients
with coronary heart disease. Studies of victims of out-of-hospital cardiac
arrest indicate that those who had transmural myocardial infarction or
enzyme evidence of myocardial necrosis did better than those who lacked
such evidence. In our study, the one and two year survival rates for all
patients with coronary heart disease of 84% and 67% are almost identical to
those reported by Cobb *et al.* (1975). We observed poorer one year and two
year survival rates in our AMI group (89% and 71%) than Cobb *et al.* (96%
and 89%). We cannot explain this for our classification of AMI victims
appears to be similar to theirs (Cobb *et al.*, 1975). AMI survival in our study
is similar, however, to that of patients with AMI who sustain ventricular
fibrillation while under coronary care.

The risk of subsequent mortality in populations with previously identified
coronary heart disease has been shown to be due to multiple variables

(Bigger *et al.*, 1978; Davis *et al.*, 1979). To describe a prognostic model of the natural history of out-of-hospital cardiac arrest victims in which therapeutic interventions can be tested, we examined our population with over 40 variables considered to be descriptive of history of disease, the event itself, and myocardial damage associated with the entry event. The presence of digitalis therapy before entry and pulmonary congestion associated with the event identified patients at high risk of subsequent mortality. BUN elevation was also a significant descriptor and is probably related to both cardiac and renal dysfunction. A separation of these two factors was not possible within the scope of investigation. In this model, BUN was used as a continuous variable that was highly predictive of recurrent arrest for values greater than 35 mg%. Left ventricular dysfunction and BUN elevation (Bigger *et al.*, 1978; Davis *et al.*, 1979) after AMI have been associated with increased mortality. A myocardial infarction associated with the arrest event has been noted to improve survival rates (Cobb *et al.*, 1975). Of particular interest was the relationship of IE group to the low-risk group. Although the IE group represented as intermediate position on the unadjusted survival curve (Fig. 3) when the data were adjusted for the covariate related to left ventricular function and BUN elevation, it became part of the low-risk subgroup. The adjusted survival curve for the low-risk group was almost identical to the unadjusted survival curve for the AMI alone, since left ventricular dysfunction was infrequent in this group. This low-risk group made up of the AMI and the IE group comprises 78% of our total population. This model, however, must be tested in subsequent populations in order to be validated.

Resuscitated out-of-hospital cardiac arrest victims and other patients with coronary heart disease show a similar variability in the clinical manifestation of their disease. Therapeutic attempts directed at decreasing the mortality of coronary heart disease should take this information into consideration when testing the effectiveness of these interventions.

References

Baum, R. S., Alvarez, H., III and Cobb, L. A. (1974). *Circulation* **50**, 1231.

Bigger, J. T., Heller, C. A., Wenger, T. L. and Weld, F. M. (1978). *Am. J. Cardiol.* **42**, 202.

Breslow, N. (1975). *Rev. int. Stat. Inst.* **43**, 45.

Cobb, L. A., Conn, R. D. and Sampson, W. E. (1971). *Circulation* **44**, II-45.

Cobb, L. A., Baum, R. S., Alvarez H., III and Schaffer, W. A. (1975). *Circulation* **52**, III-223.

Cox, D. R. (1972). *J. Roy. Stat. Soc.* **34**, 187.

Davis, H. T., DeCamilla, J., Bayer, L. W. and Moss, A. J. (1979). *Circulation* **60**, 1252.

Goldstein, S., Landis, V. R., Leighton, R., Ritter, G., Vasu, C. M., Lantis, A. and Serokman, R. (1981). *Circulation* **64**, 977.

Gordon, T. and Kannel, W. B. (1971). *JAMA* **215**, 1617.

Liberthson, R. R., Nagel, E. L., Hirschman, J. G. and Nussenfeld, S. R. (1974a). *N. Engl. J. Med* **293**, 317.
Liberthson, R. R., Nagel, E. L., Hirschman, J. G. and Nussenfeld, S. R. (1974b). *Circulation* **49**, 790.
Lovegrove, T. and Thompson, P. (1978). *Am. Heart J.* **96**, 711.
Myerburg, R. J., Conde, C. A., Sung, R. J., Mayorga-Cortes, A., Mallon, S. M., Sheps, D. S., Appel, R. A. and Castellanos, A. (1980). *Am. J. Med.* **68**, 568.
Rissanen, M., Romo, M. and Siltanen, P. (1978) *Br. Heart J.* **40**, 1025.
Schaffer, W. A. and Cobb, L. A. (1975). *N. Engl. J. Med.* **293**, 259.

The Epidemiology of Ischaemic Heart Disease Revisited: Synopsis

R. SARACCI

Section of Epidemiology and Biostatistics,
Institute of Clinical Physiology, CNR, Pisa, Italy
and International Agency for Research on
Cancer, Lyon, France

Two elements can be selected as particularly prominent in the scene of IHD epidemiology at the beginning of the eighties:

(a) the decrease in mortality which is, at a variable pace, underway in a number of countries in different continents: USA, Canada, Australia, New Zealand, Belgium, Finland, Switzerland and Israel. In other countries, particularly in Central–Eastern Europe, mortality rates have, on the contrary, shown in the last 10–15 years a marked increase, while in countries of North and Western Europe rates tended to remain stable, generally at "high" levels. These sharply diverging time trends apply to male mortality rates, while females rates are comparatively more even and smoothly changing. The decrease in mortality in countries like the US appears to be real (i.e. not a statistical artefact), started in the late sixties–early seventies, but due to the inevitable time lag in the processing of the relevant data, its full extent has become appreciated (not without surprise) only recently.

(b) the shifting attitudes, from negative–sceptical to more positive–

optimist, towards the interpretation of the available evidence on the efficacy of interventions directed either at preventing IHD development and clinical manifestation (through risk factors modification) or at treating its clinical course. There is little question that direct and unambiguous experimental evidence in man (through randomized trials) of a beneficial effect, particularly in terms of mortality reduction, is still missing for *any* of the interventions in current and wide use in the seventies, be they preventive or corrective, with the notable exceptions of hypertension control and, limited to subgroups of advanced IHD patients, coronary bypass surgery. Hypertension in particular is the factor for which the clearest experimental evidence in man (from well-conducted randomized trials) exists of a reduction both in all-causes mortality and in IHD mortality as an effect of adequate control. Unless the decreases in IHD mortality rates observed in the seventies in several different populations are *all* and *entirely* due to a better control of hypertension and to bypass surgery (which seems unlikely) and/or to unknown factors (an explanation to be invoked only after ruling out all others), one is lead to accept the interpretation that some or all of the other factors for which the experimental evidence is still inadequate have in fact been playing a beneficial role (of such factors cigarette smoking is undoubtedly the one for which the soundest non-experimental evidence of a causal relationship with IHD and of benefit following cessation does exist).

To unravel their relative contributions promises to be a job which will guide much research effort, particularly by epidemiologists, in the coming decade. This research pursuit is best viewed against the criteria of need and feasibility, i.e.

(1) What is needed and may be feasible

to monitor in selected areas IHD incidence, mortality and fatality rates, as well as, if at all possible, risk factors and treatment practices;

to refine more systematically than hitherto done both the measurements of exposure variables (e.g. stress indicators etc.) and end-point variables (the different clinical *and* pathological entities lumped under the IHD label); this may help – among other things – to go deeper than the concept of "risk factor" which is pragmatically most valuable but should not become a permanent surrogate for aetiological understanding;

to work out analytically, for each plan of large scale organized attack, against IHD at local/national level, the expected costs and benefits of alternative strategies (preventive and therapeutic), taking into account whatever uncertainties still surround the efficacy of each particular intervention (i.e. to perform "policy research" explorations).

(2) What is needed and may not be feasible

to obtain all evidence on efficacy of interventions through randomized trials, however hard one may strive to get them done;

to detect "small" beneficial effects, which may however be quite important in public health terms, by epidemiological studies;

to find out some criterion, simple or composite, which will allow to predict nearly 100% of IHD cases.

If a single message may be retained from this it is that in the last decade we (i.e. people in a number of countries) have been doing, intentionally or not, "something" which appears to substantially lower IHD mortality. In looking for new ways of attacking the disease we should not forget that to discover what in fact we have been doing (and to take advantage of it) is a paramount priority.

Bibliography

The recent literature on IHD is not only huge in primary sources of information, but also rich in commentaries, critiques, reviews. A microscopic sample of six general references (*not* covering the most recently debated aspects of MI secondary prevention, in particular the aspirin/dipyridamole/sulphinpyrazone trials):

Borhani, N. O. (1977). *Am. J. Cardiol.* **40**, 251–259.
Kuller, L. H. (1980). *Circulation* **61**, 26–28.
   (Two balanced commentary articles, the first one obviously less up-to-date but more detailed.)
Havlik, R. J. and Feinleib, M. (Eds) (1979). Proceedings of the conference on the decline in coronary heart disease mortality, US DHEW, NIH publication ns. 79–1610, Washington D.C.
   (May be used as an entry point to the problem as well as to the discussion of several risk factors and treatment practices.)
Jenkins, C. D. (1976a,b). *New Engl. J. Med.* **294**, 987–994 and 1033–1038.
Haynes, S. G., Feinleib, M. and Kannel, W. B. (1980). *Am. J. Epid.* **III**, 37–58.
   (These three papers cover one aspect not included in ref. 3.)
Berwick, D. M., Cretin, S. and Keeler, S. (1980). "Cholesterol, children and heart disease: an analysis of alternatives". Oxford University Press, New York.
   (Illustrates the "policy research" approach; several parts may make tough reading for someone with scarce statistical background: still it is well worth for anyone wishing to plan organized community interventions.)

Active and Quiescent Phases of Coronary Disease: A Variable Susceptibility to Dynamic Obstructions May Represent The Elusive Link Between Atherosclerosis and Ischaemic Events

A. MASERI

Royal Postgraduate Medical School, University of London, Cardiovascular Research Unit, Hammersmith Hospital, London, UK

In the attempt to formulate a perspective of our understanding of ischaemic heart disease for the eighties, I will resort to speculations derived from clinical experience, research and thoughts developed during the seventies.

The working hypothesis that I wish to present cannot be expected to be fully documented for the very reason that it is a perspective but I hope it will be useful as a point of reflection and of stimulus of further thought and research.

Frontiers Cardiol. for the 80s.
0-12-220680-0

Key Questions

With the exception of angina in stationary phases, ischaemic events are typically episodic. Why do events occur in some individuals, but not in others with similar or greater severity of coronary atherosclerosis? Why do they occur at a certain time, usually unpredictably and are often followed by asymptomatic periods lasting sometimes several years? Do they occur as a result of a slow, gradual process of narrowing of the coronary arteries, eventually reaching a critical threshold, or as a result of sudden narrowing of the lumen that may disappear after the acute events?

These general questions are not new, but they are too often overlooked in the desire to have a readily available, single culprit against which appropriate action could be attempted.

The Available Evidence

In the search for a single common denominator, coronary atherosclerosis stands out as the most obvious correlate of angina, infarction and sudden death. However, post-mortem and arteriographic findings reveal an extremely wide scattering in the relation between severity of coronary atherosclerotic obstructions and signs or symptoms of ischaemic heart disease. Coronary arteriographic findings are similar in "stable" and "unstable" angina, do not change when the waxing phase of symptoms is over and are highly variable in patients with recent infarction. No critical narrowings are found in about 10% of patients with proven "unstable" angina and a similar percentage had to be excluded from the NIH trial of medical vs surgical treatment of "unstable" angina, for this reason. The occurrence of angina and infarction is now documented beyond doubt in patients without appreciable coronary obstructions. At the other extreme, the prevalence of coronary atherosclerosis in the population is about ten times higher than the prevalence of ischaemic heart disease and some patients with critical obstructions have a normal exercise tolerance so that their stress test is defined "false" negative.

The discrepancy between coronary atherosclerosis and clinical manifestations of ischaemic heart disease cannot be simplistically dismissed as an artefact resulting from inaccurate assessment of coronary anatomy or of the signs of ischaemia, because it is just too large and obvious (Maseri, 1980, 1982; Maseri et al., 1980).

A Working Hypothesis

I believe that enough evidence has been gathered to move the focus from fixed atherosclerotic narrowings to dynamic stenoses resulting from a variable combination of arterial wall lesions, vasoconstriction and increased thrombotic tendency. It is attractive to speculate that, at a certain time, in some individuals, but not necessarily in others with similar degrees of atherosclerotic narrowings, coronary arteries may develop a variable and changing susceptibility to dynamic obstructions. These dynamic obstructions are largely responsible for the onset and for the waxing of symptoms. They heavily influence prognosis in association with the severity of pre-existing fixed atherosclerotic obstructions and myocardial damage, thus representing an important, though elusive, link between coronary atherosclerosis and ischaemic events (Maseri, 1980; Maseri, *et al.*, 1983). Conversely, in quiescent phases, when coronaries are scarcely susceptible to dynamic obstructions, atherosclerotic stenoses carry a much better prognosis: they do not cause ischaemia unless myocardial demand is increased beyond a fixed level, set by the overall chronic impairment of coronary flow reserve which results from the balance between extent of obstruction and of collateral development (Maseri, 1980).

Physiological changes in vasomotor tone around an eccentric stenosis, abnormal response or abnormal stimuli of the smooth muscle and intravascular plugging by blood elements all are potential and interrelated elements of dynamic obstructions. The understanding of the mechanisms responsible for the variable and changing susceptibility of coronary arteries to dynamic obstructions can open additional important avenues for the management and prevention of ischaemic heart disease.

Bibliography

Maseri, A. (1980). *Br. Heart J.* **43**, 648.
Maseri, A. (1982). *Clin. Sci.* **62** (2), 119.
Maseri, A., Chierchia, S. and L'Abbate, A. (1980). *Circulation* **62**, Suppl V, 3.
Maseri, A., Chierchia, S., Davies, G., Crea, F. and Fox, K. M. (1983). *Am. J. Cardiol.* (in press).

III. Progress in Clinical Pharmacology

Antihypertensive Drugs and Autonomic Nervous System

G. MANCIA

Institute of Clinica Medica IV, University of Milan and Centre of Clinical Physiology and Hypertension, Ospedale Maggiore, Milan, Italy

Drugs that interfere with the sympathetic nervous system play an important role in the therapy of hypertension. This presentation will briefly review these drugs, focusing on some haemodynamic features that characterize their effect and make them more or less beneficial.

The first drugs that were shown to be truly effective in reducing elevated blood pressure values were ganglionic blocking agents, and indeed it was from their use that the successful history of antihypertensive treatment began. However, the haemodynamic actions of these agents were far from being ideal. Besides reducing peripheral vascular resistances ganglion blockers caused a reduction in cardiac output thereby acting on a variable that is normally unaltered in established hypertension. Furthermore, the hypotensive action was evident in the upright but much less so in the lying position. Finally, and most importantly, there was with these agents a severe impairment of cardiovascular adjustments to nonresting conditions that produced hypotension and collapse during orthostasis and exercise (Organe et al., 1949; Taylor, 1980). This feature prevented widespread use of ganglion blockers in ambulant hypertensive subjects and also introduced a dilemma. Although effective in lowering blood pressure, pharmacological interference with the sympathetic nervous system may have a limited value

Frontiers Cardiol. for the 80s.
0-12-220680-0

because of its impairment of an essential mechanism for circulatory homeo-stasis. This dilemma persisted with the synthesis and the clinical use of antihypertensive drugs such as guanethydine, bretylium and phentolamine, which interfered with the sympathetic function at the nerve terminals or at the receptor level (Moyer and Caplovitz, 1953; Sonnershedt and Conway, 1970; Goldberg and Raftery, 1976). The dilemma, however, turned out to be avoidable when methyldopa and clonidine, whose sympathetic inter-ference was mainly within the central nervous system (van Zwieten, 1976), were synthetized. Although effectively antihypertensive, these drugs (1) exerted their haemodynamic action through a reduction in vascular resistance with no substantial change in cardiac output; (2) did not have as a main feature orthostatic hypotension; (3) did not cause impairment in the cardio-vascular adjustment to exercise or other conditions that departed from rest (Safar *et al.*, 1979; Mancia *et al.*, 1979, 1980).

Furthermore, both methyldopa and clonidine caused little or no impair-ment of arterial baroreflexes (Mancia *et al.*, 1979, 1980). Figure 1 refers to hypertensive subjects in whom the blood pressure control exerted by the carotid baroreceptors was studied (neck chamber technique) before and

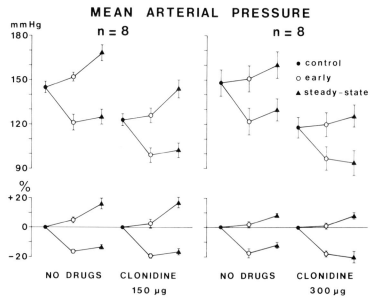

Figure 1. Pressor and depressor effects of carotid baroreceptor deactivation and stimulation before and after 150 µg or 300 µg of clonidine administered i.v. Early and steady-state refer to the reflex responses measured respectively early after the beginning of the stimulus and in a later phase when stabilization had been achieved. Data from subjects with essential hypertension in which similar baro-receptor manipulations were applied, before and after clonidine (From Mancia et al. (1979a), with permission.)

after i.v. administration of 150 μg and 300 μg of clonidine. The pressor responses to baroreceptor deactivation and the depressor responses to baroreceptor stimulation (with regard to the tonic level of baroreceptor activity) were identical before and after the clonidine-induced therapeutical effect indicating (1) no reduction in sensitivity of this important baroreflex function and (2) a reversal of the resetting that is known to affect the baroreflex in hypertension, towards the lowered blood pressure values. This suggests that whatever is responsible for this resetting has a strong functional component (Mancia and Mark, 1983). It also suggests that with clonidine (as well as with methyldopa) this homeostatic mechanism acts to stabilize and defend the hypotension achieved. Recently the 24 h variation coefficient for blood pressure (continuous blood pressure recording in ambulant patients) has been found to be similar before and during the hypotension induced by clonidine (Mancia *et al.*, 1981). This confirms in a more practical set-up the preservation of the antioscillatory role of the baroreflexes.

Methyldopa and clonidine undoubtedly represented a great progress in antihypertensive treatment. They combined the ability to reduce sympathetic vasoconstrictor tone and to preserve the phasic homeostatic variations

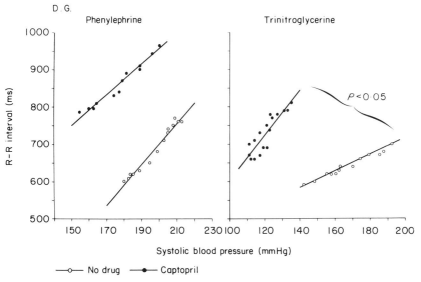

Figure 2. Bradycardic and tachycardic effects of arterial baroreceptor stimulation and deactivation before and after oral administration of 50 mg captopril. The data are shown as linear regressions between the rise or the fall in systolic blood pressure (induced by i.v. phenylephrine or trinitroglycerine) and the resulting lengthening or shortening of the R–R interval. Note that despite the hypotension the slope of the regression with baroreceptor deactivation is greater (the reflex sensibility is greater) after the administration of the drug. Data from a subject with essential hypertension.

of this tone around its reduced value. Although the mechanisms through which this was obtained were (and remain) unknown, it was assumed that they stemmed from the central site of action of these drugs. However, recent observations on another antihypertensive agent, prazosin, have demonstrated that also drugs with a peripheral action on the sympathetic nervous system can behave in a similar fashion. Prazosin owes its hypotensive effect to blockade of alpha-adrenergic receptors (Graham and Pettinger, 1979). Yet (and unlike other alpha-blocking agents) the hypotension induced by prazosin also is accompanied by no reduction in cardiac output, no impairment of sympathetic cardiovascular regulation, and by no impairment of the baroreceptor-blood pressure control (Mancia *et al.*, 1980). It is likely that these features depend at least in part on the selective alpha-blocking properties of this drug (Darcy, 1980; Zanchetti, 1981) i.e. by the fact that the blockade is limited to only a fraction of all alpha-receptor population (alpha$_1$ but not alpha$_2$ pre- and post-synaptic receptors). What is important to emphasize, however, is that hypotension and preservation of circulatory homeostasis can now be achieved through peripheral as well as central "antisympathetic" agents.

Two further examples of autonomic effects of cardiovascular drugs will be given. The former example refers to the mechanisms of the antihypertensive

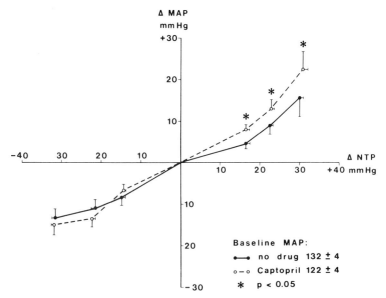

Figure 3. Pressor and depressor responses to carotid baroreceptor deactivation and stimulation obtained via application of positive and negative neck pressures respectively both before and after oral administration of 50 mg captopril. The pressor responses were all significantly greater after captopril. Data from eight subjects with essential hypertension. (From Mancia et al. (1982), with permission.)

action of captopril, a drug that inhibits the converting enzyme thereby reducing the formation of angiotensin II and aldosterone from angiotensin I. This action, however, does not explain entirely the hypotension induced by captopril and other mechanisms have been proposed (Marks *et al.*, 1980). We have shown that one of them may be potentiation of arterial baroreflexes (Mancia *et al.*, 1982). In eight subjects with essential hypertension the baroreceptor control of heart rate was examined by varying the arterial baroreceptor stimulus through injection of vasoactive drugs and the baroreceptor control of blood pressure by varying the carotid baroreceptor stimulus through a neck chanber (Figs 2 and 3). The heart rate and blood pressure responses to baroreceptor deactivation were enhanced after administration of a hypotensive dose of captopril, indicating that although the baroreceptor activity might be expected to be reduced (because of the blood pressure reduction) the reflex exerted more rather than less tonic restraint on the cardiovascular system. This phenomenon may account, at

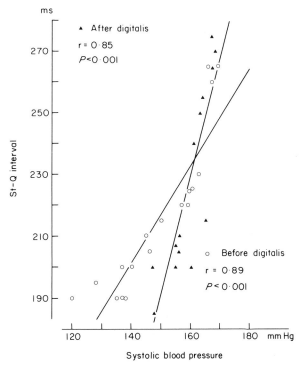

Figure 4. Reduction in atrio-ventricular conduction rate induced by arterial baro-receptor stimulation before and after 0·8 mg lanatoside C i.v. The data are shown as linear regressions between the rise in systolic blood pressure (induced by i.v. phenylephrine) and the resulting lengthening in the St–Q interval of a subject with atrial pacing. Note that the slope of the regression is greater after digitalis.

least in part, for the reduction in pressure obtained with this drug, and also explain the common observation that this reduction is achieved without tachycardia and rise in plasma catecholamines. The baroreflex potentiation induced by captopril may also imply that in hypertension angiotensin II affects neural and reflex cardiovascular regulation, perhaps via an influence at a central level (Ferrario *et al.*, 1979). The latter example refers to digitalis. We have found (Ferrari *et al.*, 1981) that (1) clinical doses of this drug markedly potentiate both in normotensive and hypertensive subjects the arterial baroreceptor control of heart rate and blood pressure, (2) the potentiation involves both the vagal and the sympathetic components of the reflex and (3) this phenomenon is particularly marked for the reflex control of atrio-ventricular conduction time (Mancia *et al.*, 1979; Ferrari *et al.*, in preparation) (Fig. 4). The digitalis-induced potentiation of the baroreflex may play an important role in determining some of the major clinical actions of the drug, for example slowing of ventricular rate. It may also determine some of its ancillary features (reduction in atrial rate, increase in diuresis, etc.).

References

Darcy, M. J. (1980). *J. cardiovasc. Pharmacol.* **2** (suppl. 3), s287.

Ferrari, A. *et al.* (1981). *Circulation* **63**, 279.

Ferrari, A. *et al.* (1983). *Cardiovasc. Res.* (in press).

Ferrario, C. *et al.* (1979). *Hypertension* **1**, 235.

Goldberg, A. D. and Raftery, E. B. (1976). *Lancet* **ii**, 1052.

Graham, R. M. and Pettinger, W. A. (1979). *N. Engl. J. Med.* **300**, 232.

Ludbrook, J. *et al.* (1977). *Clin. Sci. mol. Med.* **53**, 165.

Mancia, G. and Mark, A. (1983). *In* "Handbook of Physiology, Circulation", Vol. 3 (Shepherd, J. T. and Abboud, F., eds). American Physiological Society, Washington D.C., (In press.)

Mancia, G. *et al.* (1979a). *Hypertension* **1**, 362.

Mancia, G. *et al.* (1979b). *Circ. Res.* **44**, 752.

Mancia, G. *et al.* (1980a). *Am. J. Cardiol.* **45**, 1237.

Mancia, G. *et al.* (1980b). *Hypertension* **2**, 700.

Mancia, G. *et al.* (1981). *J. cardiovasc. Pharmacol.* **3**, 1193.

Mancia, G. *et al.* (1982). *Am. J. Cardiol.* **49**, 1415.

Marks, E. S. *et al.* (1980). *Clin. Sci.* **58**, 1.

Moyer, J. H. and Caplovitz, C. (1953). *Am. Heart J.* **45**, 602.

Organe, G., Paton, W. D. M. and Zaimis, E. J. (1949). *Lancet* **i**, 21.

Safar, M. E. *et al.* (1979). *Clin. Pharmacol. Ther.* **25**, 266.

Sannerstedt, R. and Conway, J. (1970). *Am. Heart J.* **79**, 122.

Taylor, P. (1980). *In* "The Pharmacological Basis of Therapeutics", (Goodman, A. and Gilman, A., eds), p. 211. Macmillan, New York.

Van Zwieten, P. A. (1976). *In* "Hypertension: determinants, complications and intervention" (Onesti, G. and Klimt, C. R., eds), p. 295. Grune & Stratton, New York.

Zanchetti, A. (1981). Atti 82° Congresso Medicina Interna, Pozzi L., Roma, p. 513.

Beta-Blockers: Increase in Target/Non-Target Effect Ratio

C. T. DOLLERY

Royal Postgraduate Medical School, University of London, Department of Clinical Pharmacology, Hammersmith Hospital, London, UK

Existing beta-adrenergic antagonists such as propranolol are capable of shifting the isoprenaline dose ratio more than 300-fold when used in high doses. These doses probably produce greater than 95% inhibition of endogenous beta receptor mediated responses. Thus in terms of absolute efficacy there is limited scope for further improvement. All the beta-blockers in clinical use are competitive antagonists and their effect is rapidly reversible when the plasma concentration falls. As the plasma half-life of different drugs such as propranolol and atenolol varies between about three and eight hours the duration of action is limited. New beta adrenergic blocking drugs are being developed with much longer duration of action. One example is FM24 which contains the highly rigid norbenyl ring. This drug dissociates only slowly from the beta receptor and appreciable inhibition of exercise tachycardia is demonstrable as long as seven days after a single dose. Drugs of this kind may permit a more even degree of beta-blockade during the 24 h or alternatively dosing less frequently than once per day.

Frontiers Cardiol. for the 80s.
0-12-220680-0

Specific Targeting

Efforts to direct drugs towards specific organs by using carriers such as liposomes have had very limited success and the only method of achieving greater specificity is if the receptor itself has different characteristics. These differences in characteristics are most evident between the beta$_1$ and beta$_2$ subtypes. Both radioligand binding techniques with substances such as tritiated dihydroalprenolol and dose-response curves have shown that substances such as prenalterol and dobutamine are selective agonists at the beta$_1$ receptor and atenolol, metoprolol and acebutalol are competitive antagonists at this receptor. The corresponding agonists for the beta$_2$ receptor include salbutamol and terbutaline. Selective antagonists for the beta$_2$ receptors are not in general use.

These agents are selective but they are not completely specific. High doses of an agonist or antagonist which is selective for one type of receptor will inevitably affect the other type. This is the reason why asthma can be worsened by drugs like atenolol and metoprolol. Further improvements in selectivity are probably possible but it is doubtful whether absolute specificity will ever be achieved.

The most useful conceptualization of the difference between the beta$_1$ and beta$_2$ receptors is that due to Ariens (1981) who suggested the beta$_1$ receptor is the noradrenaline receptor for neurally released transmitter while the beta$_2$ receptor is a hormone receptor for circulating adrenaline. The distinction can be seen most clearly in tissues like the ventricular myocardium which is richly innervated by adrenergic nerve endings and has receptors entirely of the beta$_1$ type compared with the peripheral lung tissue which has no discernible sympathetic nerve supply and whose adrenergic receptors are almost entirely of the beta$_2$ type.

Therapeutic Applications

The great majority of therapeutic applications with beta-blockers require inhibition of the beta$_1$ receptors. These include angina, arrhythmia and hypertension. Direct applications of beta$_2$ inhibition are few and may include migraine and essential tremor.

Beta receptors on cardiac and smooth muscle cells are familiar but those on adipocytes, hepatocytes, mast cells, endocrine tissues etc. should not be forgotten. These receptors are important in mediating the rise in free fatty acids and fall in serum potassium when adrenaline is released, the recovery from hypoglycaemia and the modulation of release of mediators by mast cell. The action of beta receptor blocking drugs on these receptors is an important area for furture pharmacological research and has implications for therapeutics.

Bibliography

Ariens, E. J. (1981). *Trends in the Pharmacological Sciences* **2**, 170–1.
Daly, M. J. (1981). *Trends in the Pharmacological Sciences* **2**, 168–9.
Dollery, C. T. (1980). *Primary Cardiology Supplement* **1**, 8–14.

Cardiac Alpha Adrenergic Receptors: Do They Have a Role?

A. GIOTTI, F. LEDDA,
F. FRANCONI, L. MANTELLI
and A. MUGELLI

Department of Pharmacology and
Toxicology, University of Florence,
Florence, Italy

Non-beta adrenergic mechanisms have been documented in myocardial fibres (Kunos, 1978; Benfey, 1980; Scholz, 1980; Szekeres and Papp, 1980; Boucher, 1981).

These mechanisms are operated by receptors which show similarities to the classical alpha-adrenoceptors present in vascular smooth muscle cells, at least as far as the antagonists are concerned.

While waiting for direct data, it may be advisable to use the term "cardiac alpha-adrenergic effects" rather than "cardiac alpha-receptors". In fact, in spite of very carefully-conducted experiments, the possible "aspecific effects" of the drugs used to reveal the receptors' presence, have not yet been ruled out.

The "non-beta adrenergic effects" can be evoked by mixed physiological agonists, however their presence can be shown more clearly by comparing relatively pure alpha-agonists (i.e. phenylephrine) with relatively pure beta-agonists (i.e. isoproterenol).

The relative potency of physiological agonists on cardiac alpha-adrenergic mechanisms, as well as the relationships between the alpha-activated component of inotropism (Govier, 1967), the alpha-increase in the refractory

Frontiers Cardiol. for the 80s.
0-12-220680-0

period (Govier et al., 1966), the alpha-inhibitory action on automatic activity (Posner et al., 1976), the alpha-prolongation of action potential duration (Giotti et al., 1968, 1973; Pappano, 1971) the alpha-decrease in ^{42}K uptake (Posner and Vassalle, 1971), the alpha-metabolic activation (Clark and Patten, 1981) require further studies.

Alpha-adrenergic mechanisms could be relevant to some pathological conditions, though we must not forget the interesting studies done on the so-called adrenergic receptor interconversion (Kunos, 1977). One of the pathophysiological conditions which may be particularly relevant to clinical practice is the possible use of alpha-antagonist agents to suppress ventricular dysrhythmia, either present or evoked by adrenergic stimulation in ischaemic or post-ischaemic cardiac fibres (Sheridan et al., 1980). The effects of alpha-blockers may be synergistic with beta-blockade (Chiarello et al., 1980).

The arrhythmogenic properties of mixed adrenergic agonists can easily be shown in simplified models in vitro. In spontaneously-beating Purkinje fibres in Tyrode solution at 37°C in 0·9 mM $CaCl_2$ in the presence of noradrenaline $5 \cdot 10^{-6}g/ml$, the APD prolongation is followed by oscillations at plateau level which eventually become the only electrical activity. This effect of noradrenaline is not shared by pure beta agonists such as isoprenaline; it disappears at low-temperatures and is specifically blocked by phentolamine $2 \cdot 10^{-6}g/ml$ (Giotti and Ledda, unpublished results). The arrhythmogenic properties of noradrenaline are also easily shown in preparations where the membrane potential is made to oscillate at nearly normal values by unphysiological ions like Ba^{2+} (Mugelli et al., 1981a). In this case, norepinephrine strikingly potentiates the arrhythmogenic properties of Ba^{2+} ions, an effect which can still be obtained in the presence of practolol (Mugelli et al., 1981b). The fact that alpha-adrenergic arrhythmogenic effects can be shown in vivo in post-ischaemic conditions as well as in vitro in perfused preparations at physiological temperature, reinforces the view that the in vitro model preparations at physiological temperature are in fact metabolically similar to reperfused post-ischaemic preparations.

The complex relationship both at intracellular and membrane level between adrenergic agonists, Ca^{2+} ions, calcium blocking agents (Posner et al., 1976; Glossmann et al., 1980) and other known (and unknown) physiological substances (see e.g. taurine) (Franconi et al., unpublished results), indicate the need for intensive integrated biochemical–physiological research in the field of adrenergic alpha – beta regulation of cardiac function.

The presence of alpha-receptors outside myocardial cells but on cells functionally integrated with myocardium (e.g. presynaptic alpha-receptors on cardiac nerve fibres, mast cells, coronary smooth muscle cells, etc.) makes interpretation of alpha-mediated effects at an integrated level (in vivo experiments) a particularly difficult task. The need for further experiments in simplified conditions, aimed at unravelling the electrophysiological basis of alpha-activated dysrhythmias, should be stressed.

References

Benfey, B. G. (1980). *Can. J. Physiol. Pharmacol.* **58**, 1145–1157.

Boucher, M. (1981). *J. Pharmacol. (Paris)* **12**, 111–121.

Chiarello, M., Brevetti, G., DeRosa, G., Acunzo, R., Petillo, F., Rengo, F. and Condorelli, M. (1980). *Am. J. Cardiol.* **46**, 249–254.

Clark, M. G. and Patten, G. S. (1981). *Nature* **292**, 461–463.

Franconi, F., Giotti, A., Ledda, F., Mantelli, L. and Mugelli, A. (Unpublished results).

Giotti, A. and Ledda, F. Unpublished results.

Giotti, A., Ledda, F. and Mannaioni, P. F. (1968). *Br. J. Pharmacol.* **34**, 695P.

Giotti, A., Ledda, F. and Mannaioni, P. F. (1973). *J. Physiol.* **229**, 99–113.

Glossmann, H., Hornung, R. and Presek, P. (1980). *J. cardiovasc. Pharmacol.* **2**, (suppl. 3) 303–324.

Govier, W. C. (1967). *Life Sci.* **6**, 1361–1365.

Govier, W. C., Mosal, N. C., Whittington, P. and Broom, A. H. (1966). *J. Pharmacol. Exp. Ther.* **154**, 255–263.

Kunos, G. (1977). *Br. J. Pharmacol.* **59**, 177–189.

Kunos, G. (1978). *Ann. Rev. Pharmacol. Toxicol.* **18**, 291–311.

Mugelli, A., Amerini, S., Piazzesi, G. and Giotti, A. (1981a). *J. mol. Cell. Cardiol.* **13**, (suppl. 1) 62 (abstr.).

Mugelli, A., Amerini, S., Piazzesi, G. and Giotti, A. (1981b). Unpublished results.

Pappano, A. J. (1971). *J. Pharmacol. Exp. Ther.* **177**, 85–95.

Posner, P. and Vassalle, M. (1971). *J. Life Sci.* **1**, 67–78.

Posner, P., Farrar, E. L. and Lambert, C. R. (1976). *Am. J. Physiol.* **231**, 1415–1420.

Scholz, H. (1980). *In* "Handbook of Experimental Pharmacology" (Ed. L. Szekeres), **54**, 651–733. Springer Verlag, Berlin, Heidelberg and New York.

Sheridan, D. J., Penkoske, P. A., Sobel, B. E. and Corr, P. B. (1980). *J. clin. Invest.* **65**, 161–171.

Szekeres, L. and Papp, J. G. Y. (1980). *In* "Handbook of Experimental Pharmacology", (Ed. L. Szekeres), **54**, 598–650. Springer Verlag, Berlin, Heidelberg and New York.

Calcium Antagonists: Differential Properties

R. KREBS

Pharma Research Centre,
Department of Medicine, Bayer AG,
Wuppertal, West Germany

Subsumed under the terms calcium antagonists, calcium channel blocking agents or slow channel blockers have been a number of drugs that inhibit the slow inward current of calcium into heart and vascular smooth muscle cells (verapamil, gallopamil, nifedipine, niludipine, nimodipine, nisoldipine, nitrendipine, diltiazem, nicardipine).

On the basis of recent results (Church and Zsoter, 1980; Boström et al., 1981) it has been suggested that the basic mechanism of action of Ca-blockers may be an interaction of these drugs with the intracellular Ca^{2+}-binding. In these investigations it has been clearly demonstrated that organic Ca-antagonists in contrast to La^{3+} do not impair 45 Ca^{2+}- uptake (Church and Zsoter, 1980; Boström et al., 1981) but decrease the number of Ca^{2+} binding sites of calmodulin (Boström et al., 1981).

From the clinical experience obtained mainly with verapamil and nifedipine it is obvious that these compounds are of great value in the treatment of numerous cardiovascular disorders. But animal experiments as well as clinical experience have also demonstrated differences amongst these agents on which I will concentrate solely.

Strength of Effects

A comparison on a molar basis of verapamil, nifedipine and diltiazem *in vitro* reveals nifedipine to be the most potent of these drugs concerning

Frontiers Cardiol. for the 80s.
0-12-220680-0

coronary vasodilation (Table 1). In the same model of K-depolarized pig coronary arteries verapamil and diltiazem are active in the same molar concentration range (Fleckenstein, 1977) (Table 1). Concerning the negative inotropic effect the threshold concentration for nifedipine also seems to be lower than that for verapamil and diltiazem (Table 1). However, comparing both the effects the difference is lowest with verapamil and at least ten times higher for nifedipine. This is confirmed by comparing the quantitative

Table 1

Generic name	Trade name	ED_{50} (appr.) Pig coronaries	Negative inotropic effect (threshold concentration)	Difference
Verapamil	Isoptin	2×10^{-7} M	5×10^{-7} M	2·5
Nifedipine	Adalat	8×10^{-9} M	2×10^{-7} M	> 10
Diltiazem	Herbesser	$2·5 \times 10^{-7}$ M	1×10^{-6} M	4

According to Fleckenstein, 1977.

differences between nifedipine (taken as 100%), verapamil and diltiazem on a weight basis (Table 2). When administered in equal doses by weight the vasodilation by verapamil and diltiazem is much less compared with that of nifedipine (8% resp. 4%). The negative inotropic effect caused by these drugs is in the same range for verapamil but seems to be somewhat less for diltiazem as compared to verapamil if one takes the main effect, the vasodilation as basis for assessment. Both verapamil as well as diltiazem have much stronger negative chronotropic as well as negative dromotropic effects.

Because nifedipine is the most potent vasodilator amongst all these drugs it produces a strong reflex–adrenergic response *in vivo* which in turn counterbalances its negative inotropic, chronotropic and dromotropic effects. The net result is that of a relatively pure vasodilation with little

Table 2   Effects (%) of verapamil and diltiazem on some cardiovascular parameters (in vitro) in comparison to nifedipine (= 100%)

	Verapamil	Diltiazem
Vasodilatation	8	4
Negative inotropic effect	8	2·5
Negative chronotropic effect	100	33
Negative dromotropic effect	50	50

Calculated from Ono and Hashimoto, 1979.

resultant electrophysiologic or inotropic effects. In contrast, the same degree of vasodilation produced by verapamil is in man accompanied by a greater negative dromotropic effect (Rowland *et al.*, 1979) and reflex induced adrenergic activity does usually not completely upset the direct electrophysiologic effects of verapamil (Henry, 1980). Consequently, in an experimental set-up in which nifedipine, verapamil and diltiazem were injected into the posterior septal artery of dogs in doses which doubled blood flow verapamil and diltiazem but not nifedipine increased AV conduction time (Taira *et al.*, 1980). The conclusion from these experiments was that the coronary vasculature and the AV node were both affected by verapamil and diltiazem within the same dose range. In contrast nifedipine was about nine times as selective for the coronary vasculature as for the AV node. This selectivity of action seems to be characteristic of the class of dihydropyridine compounds. The differences amongst the calcium channel blocking agents in this regard as well as in others may reflect the different chemical structures associated with distinct differences on various electrophysiologic parameters.

Electrophysiological Properties

The fact that reentrant tachyarrhythmias can be effectively terminated by verapamil but not by nifedipine stimulated more sophisticated investigations on the electrophysiological properties of both the drugs (Table 3). Using the voltage clamp technique it has been shown that the influence of verapamil on some electrophysiological parameters is, in clear contrast to nifedipine, rate-dependent. The depression of the slow inward current by nifedipine was found to be clearly dose-dependent (Bayer and Ehara, 1977; Bayer *et al.*, 1977; Ehara and Kaufmann, 1978, 1980) whereas that of verapamil was dominantly dependent on frequency (Ehara and Kaufmann, 1978) and markedly enhanced by prolonged incubation (Kass and Tsien, 1975; Nawrath *et al.*, 1977; Ehara and Kaufmann, 1978). From these experiments the conclusion was drawn that both verapamil and nifedipine reduce the number of operating slow inward channels (Table 3). However, in contrast to nifedipine, verapamil has additionally an influence on the kinetics of the still operating channels so that the activation and more dominantly the recovery from inactivation are slowed down by verapamil but not by nifedipine (Kohlhardt and Flekenstein, 1977; Antman *et al.*, 1980 Henry, 1980). Furthermore verapamil (Ehara and Kaufmann, 1978) and D600 (Kass and Tsien, 1975; (Nawrath *et al.*, 1977) but not nifedipine (Kohlhardt and Fleckenstein, 1977) have been found to reduce the outward current under certain circumstances. From these findings Henry (1980) concluded that verapamil is not a selective channel blocker but has complex electrophysiological effects. For diltiazem voltage clamp experiments are not yet available. However, concerning its effects on the monophasic action

Table 3 *Electrophysiological properties of nifedipine and verapamil*

| | Slow inward (Ca^{++}) current channel | | Fast inward (Na^{+}) current | Channel reactivation | K^{+} outward current | Rate dependency |
	number	kinetics				
nifedipine (10^{-7} – 10^{-5} M)	+	–	–	–	increased	–
verapamil (10^{-7} – 10^{-6} M)	+	+	+ at high concentration	delayed	decreased	+

potential this drug resembles verapamil (Sailcawa *et al.*, 1977). This simil-arity is confirmed by the fact that both verapamil (Bayer *et al.*, 1975; Kaufmann and Uchitel, 1976; Kaufmann, 1977) and diltiazem (Nakajima *et al.*, 1975; Nabata, 1977; Saikawa *et al.*, 1977) in contrast to nifedipine (Kohlhardt and Fleckenstein, 1977) exert fast channel blocking effects at high concentrations. As a result in the clinical situation verapamil and diltiazem may delay AV conduction (Autman *et al.*, 1980; Henry, 1980; Stone *et al.*, 1980).

In humans the effective and functional refractory periods of the AV node are increased by diltiazem and verapamil but decreased by nifedipine (Kawai *et al.*, 1981). This effect of nifedipine is explained on the basis of a reflex increase in sympathetic tone caused by the stronger and faster decline in systemic arterial pressure produced by nifedipine as compared with other Ca^{2+} antagonists.

Differences Due to Tissue Specificity

The fact that the contractility of the heart and its conduction system (especi-ally AV conduction) in animal experiments as well as in humans are affected by nifedipine only when the drug is applied in a dose or concentration exceeding the therapeutic range by more than 10 but can be affected by verapamil within its therapeutic dose range shows different features of both the drugs concerning tissue sensitivity (Autman *et al.*, 1980; Henry, 1980). The resultant advantage of verapamil is its high effectiveness in blocking reentrant tachyarrhythmias which made it to the drug of choice for these conditions. On the other hand the lack of nifedipine to precipitate AV block permits its combination with drugs like beta-receptor blockers and digitalis compounds (Henry, 1980; Stone *et al.*, 1980).

It has been reported that the efficacy of calcium antagonists in releaving K-contractures is more pronounced than releaving contractures due to stimulation by norepinephrine or serotonin (Massingham, 1973; Nguyen Duong and Brecht, 1977). The inability of calcium antagonistic drugs to block specifically the alpha-adrenergic effects of norepinephrine or phenylephrine may be the basis for the fact that postural hypotension in humans has so far been reported for neither drugs. This has also been confirmed for the dihydropyridine compound nimodipine on femoral artery (Table 4). However, the effects on nimodipine found on the basilar artery differed quantitatively reflecting different sensitivities or regulatory mechanisms for contraction in the response of both the arteries (Allen, 1980; Towart and Kazda, 1980). In contrast to the femoral artery on which only weak effects were observed nimodipine effectively prevented an increase in tonus due to stimulation by phenylephrine and serotonin on the basilar artery (Allen, 1980; Towart and Kazda, 1980).

In accordance with the concept of differing tissue resp. organ sensitivity,

Table 4   Effects of nimodipine on basilar artery
and femoral artery in vitro

	Nimodipine (8×10^{-9} M)	
	Basilar	Femoral
Phenylephrine	Strong ↓	Weak ↓
Serotonin	Strong ↓	Weak ↓
KCl	Strong ↓	Strong ↓

From Allen, 1980 and Towart and Kazda, 1980.

is the result that the calcium-dependent release of norepinephrine from sympathetic nerve endings is not inhibited at therapeutic plasma concentrations by either nifedipine (Starke and Schümann, 1973) or verapamil (Haeusler, 1971).

One of the approaches for the development of calcium antagonistic drugs in future may be to select compounds with a high specificity for selected target organs. As an example may serve the development of the dihydropyridine compound nisoldipine. Pharmacologically it differs from nifedipine if compared on a molar basis by a much more selective effect on venous smooth muscle (Kazda et al., 1980). In contrast to nifedipine for which all vessels tested the portal vein is the least sensitive, the portal vein is the most sensitive structure affected by nisoldipine. The effect on heart muscle tissue is for both the drugs in the same molar concentration range. Therefore, the distance between the dose-response curves for both the drugs on vessel structures and heart muscle tissue is wide for nisoldipine and narrower for nifedipine. Nisoldipine is the first Ca^{2+} antagonist for which an effect on the venous system has been demonstrated. Moreover, it has been found to be the most powerful drug in preventing and releaving coronary vasospasm due to thromboxane stimulation (Okamatsu et al., 1981).

Haemodynamic Effects

Although negative inotropic effects have been described in vitro for nifedipine, verapamil and diltiazem a decrease in left-ventricular performance could not be observed in vivo within the therapeutic concentration range. This discrepancy is often attributed to baroreflex stimulated sympathetic discharge masking the direct negative inotropic effects in vivo. Indeed increases in left-ventricular end-diastolic pressure are seen if the direct negative inotropic effects are not counterbalanced by reflex events (Henry, 1980; Stone et al., 1980). Because verapamil induces less arterial hypotension than nifedipine it consequently provokes less adrenergic discharge and left-ventricular end-diastolic pressure usually rises after its administration. In contrast, after nifedipine usually a decrease of left-ventricular end-diastolic pressure has been observed.

Moreover, nifedipine produced in most of the observations even an improvement of cardiac performance (increases of stroke volume, cardiac output, dp/dt max.) which can be attributed to the drug induced pronounced decrease of afterload.

However, all the haemodynamic results reported with verapamil have been observed after i.v. application of the drug. It may well be that a too high concentration may have been present under these circumstances.

After oral application the therapeutic plasma level of all the drugs is known to be much lower than the negative inotropic threshold concentrations (Henry, 1980). A direct comparison of the three calcium channel blocking agents mentioned, nifedipine, verapamil and diltiazem, under identical conditions is not available. A difference in the haemodynamic profile for nifedipine was seen to exist between acute and chronic administration of the drug in hypertensives. In contrast to single dose studies which have always shown the existence of a dependency of the effect on dose and pretreatment value in studies of longer duration (3–12 weeks) there could not be observed a clear-cut dose-response relationship under nifedipine (Krebs *et al.*, 1981). The maximum antihypertensive as well as anti-anginal effect was seen only after several days of treatment (Krebs *et al.*, 1981). Investigation of pharmacokinetic parameters at the same time revealed essentially no change, for example in half-life, which means that this effect cannot be explained by a cumulation of the drug but rather by a pharmacodynamic effect. Accordingly in contrast to the acute effect which lasts for about 6 h discontinuation of nifedipine therapy after 4 weeks of treatment was followed by a slow increase in blood pressure, which reached the pretreatment level within 1–2 days. From these results it may be concluded that the duration of action of a single dose is prolonged after long-term treatment (Krebs, *et al.*, 1982). In contrast to the acute effects on long-term application there is a clear dissociation between pharmacokinetic and pharmacodynamic behaviour of the drug. In most of the long-term studies heart rate was reported to remain unchanged or even to decrease (Krebs *et al.*, 1981). This is in contrast to the acute effects of the drug and may well be explained by resetting of the baroreflex mechanism. Because of the well-known pharmacodynamic tolerance developing during long-term treatment with vasodilators Koch-Weser, 1974), it is important to mention that the blood pressure lowering effects of Ca-channel blockers, i.e. nifedipine, do not appear to wane during chronic therapy (Krebs *et al.*, 1981).

Pharmacokinetics

The absorption of nifedipine, verapamil and diltiazem is uniformly more than 90% (Table 5). However, because of their high metabolization vera-

Table 5   Pharmacokinetics of calcium antagonists

	Nifedipine	(±) Verapamil	Diltiazem
Dosage (oral mg/8/h)	10–20	80–160	80–120
Absorption (oral %)	> 90	> 90	> 90
Bioavailability (%)	65–70	10–22	< 20
Onset of action			
Sublingual (min)	3	. . .	. . .
Oral (min)	< 10	< 30	< 30
Protein binding (%)	90	90	80
Plasma half-time (β-phase, h)	5	3–7	4
Metabolism	Extensively metabolized to an inert free acid and lactone	Extensive 1st pass hepatic extraction (70% of oral dose)	Extensively deacetylated
Excretion			
Renal (%)	70 1st day (80 total)	50 1st day (70 total)	35 (total)
Fecal (%)	< 15	15	65

According to Henry, 1980.

pamil and diltiazem have a low biovailability whereas that of nifedipine is high (65–70%). In patients with liver diseases the liver-clearance of verapamil has been found to be reduced as much as more than 60% (Woodcock et al., 1981). In these patients the bioavailability varied between 3·8 and 64% and the t/2 β (min) was increased from 170 ± 72 to 815 ± 516 ($P < 0·05$). The onset of the effect after oral administration is faster with nifedipine (< 10 min) than after administration of verapamil and diltiazem (each < 30 min). The excretion of maternal compound and metabolites through the kidneys is in descending order nifedipine > verapamil > diltiazem and fecal excretion increases in the same order.

Indications and Contraindications

Due to the differing pharmacological properties the drugs have also some differences in their clinical indications. For reentrant tachyarrhythmias for example verapamil is the drug of choice whereas nifedipine has no effect. Inversely successful management of hypertension by oral treatment has been shown for nifedipine but is not clearly established for verapamil as well as diltiazem. For later a wide interindividual variation in their effects can be expected because of the high first pass metabolism (Midtbø and Hals, 1980). All the drugs mentioned have been shown to be efficacious in patients with angina pectoris including the variant type of angina (Henry, 1980; Stone *et al.*, 1980).

Relative or absolute contraindications (Henry, 1980; Stone *et al.*, 1980) for verapamil but not nifedipine are: sinus bradycardia, sick sinus syndrome, AV conduction defects, digitalis toxicity with AV block and heart failure. With both the drugs verapamil as well as nifedipine caution is indicated in hypotension. In contrast to beta-blockers for both the drugs bronchospasm is no contraindication. With concomitant beta-blockers therapy some care should be taken concerning verapamil.

Future Aspects

After recognition of the importance of this class of compounds has taken place by the medical community we certainly can expect a further development of new compounds. It is not anyone speculative forecasting that at the end of this decade we will have Ca^{2+}-antagonistic drugs being more selective for different target organs resp. clinical indications. Consequently, the appearance of side-effects, which are already for some of the drugs used presently well tolerable, will change qualitatively and quantitatively. With increasing our knowledge about the role of Ca^{2+} in the pathophysiology of diseases these drugs will be used also for indications we presently even do not think about. Some new indications (acute myocardial infarction, cardiac insufficiency, pulmonary hypertension, unstable angina, protection of tissues against ischaemia, prevention of reinfarction, hypertrophic cardiomyopathy) are already under clinical investigation.

References

Allen, G. S. (1980). Effects of nimodipine on basilar and femoral arteries. Personal communication.

Antman, E. M., Stone, P. H., Muller, J. E. and Braunwald, E. (1980). *Ann. intern. Med.* **93**, 875–885.

Bayer, R. and Ehara, T. (1978). *In* "The Action of Drugs on Calcium Metabolism" (Van Zwieten, P. and Schonbaum, E., Eds) 31–37. Proceedings of a symposium organized by the Division of General Pharmacology of the Dutch Pharmacological Society, The Netherlands (1977), Stuttgart 1978.

Bayer, R., Kalusche, D., Kaufmann, R. and Mannhold, R. (1975). *Naunyn Schmiedebergs Arch. Pharmacol.* **290**, 81–97.

Bayer, R., Rodenkirchen, R., Kaufmann, R., Lee, J. H. and Hennekes, R. (1977). *Naunyn Schmiedebergs Arch. Pharmacol.* **301**, 29–37.

Boström, S.-L., Ljung, B., Mardh, S., Forsen, S. and Thulini, E. (1981). *Nature* **292**, 777–778.

Church, J. and Zsoter, T. T. (1980). *Can. J. Physiol. Pharmac.* **58**, 254–264.

Ehara, T. and Kaufmann, R. (1978). *J. Pharmacol. exp. Ther.* **207**, 49–55.

Ehara, T. and Kaufmann, R. (1980). *Pfluegers Arch.* (in press).

Fleckenstein, A. (1977). *Ann. Rev. Pharmacol. Toxicol.* **17**, 149–166.

Haeusler, G. (1971). *Angiologica* (Part I) **8**, 156–160.

Henry, P. D. (1980). *Am. J. Cardiol.* **46**, 1047–1058.

Kass, R. S. and Tsien, R. W. (1975). *J. gen. Physiol.* **66**, 169–192.

Kaufmann, R. (1977). *Münch. Med. Wschr.* **199**, suppl. 1, 6–11.

Kaufmann, H. J. and Uchitel, O. D. (1976). *Naunyn Schmiedebergs Arch. Pharmacol.* **292**, 21–27.

Kawai, Ch., Konishi, T., Matsuyama, E. and Okazaki, H. (1981). *Circulation* **63**, 1035–1065.

Kazda, S., Garthoff, B., Meyer, H., Schlossmann, K., Stoepel, K. Towart, R., Vater, W. and Wehinger, E. (1980). *Arzneim. Forsch.* **30**, 2144–2162.

Koch-Weser, J. (1974). *Archs intern. Med.* **133**, 1017.

Kohlhardt, M. and Fleckenstein. A. (1977). *Naunyn Schmiedebergs Arch. Pharmacol.* **298**, 267–272.

Krebs, R., Graefe, K.-H. and Ziegler, R. (1982). *Hypertension* **44**, 271–284.

Massingham, R. (1973). *Eur. J. Pharmacol.* **22**, 75–82.

Midtbø, K. and Hals, O. (1980). *Current therap. Res.* **27**, 830.

Nabata, H. (1977). *Jan. J. Pharmacol.* **27**, 239–249.

Nakajima, H., Hoshiyama, M., Yamashita, K. and Kiyomoto, A. (1975). *Jap. J. Pharmacol.* **25**, 383–392.

Nawrath, H., Ten Eick, R. E., McDonald, T. F. and Trautwein, W. (1977). *Circ. Res.* **40**, 408–414.

Nguyen Duong, H. and Brecht, K. (1977). *Münchn. Med. Wschr.* **119**, suppl. 1, I–S 12–18.

Okamatsu, S., Peck, R. C. and Lefer, A. M. (1981). *Fed. Proc.* **40**, 727.

Ono, H. and Hashimoto, K. (1979). *Perspect. Cardiovasc. Res.* **3**, 77–88.

Rowland, E., Evans, T. and Krikler, D. (1979). *Br. Heart J.* **42**, 124–127.

Saikawa, T., Nagamoto, Y. and Arila, M. (1977). *Jap. Heart J.* **18**, 235–245.

Starke, K. and Schümann, H. J. (1973). *Arzneim. Forsch.* **23**, 193–197.

Stone, P. H., Antman, E. M., Muller, J. E. and Braunwald, E. (1980). *Ann. intern. Med.* **93**, 886–904.

Taira, N., Motomura, S., Narimatsu, A., Satoh, K. and Yanagisawa, T. (1980). *In* "Calcium-antagonism" (Fleckenstein, A. and Roskamm, H., eds), 42–43. Springer Verlag, Berlin, Heidelberg and New York.

Towart, R. and Kazda, S. (1980). *IRCS Med. Sci.* **8**, 206.

Woodcock, B. G., Rietbrock, J., Vöhringer, H. F. and Rietbrock, N. (1981). *Clin. pharmacol. Ther.* **29**, 27–34.

Calcium Antagonists: Controlled Trials

P. G. HUGENHOLTZ

Department of Cardiology, Thoraxcentre,
University Hospital, Erasmus University,
Rotterdam, The Netherlands

Introduction

As the anti-anginal action of nifedipine has become evident and accepted throughout the world, attention in the major research laboratories, still interested in nifedipine, has turned more and more towards the anti-ischaemic effects of the drug. In this regard the Thoraxcentre in Rotterdam is predicting a major, albeit still potential, role for nifedipine.

At the time of the Paris meeting of the ESC, in Summer 1980 our group (Serruys *et al.*, 1980) presented data which showed that the clinical efficacy of nifedipine in ischaemic states could largely be explained by its powerful influence on coronary vascular tone, changing both pre- and post-stenotic arterial diameter and increasing coronary bloodflow. However from other studies in that same symposium Nayler (1980) concluded that there must also be a direct oxygen sparing effect on the myocardial cell, an effect which may even be more pronounced when ischaemia is present. Recent evidence from Barry and coworkers (1981) suggests that nifedipine reduces myocardial oxygen consumption in isolated cardiac cell systems and in isolated hearts without alteration in regional myocardial function or systemic haemodynamics. Preliminary results (Verdouw *et al.*, 1982) from our laboratory indicate that this O_2-sparing effect is enhanced when low-dose nifedipine is given directly and continuously into the coronary artery in

Frontiers Cardiol. for the 80s.
0-12-220680-0

ischaemic conditions. If O_2-sparing is indeed an important factor, we must expect less ATP-breakdown during this period to fulfill Nayler's scheme (Fig. 1). In fact, de Jong *et al*. (1982) were able to show in the isolated, working Langendorff preparation that treatment by nifedipine preserved most of the high-energy phosphate energy stores during ischaemia, while under control conditions their metabolites were found in the efflux. Propanolol given in a similar dose was not able to preserve these phosphate stocks, although the combination of propanolol with nifedipine seemed to

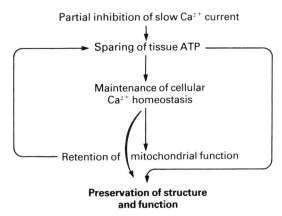

Partial inhibition of slow Ca^{2+} current

Sparing of tissue ATP

Maintenance of cellular Ca^{2+} homeostasis

Retention of mitochondrial function

Preservation of structure and function

Figure 1. Schematic representation of the mechanism whereby the Ca^{2+} antagonists protect heart muscle against the effects of ischaemia and reperfusion (from Nayler, 1980).

act even in a more protective manner than nifedipine alone. The cellular content of creatine phosphate contained in the cells upon termination of the experiment was again highest after nifedipine and the combination of nifedipine and propanolol. Verdouw *et al*. (1981) have already shown that nifedipine enhances recovery of the function of the ischaemic myocardium in regions where reperfusion with oxygenated blood was compared before and after pretreatment of nifedipine. Moreover, the incidence of ventricular arrhythmias was remarkably reduced in these ischaemic nifedipine-treated animals. There is therefore no doubt in our minds that nifedipine still has a major role to play in acute ischaemic states, such as will occur during open-heart surgery, cardioplegia and impending infarction (Verdouw *et al*., 1981; Hugenholtz *et al*., 1981; Serruys *et al*., 1981).

Recent developments in the treatment of acute myocardial infarction, i.e. immediate intervention with intra-coronary administration of thrombolytic agents, like streptokinase, have now shown that jeopardized tissue may be recovered by timely restoration of coronary bloodflow. Here, too, the protective role of nifedipine has to be investigated. The above-mentioned properties of nifedipine could markedly improve the efficacy of thrombolytic therapy, just as it recently has been shown that nitroglycerin by itself

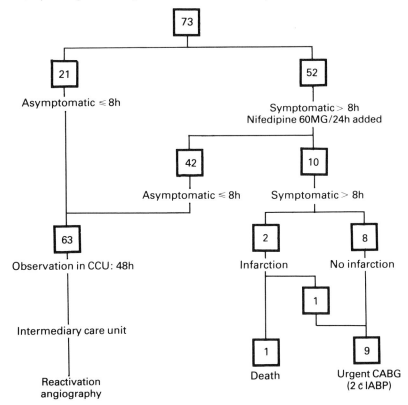

73 patients: Angina at rest, ST/T wave changes, no Q-formation, or enzyme ↑
(impending infarction), all treated ≤ 8H c̄ Bedrest, β-blockers, nitrates

73

21
Asymptomatic ≤ 8h

52
Symptomatic > 8h
Nifedipine 60MG/24h added

42
Asymptomatic ≤ 8h

10
Symptomatic > 8h

63
Observation in CCU: 48h

2
Infarction

8
No infarction

Intermediary care unit

1

1
Death

9
Urgent CABG
(2 c̄ IABP)

Reactivation
angiography

Figure 2. Data derived from a recent paper (Hugenholtz, 1982) in which it was shown that in 73 patients, all with unstable angina, observed over a one-year period out of 1563 admissions to the coronary care unit in the University Hospital in Rotterdam, 21 became asymptomatic within 8 h with conventional therapy consisting of bedrest, nitrates (oral or i.v.) and beta-blockade. Of the 52 who remained symptomatic during the first 8 h of such treatment, nifedipine was added in doses of 60 mg/24 h. In 24 of 52, usually when the second dose had been administered orally, symptoms were completely relieved. In 10 other patients, who did not experience such relief, the subsequent arteriograms showed far advanced coronary artery disease. In that study it is argued that their relief of increased vasomotor tone in patients with unstable angina was the deciding factor in explaining the clinical efficacy of this Ca^{2+} antagonistic treatment. (CABG: coronary aortic bypass graft. IABP: intraortic balloon pumping.)

affects the function of the thrombocytes (Chierchia *et al.*, 1981). Could there also be an influence of nifedipine on the thrombocytes for example by protecting ATP metabolism inside the thrombocyte? Clinical evidence from trials currently completed or in the process of being analyzed shows that its administration to patients with unstable angina and impending infarction should now be regarded as being efficacious as is evident from the data given in Fig. 2. Indeed, it has been proposed that the subset of patients in whom coronary artery spasm is suspected, whether as a primary or a secondary factor, may not benefit from beta-adrenergic blockade at all, which is currently the standard therapy throughout the world. In fact, Yasue and his colleagues (1974) have specifically argued against its use in this group of patients as clinical experience indicates a worsening of the symptoms.

Other reports also point to the failure of beta-blockade to relieve symptoms in cases with stable angina pectoris or Prinzmetal's syndrome despite its having reduced heart rate and blocked adrenergic impulses. The addition of nifedipine, or perhaps the use of nifedipine alone, may therefore be the more logical approach as suggested by Gunther *et al.* (1979). To try to identify the relative role of these drugs in unstable angina, a multicentre trial involving 600 patients is currently under way in The Netherlands. Here metoprolol is being compared to nifedipine and their combination (Fig. 3). The rationale for this large trial, which involves five University Hospitals, rests on the clinical impression derived from open studies which show that the rapidity of action of the calcium antagonists is due to the fact that they tone down the "multiplier" effect in unstable ischaemic states by inhibiting the transmembrane influx of calcium into cardiac muscle.

Reduction in the transformation of phosphate-bound energy into mechanical work by calcium-dependent myofibrillar ATP, leads to an immediate decrease in the oxidative metabolism of the heart. In recent experiments, de Jong and his colleagues (1979) showed that, even in brief periods of ischaemia promptly followed by reperfusion, there was massive release of nucleotides, indicating breakdown of high energy phosphates even when coronary bloodflow was restored within minutes after its interruption. Thus every attempt at reducing the need for oxygen may be helpful in patients with jeopardized myocardium (Clarke *et al.*, 1978; Henry *et al.*, 1979). In addition, reduction of the calcium-dependent contractile tone of the larger epicardial coronary arteries – and perhaps to some extent of the capillaries as well (dramatically illustrated by the sudden collapse of the ventricular wall thickness after intracoronary administration of the drug (Serruys *et al.*, 1981; Verdouw *et al.*, 1981)) – leads to increased flow, which in turn will promote the rapid restoration of the regional oxygen supply. Finally, dilation of large systemic arteries, may result in a further, albeit indirect, decrease in the cardiac demand for oxygen. All three mechanisms may vary in their significance, but they are essential so that when attempts at increasing venous capacitance by reducing preload (with nitrates) or at decreasing heart rate by reducing contractility (with beta-blockers) have failed, calcium antagonists provide the most direct pharmacological route of attack both for

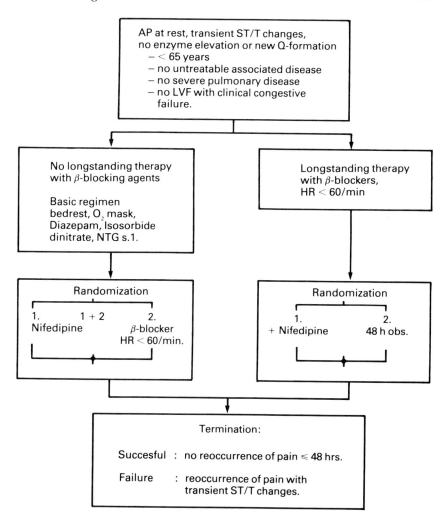

Figure 3. Flowsheet schematically indicating the procedures employed in the Inter-university trial currently under way in The Netherlands.

stable and unstable angina pectoris. Data provided by Clarke *et al.* (1979) and Henry *et al.* (1979) and by others have also indicated that when an area around an infarct is already ischaemic, the loss of such ischaemic cells can be reduced by nifedipine. These observations have led the Americans to institute a large-scale trial with nifedipine in patients with proven myocardial infarction in an effort to reduce the loss of jeopardized but still viable tissue around the infarct core. Recent studies in our laboratory have indeed shown in the pig, that in the core of the ischaemic area up to 30 min after the interruption of flow, nifedipine can increase the capillary flow and favourably alter the ratio of endocardial vs epicardial flow (Fig. 4) thus restoring wall thickness (Fig. 5) to 75% of control (Verdouw *et al.*, 1981). In terms of clinical trials, the literature is replete with studies detailing the efficacy of nifedipine (Table 1) and also of verapamil (Table 2) in the treatment of chronic stable angina pectoris. From 103 literature studies, published between 1975 and 1981, a list of 15 was selected which corresponded to the following criteria: patients with stable angina pectoris, only observations on at least 24 patients in each report,* a double-blind study design, placebo control and random assignment to therapy. When one applies these criteria, 886 patients remained, 524 were studied with nifedipine, 312 with verapamil and 50 with perhexilin treatment. Undoubtedly, this list is incomplete as the data were obtained with the help of a computer, the completeness of which, in terms of input, can only be assumed. All studies took place between 1976 and 1980 and generally provide evidence that when nifedipine is compared to placebo, the frequency of angina pectoris attacks was decreased and the extent of ischaemia on the electrocardiogram reduced, while the haemodynamic performance during exercise testing was improved.

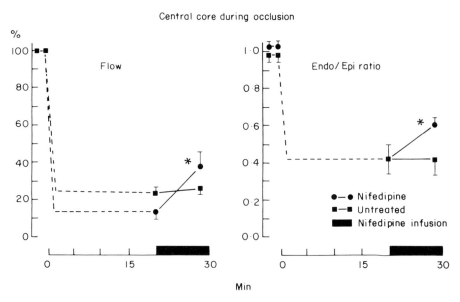

Figure 4. The ratio between endocardial vs epicardial capillary bloodflow is favourably altered after nifedipine, even in the ischaemic core. This would favour the protection of the most threatened area during ischaemia: the endocardium.

* One exception, the study conducted by Lohmolle (1979) contains only 16 patients.

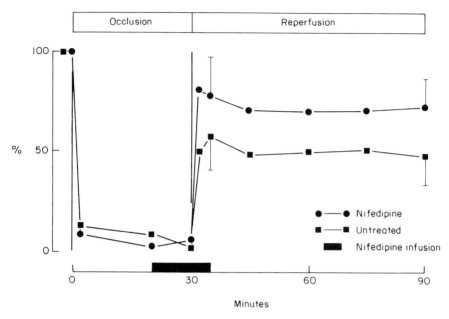

Figure 5. Along the vertical axis in percentages is given the extent of wall-thickening during systole. Before occlusion wall-thickening nearly ceases. After reperfusion it is clearly seen that the ventricular wall pre-treated with nifedipine just prior to reperfusion shows a greater return towards control values than the untreated ventricular wall. Average of 12 animal studies. Note that in the untreated animal recovery is only 50% of control, in the treated animal 75% of control.

Some studies compared the drug also to beta-blockade or to a combination of nifedipine with beta-blockade. At least five reports lead to the conclusion that the combination is the best combination to reduce severe symptoms. Similar analyses are reported for verapamil although it is remarkable that the number of studies on the latter drug is much less. The latest study to be published (Dargie *et al.*, 1980) provides the most conclusive evidence from a double blind, crossover trial that the combination of nifedipine and propanolol, as assessed in chronic stable angina, is better than either drug. An extensive overview is produced by Stone *et al.* (1980). In contrast much less is available in the literature regarding nifedipine in unstable angina pectoris. In fact only two references were produced by computer-search in addition to our own work. Similarly for verapamil few controlled studies are available (Table 2). Only the study of Parodi *et al.* (1979) shows in unstable angina, an efficacy which resembles that of nifedipine. The conclusion can be drawn that from properly controlled trials, evidence is now accruing that for the control of unstable angina or crescendo

Table 1 Double-blind/randomized/placebo-controlled studies with nifedipine in stable angina pectoris

Name	Year	City	Patients	Main conclusion
Bidoggia	1976	Buenos Aires	46	N > Placebo in Sx
Gomez	1976	Mexico	25	N > Placebo in ExTol
Stein	1976	Hamburg	72	↑ExTol
Menna	1976	Buenos Aires	33	↓Sx, ↑ExTol, ↓ST p N
Manca	1977	Parma	24	↓Sx, ↑ExTol, ↓ST p N
Adanska Dyniewska	1977	Lodz	60	↓Sx, ↑ExTol
Condorelli	1978	Napoli	30	↓Sx in proven CAD
Scardi	1978	Udine	26	N + Oxprenolol best
di Ponti	1978	Milano	48	4 drug comparison, P worst
Folli	1978	Milano	27	↓Sx, ↑ExTol
Cocco	1979	Ferrara	42	↓use of Nitro, Pindolol = N
Twaddel	1979	Glasgow	25	↑ExTol when N + P
Hopf	1979	Frankfurt	24	↓ST, ↓AP, N = V = Iso
Lohmolle	1979	München	26	↓AP, ↓PCP, ↓ST, N > P
Dargie	1980	London	16	N + Propanolol best bet

Sx = Symptoms, ExTol = Exercise Tolerance, N = Nifedipine, P = Propanolol, V = Verapamil, Iso = Isosorbidedinitrate, AP = Angina Pectoris, PCP = Pulmonary capillary pressure, ST = Ischaemic ST segment changes, ↓ = less, ↑ = more.

Table 2 *Double-blind/randomized/placebo-controlled studies with verapamil*

Name	Year	City	Patients	Main conclusion
		I: In stable angina pectoris		
Mashfold	1977	Melbourne	24	↓AP
Mir	1978	Manchester	28	↓AP, particularly in non-responders to blockers
BalaSubramanian	1980	Harrow	100	↓AP, ↑ExTol, ↓ST
di Ponti	1980	Milano	35	↓AP, ↑ExTol
Lessem	1980	Malmö	32	V + β-blockers > Placebo
Rafles	1980	Sydney	93	V > β-blockers
Epstein	1981	Bethesda	?	Comparison of P and V
		II: In myocardial infarction		
Mellengaard	1979	Copenhagen	1500	in progress
		III: In unstable angina pectoris		
Parodi	1980	Pisa	12	↓AP, ↓ST
Hillis	1981	Dallas	?	in progress

ExTol = Exercise Tolerance, P = Propanolol, V = Verapamil. AP = Angina Pectoris, ST = Segment changes, ↓ = less, ↑ = more.

angina, these drugs, and in particular nifedipine, have a major role to play. The major trial currently underway in unstable angina patients as a co-operative effort between five University Hospitals in The Netherlands should provide the most definitive answer of the relative roles of beta-blockade by metoprolol, nifedipine, and their combination vs placebo (Fig. 3.). Finally in terms of controlled trials for the salvage of jeopardized myocardium during acute ischaemia such as during cardiopulmonary bypass or during outright myocardial infarction, here plans are being formulated.

A number of centres in Europe will compare the use of a nifedipine infusion to the currently conventional cold-cardioplegia, while another large trial is currently underway, in a number of East Coast US hospitals in patients with proven myocardial infarction. These three large-scale trials should in the next years provide us with the necessary evidence to the efficacy of this approach in patients with various acute ischaemic cardiac conditions.

References

Bala Subramanian, V., Raramavisan, R., Lahira, A. and Raftery, E. B. (1980). *Lancet* i, 841–844.

Bairy, W. H. Biedert, S., Miura, D. S. and Smith, T. W. (1981). *Circ. Res.* **49**, 141–149.

Brower, R. W., De Jong, J. W., Haalebos, N., Simoons, M. L., Van den Bos, A., De Jong, D. S., Bos, E. and Hugenholtz, P. G. (1982). *In* "Kalziumantagonisten zur Kardioplegie und Myokardproduktion in der offenen Herzchirurgie (Eds. H. A. Tschirkov and V. Schlosser), p. 69. George Thieme Verlag, Stuttgart and New York.

Chierchia, S., De Caterina, R., Crea, F., Bernini, W., Giannessi, D., Gazzetti, P. and Maseri, A. (1981). *Circulation* **64**, suppl IV, 191, (abstr.).

Clarke, R. E., Christlieb, I. V., Henry, P. D., Fischer, A. E., Nora, I. D., Williamson, J. R. and Sobel, B. E.. (1979). *Am. J. Cardiol.* **44**, 825–831.

Dargie, M. J., Lynch, P., Krikler, D. M. and Krikler, S. (1980). *Br. Heart J.* **43**, 724 (abstr.).

Gunther, S., Green, L., Muller, J. E., Mudge, G. H. and Grossman, W. (1979). *Am. J. Cardiol.* **44**, 793–797.

Henry, P. D., Shuchleib, R., Clark, R. E. and Perez, J. E. (1979). *Am. J. Cardiol.* **44**, 817–824.

Hugenholtz, P. R., Michels, H. R., Serruys, P. W. and Brower, R. W. (1981). *Am. J. Cardiol.* **47**, 163–173.

Hugenholtz, P. G., Serruys, P. W. and Balakumaran, K. (1983). *J. Cardiovasc. Med.* **7**.

De Jong, J. W. (1979). *In* "Pathophysiology of Myocardial Perfusion", (Ed. W. Schaper), 719–750. Biomed. Press, Amsterdam.

De Jong, J. W. Harmsen, E., De Tombe, P. P. and Keijzer, E. (1983) *Eur. J. Pharmacol.* (in press).

Mellengaard, K. (1980). Proceedings of the Int. Symposium on Calcium Antagonism in Cardiovascular Therapy (Eds, A. Zanchetti and D. M. Krikler), p. 301. Excerpta Medica, Amsterdam, Oxford and Princeton.

Nayler, W. F. (1980). *Eur. Heart J.* **1**, suppl. B. 5–14.

Parodi, O., Maseri, A. and Simonetti, I. (1979). *Br. Heart J.* **41**, 167–174.

Serruys, P. W. Steward, R., Booman, F., Michels, R., Reiber, J. H. C. and Hugenholtz, P. G. (1980). *Eur. Heart J.* **1** suppl B, 71–85.

Serruys, P. W., Brower, R. W., Ten Katen, H. J., Bom, A. H. and Hugenholtz, P. G. (1981). *Circulation* **63**, 584–591.

Stone, P. H., Antman, E. M. Muller, J. E. and Braunwald, E. (1980). *Ann. intern. Med.* **93**, 886–904.

Verdouw, P. D., Hartog, J. M., Ten Cate, F. J., Schamhardt, H. D., Bastianns, O. L., Van Bremen, R. H., Serruys, P. W. and Hugenholtz, P. G. (1981). *In* "Drug Treatment of Myocardial Infarction" (Eds P. A. van Zwieten, P. G. Hugenholtz and E. Schönbaum). *Progr. in Pharmacol.* **4**, 91–100.

Verdouw, P. D., Ten Cate, F. J., Hartog, J. M., Scheffer, M. G. and Stam, H. (1982). *Basic Res. Cardiol.* **77**, 26–33.

Yasue, M., Touyama, M. and Shimamoto, M. (1974). *Circulation* **50**, 534–539.

Controlled Clinical Trials in Angina Pectoris

O. PARODI, I. SIMONETTI,
M. LAZZARI, S. SEVERI
and A. L'ABBATE

Institute of Clinical Physiology, CNR and
Institute of Patologia Medica, University of
Pisa, Pisa, Italy

Angina pectoris is a clinical syndrome characterized by a sudden, transient, reversible imbalance between myocardial oxygen requirements and blood supply.

It is now possible to distinguish:

(1) Classical effort angina with a fixed ischaemic threshold, in which an atherosclerotic organic stenosis limits the increase in regional myocardial blood flow (Friedberg, 1966).
(2) Angina at rest characterized by ischaemic episodes without any apparent cause and triggered by a coronary vasospasm (Maseri et al., 1975; Maseri, 1977; Maseri, 1980a).
(3) Mixed forms of angina, with transient ischaemic episodes both at rest and on effort in which functional and organic factors interact, in a complex way (angina on cold exposure, angina on emotion, angina on effort with widely variable ischaemic threshold) (Mudge et al., 1976; Schang and Pepine, 1977; Brunelli et al., 1981).

Therefore different pathophysiologic mechanisms are responsible for these different clinical conditions (Maseri, 1980b). Moreover, the incidence of the second and third form of angina is, according to the experience of the last years, larger than the one of classical pure effort angina (Maseri *et al.*, 1978). For these reasons a correct evaluation of antianginal drugs should be based on a careful selection of groups of patients as well as on the use of different experimental protocols designed according to the type of angina under study.

Angina at Rest

General Considerations

There are several factors conditioning the design of pharmacological trials in patients with angina at rest:

(1) The spontaneous variability in frequency and severity of ischaemic episodes (Biagini *et al.*, 1981), requiring short-term multiple cross-over placebo-controlled trials.

(2) The high incidence of asymptomatic episodes (40–80% of the ischaemic episodes), which accounts for the opportunity of an objective, unbiased evaluation of the ischaemic events, possible by continuous electrocardiographic monitoring (Schang and Pepine, 1977; Chierchia *et al.*, 1981). This also gives the reason for the inadequacy of the computation of nitroglycerin consumption in the evaluation of the drug response.

(3) The potential seriousness of this syndrome, easily evolving into more severe clinical pictures: this sometimes makes a complex ethical problem to ensue, not easy to resolve and requiring strict criteria for the selection of patients as well as the opportunity to perform the trial in a Coronary Care Unit.

(4) The possibility of interindividual differences in drug absorption, bioavailability and kinetics, very difficult to overcome and requiring the use of sustained doses of the tested drugs as well as several blood samples in various phases of the trial to assess their blood level.

(5) The possible attenuation of the antianginal property of the drug (Abrams, 1980) which can be assessed only by means of an adequate long-term follow-up.

Selection of the Patients

To be included in the study, the patients should have a minimum of ischaemic episodes per day, symptomatic or asymptomatic, sufficient for a correct statistical evaluation; at least not less than 3–4 per day. At the same time, patients should not have met any of the following exclusion criteria:

(1) Very frequent and prolonged ischaemic attacks, unresponsive to symptomatic therapy.
(2) Dangerous arrhythmias (ventricular tachycardia, ventricular fibrillation, complete A–V block) or acute left ventricular failure during the ischaemic episodes.
(3) Clinical and/or radiologic criteria of congestive heart failure.
(4) Clinical and/or electrocardiographic and/or enzymatical criteria of acute myocardial necrosis or a history of recent (< 2 months) myocardial infarction.
(5) Electrocardiographic and/or angiographic findings of left main trunk disease.
(6) Large old myocardial infarction.
(7) Presence in a same ischaemic episode or in different episodes of electrocardiographic alterations in different leads, suggesting spasms on more than one vessel.
(8) Age superior to 70 years.
(9) Possible dangerous interactions with other essential drugs.

Experimental Design

Patients should be in the Coronary Care Unit, under continuous visual and graphic electrocardiographic monitoring. The number of anginal episodes and the number of electrocardiographic episodes with or without pain (ST segment displacement should permit unequivocal interpretation of tracings) should be noted.

Angina on Effort

The efficacy of antianginal drugs in improving exercise tolerance may actually be evaluated only in patients with stable angina on effort. This evaluation needs the following prerequisites:

(1) A carefully recorded medical history revealing the clinical picture of angina on effort with a fixed anginal threshold.
(2) Exclusion of patients with a functional impairment of myocardial blood flow, namely patients who showed a positive ergonovine test and/or ischaemic episodes ensuing at rest revealed by continuous electrocardiographic monitoring and/or a coronary vasospasm during coronary angiography.
(3) Repeated exercise stress-tests should provide the demonstration of a fixed ischaemic threshold. An instrumentation able to guarantee a reproducible work-load for each step should be available. Continuous monitoring of multiple electrocardiographic leads should allow the immediate recognition of the electrocardiographic ischaemic changes

(Bruce *et al.*, 1963). Frequent measurements of arterial blood pressure, i.e. every minute, should be performed in order to assess the pressure–rate product. Exercise tolerance should be assessed on the basis of the total work load, duration of the exercise and systolic pressure–heart rate product at the appearance of undebatable electrocardiographic ischaemic signs (i.e. $\geq 1·5$ mm ST segment displacement) (Brunelli *et al.*, 1982).

This procedure will certainly limit the number of patients enrolled (angina only on fixed limited effort is a rare syndrome!), but it is mandatory to exclude that possible coronary vasoconstriction elicited by effort (Specchia *et al.*, 1979; Brunelli *et al.*, 1981) could induce variable responses to exercise, independent from the actual drug effectiveness.

After this assessment, the evaluation of the effect of drugs on exercise tolerance at short term should be assessed by a crossover design in which patients perform repeated stress tests under the tested drugs and under placebo, in the same general conditions (hour of the day, room temperature, time distance from meal, etc.). A long-term follow-up consisting of periodically repeated exercise tests will confirm or not the persistence of the drug efficacy.

Mixed Form of Angina

This clinical picture characterizes a group of patients whose symptomatology may involve different pathogenetic mechanisms.

A therapeutical trial in this particular set of patients should take into account: (a) the presence of functional factors, responsible for the ischaemic episodes at rest; (b) the presence of atherosclerotic coronary artery lesions limiting the exercise tolerance; (c) the variable combination of functional and organic mechanisms responsible, for example, for a widely variable response to physical stress. This bizarre combination of different pathogenetic mechanisms creates difficulties not easy to solve in the evaluation of the clinical response to drugs exclusively or prevalently acting on only one of them.

Long-Term Study

A long-term follow-up is required for a complete evaluation of antianginal drugs to verify: (1) the persistence of the drug efficacy at a distance of time; (2) the incidence of myocardial infarction and cardiac death in the treated population; and (3) the tolerance of the drug and the eventual appearance of side-effects.

The persistence of the drug efficacy should be easily assessed in patients with stable angina by means of periodic exercise stress tests, while in angina at rest Holter monitoring is useful, in order to detect asymptomatic ischaemic episodes and following drug discontinuation to exclude a spontaneous remission of the disease.

For a proper, correct evaluation of the incidence of myocardial infarction and cardiac death in a patient-population under a certain medical treatment, a control-population under placebo is needed. The two groups of patients should be selected on the basis of the same inclusion/exclusion criteria and randomly assigned to the one or the other treatment.

But this approach, mainly in symptomatic patients, is greatly limited by ethical problems, so that the evaluation of the anginal patients can be performed only comparing the drug under investigation to another drug, with proven and well quantified efficacy in the prevention of myocardial infarction and cardiac death. This implies the enrollment of a larger population of patients and a more prolonged period of follow-up, so that the results can reach statistical significance.

Another important point is that the selection of the patients should be based on homogenous criteria with regard to the pathogenetic mechanisms of their anginal syndrome. The drug-tolerance and eventual side-effects can be assessed by periodical clinical controls, in which at least a basal electrocardiogram, a chest X-ray and a complete blood-chemistry and urinary-analysis should be performed.

Controlled Clinical Trials in Patients with Angina at Rest by a Double-blind Double Crossover Study

Because of several factors, previously analysed, influencing the study of patients with angina at rest, a double-blind double crossover design is mandatory in these patients.

In the last few years, short-term crossover trials with continuous electrocardiographic monitoring in CCU were performed in order to assess the efficacy of verapamil (Parodi *et al.* 1979, 1980), isosorbide dinitrate (Distante *et al.*, 1979), nifedipine (Previtali *et al.*, 1980) against placebo, and of verapamil against propranolol (Parodi *et al.*, 1982) in patients with angina at rest. We report our personal experience with verapamil, the efficacy of which was compared with that of placebo and of propranolol.

Verapamil vs Placebo

Twelve patients with frequent, daily episodes of angina were included in the study and evaluated during two treatment periods alternating with two placebo periods, with the aim of comparing the extent and the consistency of the response of the individual patients with that of the group as a whole. Of the nine patients angiographically evaluated, two showed single-vessel, four double-vessel and three triple-vessel disease.

The study consisted of four 2-day treatment periods, organized according to the following plan:

Treatment A_1: verapamil (80 mg) 1 tablet every 4 h for 2 days (480 mg/24 h).

Treatment B_1: placebo 1 tablet every 4 h for 2 days.

Treatment A_2 and B_2 were respectively as A_1 and B_1. The two sequences of treatments A_1, B_1, A_2, B_2, or B_1, A_1, B_2, A_2, were randomized. All episodes of angina with ST-segment elevation or depression were recorded by continuous monitoring in the CCU and submitted to statistical analysis.

We selected 48-h periods and frequent drug administration (1 tablet every 4 h), because of the 2–3 hour half-life in blood of verapamil after its oral administration and because of possible carryover effects of the drug.

For the group as a whole, the number of episodes during the 48-h run-in period was not statistically different from that during the placebo periods (128 vs 123 and 130). In contrast, during each period of verapamil treatment, a highly significant reduction in the number of episodes was observed (31 and 23, $P < 0.006$, $P < 0.003$). The reduction was similar for the number of episodes with ST-segment elevation and depression and for symptomatic and asymptomatic episodes (Parodi et al., 1979). While in the first 11 patients verapamil appears to be consistently effective in reducing the number of ischaemic episodes (no episodes were observed during both periods of treatment in two patients and during one of the two periods in four), for the last patient studied verapamil failed to improve his clinical situation during the first 48 h of treatment.

We could not find an evident explanation for the inconsistent effects observed in this case, but we observed that in some patients it is not possible to prevent ischaemic attacks completely, probably because of the very acute phase of their disease. In spite of the vigorous therapeutic management performed, some of these attacks evolve into myocardial infarction.

Verapamil vs Propranolol

After the objective demonstrated of the effectiveness of verapamil in the prevention of ischaemic attacks at rest, we turned our interest to compare the relative efficacies of verapamil and propranolol in this form of angina. In many countries (USA, Canada) beta-blockers are the drug of choice for treatment of angina pectoris, either effort induced or resting angina. In particular, propranolol associated to nitrates is considered to be the best "medical reference" for comparison between medical and surgical therapy (Pugh et al., 1978).

Eight patients with more than six attacks of angina at rest per day had been until now selected for the study. Four showed ST-segment elevation and the other four ST-segment depression during the spontaneous attacks.

None of them had previous or recent myocardial infarction. One had normal coronary arteries, two single-vessel disease, five double- or triple-vessel disease.

The study was single-blind, double crossover. When planning it, consideration was given to the possibility of doing it in a double-blind manner. The multiple crossover, double-placebo design, the objective nature of the main parameters of efficacy (electrocardiographic manifestations of ischaemia) and the desire to minimize the risk of the patients, weighted in favour of a single-blind trial.

The oral dose of propranolol was 300 mg per day, while the dose of verapamil was 400 mg per day. Each period lasted 48 h and between the two active drugs, a 48 h placebo period was intermitted with the aim of avoiding the carry-over effect of the two active drugs and to assess the natural course of symptoms. Figure 1 shows the results in the first eight patients studied (after randomization, four started with verapamil and the other four with propranolol).

The number of ischaemic events recorded during beta-blocker treatments was not significantly different from that observed during each relative placebo period. By contrast, during the verapamil periods a marked reduction of the ischaemic episodes was observed, mainly in the second 24 h, after that an adequate blood concentration of the drug was reached. The interposition of placebo periods between each active drug has demonstrated that, in all patients studied, the acute phase of the disease was maintained for the whole duration of the trial. Looking at these data, it is not surprising that a lot of patients with resting angina are handed-over to surgery because of failure of medical therapy, if medical treatment is represented by a beta-blocker.

The ineffectiveness of propranolol, as demonstrated by this clinical controlled study, is in agreement with the new physiopathologic views on angina pectoris (Maseri *et al.*, 1978; Maseri, 1980) and strengthen the rationale for the desuetude of beta-blockers in vasospastic angina.

It is also important to recognize that although the average effective daily dose of propranolol is of the order of 240 mg, it may vary from 50 to 800 mg (Guazzi *et al.*, 1975). Some patients have improvement at a lower dose, in others significant additional benefit is frequently observed at levels of higher dosage.

Thus, controlled clinical trials on a fixed dose, like that used in our study, do not permit us to evaluate the best response at the maximal tolerated dosage and may, indeed underestimate the antianginal properties of the drug.

Conclusions

Recent acquisitions on the pathophysiology of ischaemic heart disease demonstrate that the pathogenesis of angina pectoris is not unifocal. Dif-

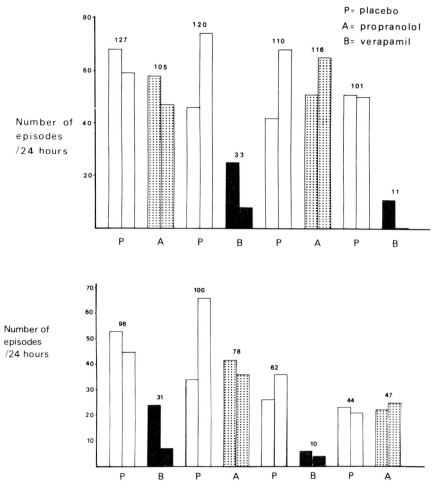

Figure 1. Results of the comparison between propranolol (A) and verapamil (B) in eight patients with angina at rest treated with the two drugs in a single-blind, double crossover trial. Every 48-h period is divided in two columns of 24-h duration each. A placebo period of the same duration was always interposed between the two drug-periods. The upper section shows the results of the four patients who started with propranolol. The lower section shows the results of the four patients who started with verapamil. The number of episodes recorded during the beta-blocker-periods does not significantly differ from that observed during the corresponding placebo-periods. On the contrary, during verapamil a drastic reduction of ischaemic episodes was observed. The high number of episodes during all placebo periods (P) demonstrates in these patients that symptomatology was always in a "hot phase" during the whole trial.

ferent forms of angina need different methodological approaches for the detection of ischaemia as well as appropriate clinical trials to assess the response to therapy. *Ad hoc* designed trials for angina pectoris at rest have documented that nitrates and calcium-entryblockers are remarkably effective in the prevention of ischaemic attacks while beta-blockers appear to be no different from placebo.

References

Abrams, J. (1980). *Am. J. Cardiol.* **99**, 113–123.

Biagini, A., Carpeggiani, C., Mazzei, M., Testa, R., Michelassi, C., Antonelli, R., L'Abbate, A. and Maseri, A. (1981). *G. ital. Cardiol.* **11**, 4–11.

Bruce, R. A., Blackman, J. R., Jones, J. W. and Snrait, G. (1963). *Pediatrics* **32**, 742–747.

Brunelli, C., Lazzari, M., Simonetti, I., L'Abbate, A. and Maseri, A. (1981). *Eur. Heart J.* **2**, 155–161.

Brunelli, C., Lazzari, M., Marraccini, P. and L'Abbate, A. (1982). *In* "Atti del Congresso Nazionale di Cardiologia, Firenze 3-6 Giugno, 1982" p. 375. O.I.C. Medical Press, Firenze.

Chierchia, S., Lazzari, M. and Maseri, A. (1981). *Am. J. Cardiol.* **47**, 446.

Distante, A., Maseri, A., Severi, S., Biagini, A. and Chierchia, S. (1979). *Am. J. Cardiol.* **44**, 533–539.

Friedberg, C. K., (1966). *In* "Diseases of the Heart" (C. K. Friedberg, Ed.), p. 706. W. B. Saunders, Philadelphia.

Guazzi, M., Fiorentini, C., Polese, A., Magrini, F. and Olivari, M. (1975). *Br. Heart J.* **37**, 1235–1245.

Maseri, A. (1980a). *In* "Atherosclerosis Reviews" (R. Hegyeli, Ed.), Vol. 7, pp. 123–131. Raven Press, New York.

Maseri, A. (1980b). *Br. Heart J.* **43**, 648–660.

Maseri, A., Mimmo, R., Chierchia, S., Marchesi, C., Pesola, A. and L'Abbate A. (1975). *Chest* **68**, 625–633.

Maseri, A., Pesola, A., Marzilli, M., Severi, S., Parodi, O., L'Abbate, A., Ballestra, A. M., Maltinti, G., De Nes, M. and Biagini, A. (1977). *Lancet* **i**, 713–717.

Maseri, A., Severi, S., De Nes, D. M., L'Abbate, A., Chierchia, S., Marzilli, M., Ballestra, A. M., Parodi, O., Biagini, A. and Distante, A. (1978). *Am. J. Cardiol.* **42**, 1019–1035.

Mudge, G. H. Jr, Grossman, W., Millis, R., Lesch, M. and Braunwald, E. (1976). *N. Engl. J. Med.* **295**, 1933–1937.

Parodi, O., Maseri, A., and Simonetti, I. (1979). *Br. Heart J.* **41**, 167–174.

Parodi, O., Simonetti, I., L'Abbate, A. and Maseri, A. (1980). *Primary Cardiology* **6**, 29–38.

Parodi, O., Simonetti, I., Lazzari, M., Carpeggiani, C., Testa, R., Biagini, A., Maseri, A. and L'Abbate, A. (1982). *Am. J. Cardioi.* **49**, 930 (Abstr.).

Previtali, M., Salerno, J., Tavazzi, L., Ray, M., Medici, A., Chimienti, M., Specchia, G. and Bobba, P. (1980). *Am. J. Cardiol.* **45**, 825–830.

Pugh, B., Platt, M. R., Mills, L. J., Cremba, D., Poliner, L. R., Curry, G. C., Blomqvist, G. C., Parkey, R. W., Buja, L. M. and Willerson, J. T. (1978). *Am. J. Cardiol.* **41**, 1291–1298.
Schang, S. J. Jr and Pepine, C. J. (1977). *Am. J. Cardiol.* **39**, 396–401.
Specchia, G., De Servi, S., Falcone, C., Bramucci, E., Angoli, L., Mussini, A., Marinoni, G. P., Montemartini, C. and Bobba, P. (1979). *Circulation* **59**, 948–954.

Prostacyclin and Thromboxane A$_2$: Circulating Hormones or Locally Acting Modulators?

C. PATRONO

Department of Pharmacology, Catholic University, School of Medicine, Rome, Italy

Introduction

Arachidonic acid (AA) is metabolized to a wide variety of biologically active substances, i.e. prostaglandins (PGs), thromboxanes (TXs), hydroxy acids, and leukotrienes (LTs). These biotransformations are illustrated in Fig. 1, which also depicts some degradative pathways. The cyclooxygenase pathway of AA metabolism has been thoroughly investigated in the heart, blood vessels, kidney and platelets. At these sites AA metabolites may be physiologically involved in modulatory roles of mostly local nature. Whenever their synthesis is acutely or chronically altered, above or under a certain threshold, the same substances can become responsible for signs and symptoms of various disease states. A complete list of pathologic conditions where such association has been demonstrated or hypothesized would read as an index of internal medicine.

The enzymatic steps of the AA cascade can be affected by a number of currently employed drugs (Patrono and Patrignani, 1982), as summarized in Table 1. Moreover, new drugs are being developed to act on specific enzymes of these complex metabolic pathways.

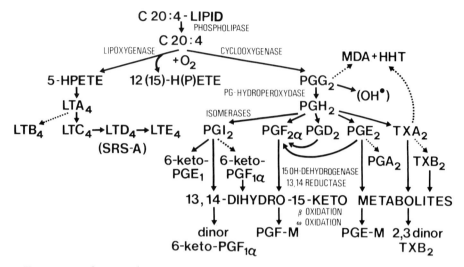

Figure 1. Pathways of arachidonic acid metabolism. C_{20}:4, arachidonic acid; PG, prostaglandin; TX, thromboxane; LT, leukotriene; H(P)ETE, hydro(per)oxy-eicosatetraenoic acid; HHT, 12L-hydroxy-5,8,10-heptadecatrienoic acid; MDA, malondialdehyde; SRS-A, slow-reacting substance of anaphylaxis; PGE-M, 7α-hydroxy-5,11-diketotetranorprostane-1,16-dioic acid; PGF-M, 5α,7α-dihydroxy-11-ketotetranorprostane-1,16-dioic acid. Broken lines represent nonenzymatic reactions.

TXA_2, a potent vasoconstrictor which induces irreversible platelet aggregation is the major cyclooxygenase product of platelet AA metabolism (Hamberg et al., 1975). Furthermore, its synthesis has been demonstrated in the lung, spleen, kidney, vessel wall and leukocytes. Prostacyclin (PGI_2), generated by the vascular wall, is a potent vasodilator and the most potent endogenous inhibitor of platelet aggregation so far discovered (Moncada et al., 1976). On these grounds, it has been suggested that physiologic control of vascular tone and platelet aggregation is influenced by the balance of TXA_2–PGI_2 production.

As the pathophysiologic and therapeutic corollaries of this concept are reviewed elsewhere in this volume, I shall restrict my discussion to some basic and controversial aspects related to the status of PGI_2 and TXA_2 in the human circulation.

Most of the evidence relating the TXA_2–PGI_2 system to control of cardio-vascular function is based on pharmacologic studies on the effects of systemically-infused natural or synthetic compounds, and on the use of selective or non selective synthesis inhibitors and antagonists (Moncada and Vane, 1980). Relatively little is known about changes in endogenous production of PGI_2, and TXA_2, because of methodologic and conceptual problems in their measurement in human body fluids.

Table 1   Drugs affecting arachidonic acid (AA) metabolism

Drug	Mechanism of action	AA metabolites affected
Corticosteroids	Macrocortin-induced inhibition of phospholipase(s)	↓PGs and TXs? ↓HETE and LTs?
BW 755c	Inhibition of cyclooxygenase and lipoxygenase	↓PGs, HETE, LTs
Aspirin	Acetylation of cyclooxygenase	↓PGs and TXs (to a variable extent in different tissues as a function of dosage)
Indomethacin and other NSADs	Selective or non-selective reversible inhibition of cyclooxygenase	↓PGs and TXs
Imidazole-derivatives Endoperoxide-analogs	Inhibition of TX-synthetase	↓TXs ↑PGs
Loop diuretics	↑AA availability? inhibition of PGDH?	↑Renal PGs and TXs
Converting-enzyme inhibitors	Bradykinin-induced activation of phospholipase(s)?	↑PGs?
Nitroglycerin, nitroprusside, hydralazine, dipyridamole	Unknown (stimulation of PGI₂-synthetase?)	↑Vascular PGI₂ ↓Platelet TXA₂?

Is PGI₂ a Circulating Substance in Man?

Although PGI_2 was initially characterized as a circulating hormone continuously released by the lungs into the arterial circulation (Gryglewski et al., 1978; Moncada et al., 1978), the validity of this concept is now questioned by a number of recent findings in healthy subjects. These include: (1) comparably low levels of 6-keto-$PGF_{1\alpha}$ (the hydrolysis product of PGI_2) in the pulmonary and brachial arterial blood (Edlund et al., 1981); (2) undetectable 6-keto-$PGF_{1\alpha}$ in peripheral venous blood (Christ-Hazelhof and Nugteren, 1981; Patrono et al., 1982); (3) low rate of endogenous secretion, i.e. $0.08–0.10$ ng/kg/min (FitzGerald et al., 1981); (4) rapid disappearance of infused PGI_2 (see Table 2). Since PGI_2 infusion rates of $2.5–5$ ng/kg/min are required in order to achieve threshold plasma concentrations for platelet and vascular effects, these data are consistent with a

Table 2   Prostacyclin in the circulation of normal man

Rate of secretion: $0.08-0.10$ ng/kg/min   (FitzGerald et al., 1981)

$T_{1/2}$: Initial phase 3.2 min   (Patrono et al., 1982)
        Slower phase 15 min

Clearance rate: 26.2 ± 4.7 ml/kg/min   (Myatt et al., 1981)
                24.4 ± 9.8 ml/kg/min   (Patrono et al., 1982)

Circulating concentration: 3.5 pg/ml calculated as $\dfrac{\text{rate of secretion}}{\text{plasma clearance}}$

< 7.5 pg/ml measured as 6-keto-PGF$_{1\alpha}$

Threshold concentration for biological effects: 100–200 pg/ml measured as 6-keto-PGF$_{1\alpha}$

local rather than systemic nature of PGI_2 action. A plasma metabolite with longer half-life, such as 13,14-dihydro-6,15-diketo-PGF$_{1\alpha}$, would probably give some long-term indication as to the amounts of acutely released PGI_2 in man (Patrono et al., 1981). Alternatively, the urinary excretion of 2,3-dinor-6-keto-PGF$_{1\alpha}$ might provide an integrated measure of daily PGI_2 production (FitzGerald et al., 1981).

PGI_2 biosynthesis has been described in human renal medullary and cortical microsomes (Hassid and Dunn, 1980), and evidence has been reported that PGI_2 is a local modulator of juxtaglomerular function in man (Patrono et al., 1982). Furosemide acutely increases renal PGI_2 production, as reflected by urinary 6-keto-PGF$_{1\alpha}$ excretion, while peripheral plasma levels of 6-keto-PGF$_{1\alpha}$ remain undetectable (Patrono et al., 1982). These results would suggest the need for further studies assessing PGI_2 production in discrete vascular districts, as modified by drugs or pathophysiologic changes.

Is Thromboxane A_2 a Circulating Substance in Man?

TXA_2 undergoes rapid nonenzymatic degradation to TXB_2 in aqueous solutions. As a great artefactual formation of the compound can be expected during blood sample collection and handling – due to platelet and leucocyte activation –, measured "peripheral plasma levels" of TXB_2 will undoubtely be very high and will not reflect the true endogenous circulating levels of the compound, if any (Granström, 1978). Moreover, daily submaximal doses of aspirin (0.45 mg/kg), which cause a selective inhibition of platelet TXA_2 formation in healthy subjects (Patrignani et al., 1982), can completely abolish "peripheral plasma levels" of TXB_2, thus suggesting a major platelet origin of this compound.

TXB₂ production during whole blood clotting represents a relatively simple tool to investigate pharmacologic effects on platelet cyclooxygenase (Patrono *et al.*, 1980). This *ex vivo* model perhaps mimics the *in vivo* situation more closely than conventional studies carried out in platelet-rich plasma with the addition of exogenous stimuli. During whole blood clotting, thrombin is the major factor responsible for platelet aggregation and release, and the time course of its formation (Schuman and Levine, 1980) is quite similar to that of TXB₂ in healthy subjects (Fig. 2).

TXB₂ synthesis has been described in the human kidney (Hassid and Dunn, 1980), and urinary TXB₂ has been suggested to reflect renal TXA₂ synthesis in healthy subjects (Ciabattoni *et al.*, 1979). The physiologic and pathophysiologic role of renal TXA₂ remains to be clarified. 2,3-dinor-TXB₂ is the major urinary metabolite of TXB₂ in man (Roberts *et al.*, 1977). To what extent it reflects platelet vs extra-platelet sources of TXA₂ has not been established.

Low-dose (0·45 mg/kg/day) aspirin can produce a cumulative and virtu-

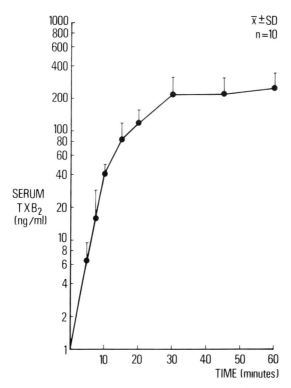

Figure 2. Time-course for the production of TXB₂ during whole blood clotting at 37°C. Each point represents the mean ± one standard deviation (s.d.) of measurements performed in 10 healthy subjects.

ally complete inhibition of platelet TXB_2 production in healthy subjects, without interfering with renal medullary and cortical sites of cyclooxygenase activity (Patrignani *et al.*, 1982). Besides its therapeutic potential, low-dose aspirin can become a useful research tool in assessing the role of platelet TXA_2 in health and disease.

Acknowledgements

The studies of the author were supported by CNR grants (78.02777.86, 79.01243.86 and 80.00351.86 of Progetto Finalizzato Tecnologie Bio-mediche, Subprogetto CHIM-2 and 80.00545.04 and 81.00321.04 of Pharmacological Research Unit). The expert editorial assistance of Ms Angelamaria Zampini is gratefully acknowledged.

References

Christ-Hazelhof, E. and Nugteren, D. H. (1981). *Prostaglandins* 22, 739–746.
Ciabattoni, G., Pugliese, F., Cinotti, G. A., Stirati, G., Ronci, R., Castrucci, G., Pierucci, A. and Patrono, C. (1979). *Eur. J. Pharmacol.* 60, 181–187.
Edlund, A., Bomfin, W., Kaijser, L., Olin, C., Patrono, C., Pinca, E. and Wennmalm, Å. (1981). *Prostaglandins* 22, 323–332.
FitzGerald, G. A., Brash, A. R., Falardeau, P. and Oates, J. A. (1981). *J. clin. Invest.* 68, 1272–1276.
Granström, E. (1978). *Prostaglandins* 15, 3–17.
Gryglewski, R. J., Korbut, R. and Ocetkiewicz, A. (1978). *Nature* 273, 765–767.
Hamberg, M., Svensson, J. and Samuelsson, B. (1975). *Proc. natn. Acad. Sci. USA* 72, 2994–2998.
Hassid, A. and Dunn, M. J. (1980). *J. biol. Chem.* 255, 2472–2475.
Moncada, S. and Vane, J. R. (1980). *In* "Adv. Prostaglandin Thromboxane Res." 6, 43–60.
Moncada, S., Gryglewski, R. J., Bunting, S. and Vane, J. R. (1976). *Nature* 263, 663–665.
Moncada, S., Korbut, R., Bunting, S. and Vane, J. R. (1978). *Nature* 273, 767–768.
Myatt, L., Jogee, M., Lewis, P. J. and Elder, M. G. (1981). *In* "The Clinical Pharmacology of Prostacyclin" (P. J. Lewis and J. O'Grady, Eds), pp. 30–42. Raven Press, London and New York.
Patrignani, P., Filabozzi, P. and Patrono, C. (1982). *J. clin. Invest.* 69, 1366–1372.
Patrono, C. and Patrignani, P. (1982). *Int. J. Immunopharmac.* 4, 127–133.
Patrono, C., Ciabattoni, G., Pinca, E., Pugliese, F., Castrucci, G., De Salvo, A., Satta, M. A. and Peskar, B. A. (1980). *Thromb. Res.* 17, 317–327.
Patrono, C., Ciabattoni, G., Peskar, B. M., Pugliese, F. and Peskar, B. A. (1981). *Clin. Res.* 29, 276A (Abstract).
Patrono, C., Pugliese, F., Ciabattoni, G., Patrignani, P., Maseri, A., Chierchia, S.,

Peskar, B. A., Cinotti, G. A., Simonetti, B. M. and Pierucci, A. (1982). *J. clin. Invest.* **69**, 231–239.
Roberts, L. J. II, Sweetman, B. J., Payne, A. N. and Oates, J. A. (1977). *J. biol. Chem.* **252**, 7415–7417.
Schuman, M. A. and Levine, S. P. (1980). *J. clin. Invest.* **65**, 307–313.

Platelet Aggregation, Vascular Wall and Ischaemic Heart Disease

J. F. MUSTARD[1],
R. L. KINLOUGH-RATHBONE[1],
and M. A. PACKHAM[2]

[1] Department of Pathology, McMaster University, Hamilton, Ontario and [2] Department of Biochemistry, University of Toronto, Toronto, Ontario, Canada

Introduction

Platelets contribute in at least two ways to the development of athero-sclerosis and its clinical complications. First, the interaction of platelets with injured vessel walls plays a part in initiating atherosclerotic lesions, and second, the thromboemboli responsible for some of the complications of vascular disease have a large platelet component (Mustard and Packham, 1975; Mustard *et al.*, 1978, 1981b; Ross and Vogel, 1978; Kinlough-Rathbone and Mustard, 1981; Ross, 1981).

The Role of Platelets in the Development of Atherosclerosis

Platelets are involved in both the early and the later stages of the develop-ment of atherosclerotic lesions. When the endothelium is lost from the surface of a normal or diseased vessel, platelets accumulate at the injury site and release factors that cause smooth muscle cell migration into the intima, and smooth muscle cell proliferation (Ross and Vogel, 1978; Ross, 1981). Experimental work in rabbits has shown that repeated injury to the endothelium can cause the development of proliferative atherosclerotic lesions which have the characteristics of advanced atherosclerosis in man (Moore, 1973). The factors controlling the proliferative response, the formation of connective tissue, the accumulation of glycosaminoglycans and lipid, the metabolism of smooth muscle cells, and the metabolism and regrowth of endothelial cells are all being studied. The glycosaminoglycans are thought to bind to low density lipoproteins (LDL) and are probably responsible for the focal accumulation of lipid in damaged vessel walls. Lipid can accumulate focally in the vessel wall in the presence of normal serum lipid concentrations, thereby contributing to the development of the lipid-rich atheromatous lesions that occur as a consequence of repeated vessel injury (Richardson et al., 1980; Moore, 1981; Minick, 1981).

The proliferative response of the smooth muscle cells following endothelial cell injury can be inhibited if animals are depleted of platelets at the time of injury (Moore et al., 1976b; Friedman and Burns, 1978). Attempts to inhibit the development of this form of atherosclerosis by the administration of drugs that inhibit platelet aggregation have been unsuccessful unless the drug also prevents platelet adhesion to the damaged wall and/or the release of granule contents from the platelets adherent to the wall, including release of the factor that is mitogenic for smooth muscle cells (Baumgartner and Studer, 1977; Clowes and Karnovsky, 1977; Mustard et al., 1981b). Since aspirin does not inhibit platelet adherence to the subendothelium or the release reaction of the adherent platelets (Kinlough-Rathbone et al., 1979; Dejana et al., 1980), it is not surprising that aspirin and other drugs that inhibit cyclo-oxygenase, do not inhibit the intimal proliferation associated with endothelial injury. In contrast, dipyridamole, which inhibits platelet adherence to the subendothelium and the release reaction of platelets adherent to the subendothelium (Weiss et al., 1981; Groves et al., 1982a), inhibits the proliferative response associated with endothelial cell injury (Harker et al., 1976).

The development of proliferative atherosclerotic lesions may also be modified by other factors, including some from the endothelial cells. Endothelial cells have been reported to form or secrete factors that inhibit smooth muscle cell proliferation (Castellot et al., 1981), but they can also release or form a factor that causes smooth muscle cell proliferation (Gajdusek et al., 1980). As endothelium grows over the smooth muscle cells, it may modify the smooth muscle cell response. Endothelial cell covering of smooth muscle cells is associated with focal accumulation of glycosaminoglycans (Richardson et al., 1980; Falcone et al., 1980).

Monocytes can be found within the lesions as they progress. Stimulated monocytes can also form and secrete a mitogen that causes smooth muscle cell proliferation (Glenn and Ross, 1981); thus, the proliferative response can be influenced by cells other than platelets and experimental proliferative lesions have been described as a consequence of factors other than those derived from platelets.

In vessels with more advanced atherosclerosis, thrombi can form on the diseased vessel surface and become organized and incorporated into the vessel wall (Duguid, 1946; Morgan, 1956; Woolf *et al.*, 1968; Crawford, 1977). Stenotic lesions may be partially a consequence of the organization of thrombi. Smooth muscle cells migrate into a thrombus (Jørgensen *et al.*, 1967b; Woolf, 1978) as a result of factors released from monocytes and platelets, and eventually a thickened intima is formed. Morphological studies have led to the conclusion that mural thrombosis is important in the development of advanced atherosclerotic lesions.

The focal nature of early and advanced atherosclerotic lesions is compatible with the concept that endothelial injury and thrombosis make major contributions to the development of atherosclerotic lesions. Haemodynamic factors influence the localization of atherosclerotic lesions (Fry, 1976; Goldsmith and Karino, 1979) because they can determine the sites of endothelial injury that are a consequence of injurious substances in the bloodstream, such as circulating antigen-antibody complexes (Kniker and Cochrane, 1968). In serum sickness, focal arteritis occurs around vessel orifices and branches (Kniker and Cochrane, 1968). The sites of maximum thrombus formation in arteries tend to be areas of disturbed blood flow such as at bifurcations, vessel orifices and sites of stenosis (Murphy *et al.*, 1962; Goldsmith, 1972; Caro, 1977; Goldsmith and Karino, 1979). In areas of high shear such as on the proximal side of a stenotic lesion, the endothelium may be disrupted (Gertz *et al.*, 1981).

Vessel Injury and Vessel Wall Reactivity

Removal of the endothelium from a normal vessel wall such as the rabbit or rat aorta leads to an initial platelet reaction with the wall, but within 1 h the surface loses its ability to cause further platelet interaction with it (Groves *et al.*, 1979). This type of injury is not associated with shortened platelet survival. However, if a normal rabbit or rat aorta is repeatedly injured, for example, by an indwelling aortic catheter, the surface is repeatedly reactive to platelets and this is associated with shortened platelet survival (Meuleman *et al.*, 1980; Kinlough-Rathbone *et al.*, 1981), even without macroscopic thrombus formation (Winocour *et al.*, 1981).

Recent studies have also shown that injury to a thickened intima in rabbits by passage of a balloon catheter through a previously damaged aorta causes the formation of platelet–fibrin thrombi as well as platelet adherence to freshly exposed connective tissue (Groves *et al.*, 1982b). Damage to the smooth muscle cells probably activates the extrinsic pathway of coagulation, leading to thrombin formation and the conversion of fibrinogen to fibrin which binds to platelets and traps them in a fibrin mesh. Evidence that much of the platelet accumulation results from thrombin and fibrin formation comes from the observation that heparin is inhibitory (Groves *et al.*, 1982b). This type of injury site also is only active for a short period of time and, as with exposure of the subendothelium, does not shorten platelet survival. Thus, a single injury to a vessel wall does not create a chronically active site, but rather, a site that is active for only a limited time. Nevertheless, such an injury is sufficient to stimulate smooth muscle cell proliferation and their growth and development into an early atherosclerotic lesion (Stemerman, 1978; Groves *et al.*, 1979). Thus, episodic injury without much thrombosis could cause extensive atherosclerosis.

An interesting practical implication of these observations is that if platelet accumulation on the surface of an injured vessel could be prevented for the period of time that it is reactive to platelets, thrombus formation would be inhibited. In one experiment in cats in which the carotid arteries were subjected to endarterectomy, heparin therapy for a period of 6 h prevented thrombus formation and during this time the injured surface became non-thrombogenic so that even when the therapy was stopped thrombus formation did not occur (Piepgras *et al.*, 1976). This may have a practical application in vascular surgery since the period of most intense therapy to inhibit platelet interaction with a damaged vessel or graft and thus prevent smooth muscle cell proliferation and thrombosis, should be during the first day following the operative procedure.

Thrombosis and the Clinical Complications of Atherosclerosis

Thrombosis of diseased arteries has been considered to be a primary cause of the clinical complications of atherosclerosis, such as heart attacks and strokes. It is becoming apparent that this concept may be too simplistic since other causes have now been recognized. Individuals who die suddenly and are found at post-mortem to have myocardial ischaemia and extensive atherosclerosis of their coronary arteries often show no sign of coronary artery thrombosis (Schwartz *et al.*, 1978; Roberts and Jones, 1979). In contrast, patients with myocardial infarction who die hours or days after the onset of symptoms usually have an occlusive thrombus in the coronary artery supplying the infarcted segment (Chandler *et al.*, 1974; Davies *et al.*, 1976, 1979). Although atherosclerosis is common to both situations, it has been proposed that different mechanisms are involved in sudden death and myocardial infarction. Occlusive thrombosis may be responsible for myocardial infarction and death of patients who do not die suddenly, but sudden death may result from other causes. Two such causes have been proposed.

(i) Embolization of mural thrombi in the coronary arteries, leading to impairment of the microcirculation, ventricular fibrillation and sudden death (Jørgensen *et al.*, 1967a; Haerem, 1978; El-Maraghi and Genton, 1980). This theory is supported by the observations of Haerem (1978) who found an increased incidence of small mural thrombi and of platelet aggregates in the microcirculation of the hearts of individuals with coronary artery disease who died suddenly, as compared with those who had died suddenly in accidents. Experiments with pigs have shown that infusion of ADP into the coronary arteries induces the formation of platelet aggregates that cause ventricular fibrillation and immediate death when they block the micro-circulation (Jørgensen *et al.*, 1967a). In addition, mural thrombi in the coronary artery of dogs caused sudden death with myocardial lesions similar to those found after sudden cardiac death in man; in contrast, in these experiments, dogs that had occlusive rather than mural thrombi tended to develop infarcts and few of them died suddenly (Moore *et al.*, 1976a). Thus, mural thrombi that embolize into the distal circulation may be a cause of sudden cardiac death although the frequency with which this occurs is unknown.

(ii) Recent observations have led to consideration of the possible role of focal coronary artery spasm in causing myocardial ischaemia and sudden death without thrombosis (Oliva and Breckenridge, 1977; Maseri *et al.*, 1980; Ganz, 1981). Spasm that persists, however, could cause myocardial infarction and thrombosis associated with the infarcted region. The associa-tion between vessel injury and spasm is well established since spasm occurs as an immediate response to vessel injury in animal experiments designed to cause thrombosis or haemostatic plug formation (Fulton *et al.*, 1953; Macfarlane, 1972). It seems reasonable to expect that injury to the lining of a coronary artery would cause spasm. Recently, Gertz and his associates (1981) showed experimentally that the high shear rate at the point where blood enters a stenotic lesion may disrupt the endothelium. If this occurs in diseased coronary arteries of man, focal spasm may ensue. Thromboxane A_2 that is formed by the platelets and white cells that adhere to the denuded site may be one of the factors responsible for vasoconstriction and spasm (Ellis *et al.*, 1976; Braunwald, 1978), whereas PGI_2 produced by a stimulated vessel wall may limit the degree and duration of spasm by causing relaxation of the smooth muscle cells (Moncada *et al.*, 1979). Obviously other mechanisms may be involved, but the possible role of thromboxane A_2 in the initiation of spasm associated with vessel injury deserves close examination. If focal injury of the vessel wall is an important factor initiating coronary artery spasm, prevention of endothelial injury should minimize the risk of spasm. This is only feasible if injury can be reduced by changes in life style (e.g. cessation of smoking, reduction of saturated fat intake, avoidance of stress). Injury caused by the haemodynamic forces generated in diseased arteries could be reduced by techniques such as angioplasty that remodel the blood vessel and lessen the stenosis.

Mechanisms in Thrombosis

Much of the original experimental work that was done to investigate the mechanisms involved in arterial thrombosis involved normal blood vessels of young animals. The results led to the conclusion that platelets interact with the exposed subendothelial structures in the vessel wall, and that collagen stimulates the platelets to form thromboxane A_2 and release their granule contents, including ADP. The ADP and thromboxane A_2 then cause the platelets that are nearby to change shape and stick to each other and to the platelets adherent to the vessel wall. The platelet mass that forms serves as a focus for the acceleration of the intrinsic pathway of coagulation through the interactions of factors VIII and IX and of factors V and X that take place in association with the platelet membrane phospholipids. The thrombin that forms causes platelet aggregation, release of granule contents, the formation of thromboxane A_2, and the formation of fibrin. The fibrin that forms around the platelet aggregate appears to stabilize it, preventing it from breaking up when the platelets deaggregate (Mustard *et al.*, 1974, 1981c; Baumgartner and Muggli, 1976; Weiss, 1978; Schafer and Handin, 1979; Packham and Mustard, 1980). This concept led to the suggestion that drugs that inhibit platelet aggregation would be possibly valuable anti-thrombotic agents in arterial disease (Weiss, 1978; Packham and Mustard, 1980).

It is now apparent that these observations which were obtained with normal blood vessels subjected to a single injury, may not be applicable when diseased vessels are injured. Recent experimental work has shown that when the thickened intima is damaged with a balloon catheter, thrombi of the type described above do not develop. Instead, the thrombi appear to be largely initiated by thrombin, (Stemerman, 1973; Packham and Mustard, 1980; Groves *et al.*, 1982b) probably formed through the extrinsic pathway of coagulation. The thrombin causes fibrin formation, and the initial thrombus is a mass of fibrin on the vessel wall, in which platelets may or may not be trapped. The growth of these thrombi may be dependent on platelets, but this too may be largely a thrombin-mediated process (Groves *et al.*, 1982b). It seems likely that in this type of thrombosis, the damaged smooth muscle cells either form or release tissue thromboplastin which rapidly activates the extrinsic coagulation pathway. The implications of these observations is that the use of drugs that inhibit platelet aggregation by inhibition of the cyclooxygenase will be relatively ineffective against thrombin. Thrombin can induce platelet aggregation and release through pathways that are independent of the arachidonate pathway and released ADP (Packham *et al.*, 1977; Kinlough-Rathbone *et al.*, 1977; Charo *et al.*, 1977). Drugs that have been used in clinical trials to prevent platelet aggregation in subjects who have had myocardial infarction include aspirin, sulphinpyrazone and dipyridamole (Elwood *et al.*, 1974; Coronary Drug Project Research Group, 1976; Elwood and Sweetnam, 1979; Breddin *et al.*, 1979; Aspirin Myocardial Infarction Study Research Group, 1980; Persantine–Aspirin Reinfarction Study Research Group, 1980; Anturane Reinfarction Trial Research Group, 1980). Both aspirin and sulphinpyrazone inhibit platelet cyclooxygenase and thereby inhibit platelet aggregation and release (Packham and Mustard, 1980). Dipyridamole inhibits platelet adherence to the vessel wall as well as platelet aggregation induced by ADP and thrombin (Cucuianu *et al.*, 1971; Packham and Mustard, 1980; Groves *et al.*, 1982a). The mechanism of its action is not clearly understood, although it is a phospho-diesterase inhibitor and therefore would contribute to an increase in platelet cyclic AMP if adenylate cyclase is stimulated (Mustard and Packham, 1978).

The results from the clinical trials with drugs that inhibit collagen-induced platelet aggregation, such as aspirin and sulphinpyrazone, have not shown particularly dramatic effects. Both aspirin and sulphinpyrazone, however, were effective inhibitors of thrombus formation in arteriovenuous shunts in man (Kaegi *et al.*, 1975; Harter *et al.*, 1979). In none of the studies of patients with coronary artery disease did aspirin produce a significant reduction in mortality, but when all the studies were grouped together, it was apparent that aspirin did reduce the incidence of myocardial infarction and this was associated with a significant reduction in mortality (Peto, 1978; Editorial, 1980). It is difficult to determine how aspirin produces this effect since sulphinpyrazone did not appear to reduce the incidence of myocardial infarction and death associated with it in the Anturane Reinfarction Trial (1980). It did, however, reduce the incidence of sudden death, probably due to a mechanism unrelated to its action on thromboembolic events (Mustard *et al.*, 1981).

There is recent evidence indicating that despite years of disfavour, anti-coagulants may indeed cause a significant reduction in mortality in post-myocardial infarction patients (Sixty Plus Reinfarction Study Research Group, 1980). This is compatible with the theory that there may be at least two mechanisms involved in the development of arterial thrombosis. One, which is largely a platelet-dependent process and therefore inhibitable by drugs such as aspirin, and another which has a significant coagulation component. These mechanisms should be considered in the light of the possibility that spasm in coronary arteries may be an important factor in the initial etiology of clinical complications, and in the development of the thrombi. Drugs which inhibit the cyclo-oxygenase pathway may, by inhibiting PGI_2 production, enhance the spasm associated with the events that occur in association with myocardial ischaemia (Friedman *et al.*, 1981).

Endothelial Injury and Risk Factors

Injury to the endothelium is important in the initiation of atherosclerosis, the development of advanced atherosclerosis, and the development of complications secondary to spasm and thrombosis. There is circumstantial evidence that some of the risk factors, such as increased low-density lipoproteins in the plasma, products of cigarette smoking, and high blood pressure, may be able to damage the endothelium (Mason *et al.*, 1977; Mustard *et al.*, 1981c). Thus, one mechanism by which the established risk factors associated with the development of atherosclerosis and their complications may contribute to the development of atherosclerosis, is through endothelial cell injury. Recently, a reduction in the incidence of coronary heart disease by cessation of smoking and lowering serum lipids has been reported in high risk subjects (Hjermann *et al.*, 1981) and in patients who have had a myocardial infarct (Kallio *et al.*, 1979).

Summary

Understanding the mechanisms that injure the endothelium should help to devise ways to control the development of atherosclerosis and its clinical complications. Vessel injury has been recognized to lead to the development of atherosclerotic lesions and thromboembolic complications. The risk factors for atherosclerosis, such as smoking, hypertension and an increase in the plasma LDL may contribute to the development of atherosclerotic lesions by their ability to damage the endothelium.

Although thromboembolism has long been thought to be a major factor in causing the clinical complications of atherosclerosis, the recent observations about the role of spasm raise interesting considerations for the future. An important point is that injury to a vessel wall is usually associated with spasm and spasm could well be responsible for the initial ischaemic events associated with sudden death for which there is little evidence of a thromboembolic process. If the spasm persists, thrombi may develop and persist after the spasm has resolved causing more permanent ischaemia, leading to myocardial infarction. If so, the control of injury and spasm may be the most important approaches to the management of clinical complications in subjects with advanced atherosclerosis.

Our understanding of the mechanisms of thrombosis has changed and it now appears that in arterial disease the diseased vessel wall can initiate thrombi that have a large coagulation component. Formation of these thrombi cannot be easily inhibited by drugs that inhibit the cyclo-oxygenase pathway. Inhibitors of thrombin generation or the effect of thrombin on platelets may be more effective in preventing the formation of this type of thrombus. Thus, the results of the clinical trials using drugs such as aspirin and sulphinpyrazone are not surprising in view of what we now know about the development of thrombosis and about coronary artery spasm.

References

The Anturane Reinfarction Trial Research Group. (1980). *N. Engl. J. Med.* **302**, 250–256.
Aspirin Myocardial Infarction Study Research Group. (1980). *JAMA* **243**, 661–669.
Baumgartner, H. R. and Muggli, R. (1976). *In* "Platelets in Biology and Pathology" (J. L. Gordon, Ed.), pp. 23–60. North-Holland Biomedical Press, Amsterdam.
Baumgartner, H. R. and Studer, A. (1977). *In* "Atherosclerosis" IV. (G. Schettler, Y. Goto, Y. Hata and G. Klose, Eds), pp. 605–609. Springer Verlag, Berlin.

Braunwald, E. (1978). *N. Engl. J. Med.* **299**, 1301–1303.
Breddin, K., Loew, D., Lechner, K., Uberla, K. and Walter, E. (1979). *Thromb. Haemostas.* **40**, 225–236.
Caro, C. G. (1977). *In* "Cardiovascular Flow Dynamics and Measurements" (N.H.C. Hwang and N.A. Normann, Eds), pp. 473–487. University Park Press, Baltimore.
Castellot, J. J. Jr, Addonizio, M. L., Rosenberg, R. and Karnovsky, M. J. (1981). *J. Cell Biol.* **90**, 372–379.
Chandler, A. B., Chapman, I., Erhardt, L. R., Roberts, W. C., Schwartz, C. J., Sinapius, D., Spain, D. M., Sherry, S., Ness, P. M. and Simon, T. L. (1974). *Am. J. Cardiol.* **34**, 823–833.
Charo, I. F., Feinman, R. D. and Detwiler, T. C. (1977). *J. clin. Invest.* **60**, 866–873.
Clowes, A. W. and Karnovsky, M. J. (1977). *Lab. Invest.* **36**, 452–464.
Coronary Drug Project Research Group. (1976). *J. chronic Dis.* **29**, 625–642.
Crawford, T. (1977). "Pathology of Ischaemic Heart Disease", pp. 1–170. Butterworths, London.
Cucuianu, M. P., Nishizawa, E. E. and Mustard, J. F. (1971). *J. Lab. clin. Med.* **77**, 958–974.
Davies, M. J., Woolf, N., and Robertson, W. B. (1976). *Br. Heart J.* **38**, 659–664.
Davies, M. J., Fulton, W. F. M. and Robertson, W. B. (1979). *J. Path.* **127**, 99–110.
Dejana, E., Cazenave, J.-P., Groves, H. M., Kinlough-Rathbone, R. L., Richardson, M., Packham, M. A. and Mustard, J. F. (1980). *Thromb. Res.* **17**, 453–464.
Duguid, J. B. (1946). *J. Pathol. Bacteriol.* **58**, 207–212.
Editorial. (1980). *Lancet* **i**, 1172–1173.
Ellis, E. F., Oelz, O., Roberts, L. J. II., Payne, N. A., Sweetman, B. J., Nies, A. S. and Oates, J. A. (1976). *Science* **193**, 1135–1137.
El-Maraghi, N. and Genton, E. (1980). *Circulation* **62**, 936–944.
Elwood, P. C. and Sweetnam, P. M. (1979). *Lancet* **ii**, 1313–1315.
Elwood, P. C., Cochrane, A. L., Burr, M. L., Sweetnam, P. M., Williams, G., Welsby, E., Hughes, S. J. and Renton, R. (1974). *Br. Med. J.* **1**, 436–440.
Falcone, D. J., Hajjar, D. P. and Minick, C. R. (1980). *Am. J. Pathol.* **99**, 81–104.
Friedman, R. J. and Burns, E. R. (1978). *In* "Progress in Hemostasis and Thrombosis" Vol. 4. (T. H. Spaet, Ed.), pp. 249–278. Grune and Stratton, New York.
Friedman, P. L., Brown, E. J., Jr., Gunther, S., Alexander, R. W., Barry, W. H., Mudge, G. H., Jr. and Grossman, W. (1981). *N. Engl. J. Med.* **305**, 1171–1175.
Fry, D. L. (1976). *In* "Cerebrovascular Diseases, Tenth Princeton Conference" (P. Sheinberg, Ed.), pp. 77–95. Raven Press, New York.
Fulton, G. P., Akers, R. P. and Lutz, B. R. (1953). *Blood* **8**, 140–152.
Gajdusek, C., Dicorleto, P., Ross, R., and Schwartz, S. M. (1980). *J. Cell Biol.* **85**, 467–472.
Ganz, W. (1981). *Circulation* **63**, 487–488.
Gertz, S. D., Uretsky, G., Wajnberg, R., Navot, N. and Gotsman, M. S. (1981). *Circulation* **63**, 476–486.
Glenn, K. and Ross, R. (1981). *Cell* **25**, 603–615.
Goldsmith, H. L. (1972). *In* "Progress in Hemostasis and Thrombosis, Vol. 1" (T. H. Spaet, Ed.), pp. 97–139. Grune and Stratton, New York.
Goldsmith, H. L. and Karino, T. (1979). *In* "Quantitive Cardiovascular Studies. Clinical and Research Applications of Engineering Principles" (N.H.C. Hwang, D. R. Gross and D. J. Patel, Eds), pp. 289–351. University Park Press, Baltimore.
Groves, H. M., Kinlough-Rathbone, R. L., Richardson, M., Moore, S. and Mustard, J. F. (1979). *Lab. Invest.* **40**, 194–200.

Groves, H. M., Kinlough-Rathbone, R. L., Cazenave, J.-P., Dejana, E., Richardson, M. and Mustard, J. F. (1982a). *J. Lab. clin. Med.* **99**, 548–558.
Groves, H. M., Kinlough-Rathbone, R. L., Richardson, M., Jorgensen, L., Moore, S. and Mustard, J. F. (1982b). *Lab. Invest.* **46**, 605–612.
Haerem, J. W. (1978). *Acta. path. microbiol. scand.* Section A, Suppl. **265**, 7–47.
Harker, L. A., Ross, R., Slichter, S. J. and Scott, C. R. (1976). *J. clin. Invest.* **58**, 731–741.
Harter, H. R., Burch, J. W., Majerus, P. W., Stanford, N., Delmez, J. A., Anderson, C. B. and Weerts, C. A. (1979). *N. Engl. J. Med.* **301**, 577–579.
Hjermann, I., Byre, K. V., Holme, I. and Leren, P. (1981). *Lancet* **ii**, 1303–1313.
Jørgensen, L., Rowsell, H. C., Hovig, T., Glynn, M. F. and Mustard, J. F. (1967a). *Lab. Invest.* **17**, 616–644.
Jørgensen, L., Rowsell, H. C., Hovig, T. and Mustard, J. F. (1967b). *Am. J. Path.* **51**, 681–719.
Kaegi, A., Pineo, G. F., Shimizu, A., Trivedi, H., Hirsh, J. and Gent, M. (1975). *Circulation* **52**, 497–499.
Kallio, V., Hämäläinen, H., Hakkila, J. and Luurila, O. J. (1979). *Lancet* **ii**, 1091–1094.
Kinlough-Rathbone, R. L. and Mustard, J. F. (1981). *Am. J. Surg.* **141**, 638–643.
Kinlough-Rathbone, R. L., Packham, M. A., Reimers, H.-J., Cazenave, J.-P. and Mustard, J. F. (1977). *J. Lab. clin. Med.* **90**, 707–719.
Kinlough-Rathbone, R. L. Cazenave, J.-P., Packham, M. A. and Mustard, J. F. (1979). *Lab. Invest.* **42**, 28–34.
Kinlough-Rathbone, R. L., Packham, M. A. and Mustard, J. F. (1981). *Thromb. Haemostas.* **46**, 248.
Kniker, W. T. and Cochrane, C. G. (1968). *J. exp. Med.* **127**, 119–135.
Macfarlane, R. G. (1972). *In* "Human Blood Coagulation, Haemostasis and Thrombosis" (R. Biggs, Ed.), pp. 543–585. Blackwell Scientific Publications, Oxford.
Maseri, A., Chierchia, S. and L'Abbate, A. (1980). *Circulation* **62**, Suppl. V, 3–13.
Mason, R. G., Sharp, D., Chuang, H. Y. K. and Mohammad, F. (1977). *Arch. Pathol. Lab. Med.* **101**, 61–64.
Meuleman, D. G., Vogel, G. M. T. and van Delft, A. M. L. (1980). *Thromb. Res.* **20**, 45–55.
Minick, C. R. (1981). *In* "Vascular Injury and Atherosclerosis" (S. Moore, Ed.), pp. 149–173. Marcel Dekker Inc., New York.
Moncada, S. and Vane, J. R. (1979). *Fed. Proc.* **38**, 66–71.
Moore, S. (1973). *Lab. Invest.* **29**, 478–487.
Moore, S. (1981). *In* "Vascular Injury and Atherosclerosis" (S. Moore, Ed.), pp. 131–148. Marcel Dekker Inc., New York.
Moore, S., Belbeck, L. W. and Evans, G. (1976a). *Circulation* **54**, Suppl. II, 202 (abstr.).
Moore, S., Friedman, R. J., Singal, D. P., Gauldie, J., Blajchman, M. A. and Roberts, R. S. (1976b). *Thromb. Haemostas.* **35**, 70–81.
Morgan, A. D. (1956). "The Pathogenesis of Coronary Occlusion". Blackwell Scientific Publications, Oxford.
Murphy, E. A., Rowsell, H. C., Downie, H. G., Robinson, G. A. and Mustard, J. F. (1962). *Can. med. Assoc. J.* **87**, 259–274.
Mustard, J. F. and Packham, M. A. (1975). *Thromb. Diath. haemorrh.* **33**, 444–456.
Mustard, J. F. and Packham, M. A. (1978). *In* "Cardiovascular Drugs" (G. S. Avery, Ed.), Vol. 3, Antithrombotic Drugs, pp. 1–83. University Park Press, Baltimore, Md.

Mustard, J. F., Kinlough-Rathbone, R. L. and Packham, M. A. (1974). *Thromb. Diath. haemorrh.* Suppl. **59**, 157–188.
Mustard, J. F., Packham, M. A. and Kinlough-Rathbone, R. L. (1978). *In* "The Thrombotic Process in Atherogenesis" *Adv. exp. med. Biol.* **104**, 127–143. (G. C. McMillan, C. B. Nelson, C. J. Schwartz and S. Wessler, Eds). Plenum Press, New York.
Mustard, J. F., Packham, M. A. and Kinlough-Rathbone, R. L. (1981a). *In* "Drug Therapeutics. Concepts for Physicians" (K. L. Melmon, Ed.), pp. 83–102. Elsevier, North-Holland and New York.
Mustard, J. F., Packham, M. A. and Kinlough-Rathbone, R. L. (1981b). *In* "Vascular Injury and Atherosclerosis" (S. Moore, Ed.), pp. 79–110. Marcel Dekker Inc., New York.
Mustard, J. F., Packham, M. A. and Kinlough-Rathbone, R. L. (1981c). *In* "Haemostasis and Thrombosis" (A. L. Bloom and D. P. Thomas, Eds), pp. 503–526. Churchill Livingstone, London.
Oliva, P. B. and Breckenridge, J. C. (1977). *Circulation* **56**, 366–374.
Packham, M. A. and Mustard, J. F. (1980). *Circulation* **62**, Supplement V. 26–41.
Packham, M. A., Kinlough-Rathbone, R. L., Reimers, H.-J., Scott, S. and Mustard, J. F. (1977). *In* "Prostaglandins in Hematology" (M. J. Silver, J. B. Smith and J. J. Kocsis, Eds), pp. 247–276. Spectrum Publications, New York.
The Persantine-Aspirin Reinfarction Study Research Group. (1980). *Circulation* **62**, 449–461.
Peto, R. (1978). *Biomedicine* **28**, 24–36.
Piepgras, D. G., Sundt, T. M., Jr. and Didisheim, P. (1976). *Stroke* **7**, 248–254.
Richardson, M., Ihnatowycz, I. and Moore, S. (1980). *Lab. Invest.* **43**, 509–516.
Roberts, W. C. and Jones, A. A. (1979). *Am. J. Cardiol.* **44**, 39–45.
Ross, R. (1981). *Arteriosclerosis* **1**, 293–311.
Ross, R. and Vogel, A. (1978). *Cell* **14**, 203–210.
Schafer, A. I. and Handin, R. I. (1979). *Prog. cardiovasc. Dis.* **22**, 31–52.
Schwartz, C. J., Chandler, A. B., Gerrity, R. G. and Naito, H. K. (1978). *In* "Adv. Exp. Med. Biol. vol. 104, The Thromboembolic Process in Atherogenesis" (A. B. Chandler, K. Eurenius, G. C. McMillan, C. B. Nelson, C. J. Schwartz and S. Wessler, Eds), pp. 111–126. Plenum Publishing Corp., New York.
Sixty Plus Reinfarction Study Research Group. (1980). *Lancet* **ii**, 989–994.
Stemerman, M. B. (1973). *Am. J. Pathol.* **73**, 7–26.
Stemerman, M. B. (1978). *In* "Adv. Exp. Med. Biol. vol. 102, Thrombosis. Animal and Clinical Models" (H. J. Day, B. A. Molony, E. E. Nishizawa and R. H. Rynbrandt, Eds), pp. 175–185. Plenum Press, New York.
Weiss, H. J. (1978). *N. Engl. J. Med.* **298**, 1344–1347, 1403–1406.
Weiss, H. J., Turitto, V. T., Vicic, W. J. and Baumgartner, H. R. (1981). *Thromb. Haemostas.* **45**, 136–141.
Winocour, P. D., Cattaneo, M., Kinlough-Rathbone, R. L. and Mustard, J. F. (1981). *Thromb. Haemostas.* **46**, 290.
Woolf, N. (1978). *Br. med. Bull.* **34**, 137–145.
Woolf, N., Bradley, J. W. P., Crawford, T. and Carstairs, K. C. (1968). *Br. J. exp. Path.* **49**, 257–264.

Changes in the Haemostatic System in Ischaemic Heart Disease: Therapeutic Implications

G. G. NERI SERNERI,
G. F. GENSINI, G. MASOTTI,
R. ABBATE, L. POGGESI,
D. PRISCO, S. FAVILLA,
A. BARTOLETTI, C. BRESCHI
and A. PANETTA

Department of Internal Medicine, University
of Florence, Florence, Italy

The concept of the haemostatic system is a functional concept derived from the experiences of these last years. During the past decade a considerably large body of data has demonstrated the existence of continuous interactions among platelets, blood clotting and the vascular wall. These observations gave rise to the concept of the haemostatic system, as an integrated functional system, which is continuously operating to maintain normal blood fluidity and normal haemostasis by multiple reciprocating mechanisms, involving feedback controls from platelets and blood clotting to blood vessels and vice versa.

Numerous investigations have documented that in ischaemic heart disease (IHD) patients as a group an increased platelet aggregation exists, but not necessarily in individual patients. Platelet aggregation is a complex reaction in which thromboxane A_2 (TxA$_2$) plays a major role, therefore it seemed interesting to investigate TxA$_2$ formation by platelets from IHD patients. Platelets from these patients when stimulated by arachidonic acid produced a larger amount of TxB$_2$, the stable derivative of TxA$_2$, in comparison to control platelets. Even when platelets were stimulated by collagen, they formed a larger amount of TxB$_2$.

These findings suggest a disorder of the arachidonic acid metabolism in platelets from IHD patients. The increased platelet aggregation and the increased TxA$_2$ formation may be by themselves enough to cause disturbances in the homeostasis of the haemostatic system. But the equilibrium between forces that maintain blood fluidity and those that promote blood clotting is further impaired in IHD patients by the presence of an hypercoagulable state and a decreased ability to produce plasma prostacyclin-like activity. The level of fibrinopeptide A (FPA) in plasma is at present the most reliable index of blood clotting activation with increased thrombin formation. In fact FPA splits quickly from fibrinogen as soon as thrombin is formed in trace amounts, and has the additional advantage of a brief half-life of $3 \cdot 5$ min.

In IHD patients a significant elevation of FPA levels in plasma (radioimmunoassay according to Hoffman and Straub, 1977) can be found, thus indicating a clear blood clotting activation. However, it is worth emphasizing that whereas no significant intergroup differences could be observed, striking differences were found when patients were examined in relation to the occurrence of spontaneous anginal attacks.

In patients with active disease, i.e. patients who were suffering from at least one anginal attack per day during the week preceding the examination, FPA levels in plasma were significantly higher than in patients with inactive disease, i.e. in patients asymptomatic at rest during the week preceding the study (Neri Serneri et al., 1981a).

Prostacyclin, the most important physiological inhibitor of platelet aggregation up to now known, is mainly produced by endothelial cells and it has been reported to be a circulating hormone. Prostacyclin can be measured by biological assay or by radioimmunoassay of 6-keto-PGF$_{1\,alpha}$, its main non-enzymatic metabolite. However, 6-keto-PGF$_{1\,alpha}$ is only one of the various metabolites of PGI$_2$ and, therefore its levels in plasma do not reflect completely the PGI$_2$ levels. For these reasons we decided to evaluate PGI$_2$ by biological assay.

By Vane's superfusion technique we measured an activity present in plasma and that produced by vessel wall under ischaemia which is provided with many of the properties of autenthic PGI$_2$. This prostacyclin-like activity in plasma and that produced by the vessel wall was identified by the following criteria:

(1) It mimics the effects of synthetic PGI$_2$ on tissues used for bio-assay (bovine coronary artery, rat stomach strip and chick rectum).

(2) It disappears in time and after warming blood which perfuses assay-tissues and after pre-treatment of the subjects with indomethacin.
(3) The activity is completely inhibited by antiserum to 5–6 dihydro-prostacyclin.

We do not know if this activity is due to PGI_2, but if it is not PGI_2 it is a very close relative.

In patients with IHD the levels of circulating PGI_2-like activity were lower than controls matched for sex, age, weight, blood pressure and smoking habits. Whereas no significant intergroup differences were observed, striking differences in PGI_2 levels could be found in relation to the activity of disease. The PGI_2-like activity was significantly lower in patients with active disease (Neri Serneri, 1979).

Also the amount of PGI_2 produced by the vessel wall after 3 min of ischaemia – a stimulus able to induce prostacyclin formation – was reduced in IHD patients. Thus, in patients with IHD and especially in patients suffering from anginal attacks, a significant imbalance in thromboregulatory mechanisms exists, with a clear-cut prevalence of the forces leading to the thrombus formation.

In the light of recent documentation giving renewed support to the role of thrombus in the genesis of myocardial infarction, it is suggested that the abnormalities of blood clotting and PGI_2 production are especially striking in patients with active disease. The decreased production of prostacyclin in patients with IHD suggests a disorder of arachidonic acid metabolism in the vessel wall. By the use of High Pressure Liquid Chromatography (HPLC) we have been able to show that homogenates of human arteries and veins are able to synthetize TxA_2 in addition to a larger amount of PGI_2 evaluated as 6-keto-$PGF_{1 alpha}$. TxA_2 is mainly produced by the media layer (Neri Serneri *et al.*, 1981b).

Thromboxane produced by the vessel wall is released into the bloodstream after appropriate stimulation such as adrenergic stimulation.

Patients were pretreated with aspirin (10 mg/kg) in order to exclude TxA_2 formation by platelets. It is worth emphasizing that aspirin administration is unable to inhibit TxB_2 production and release from the vessel wall.

In previous investigations (Neri Serneri *et al.*, 1981c) we reported that PGI_2 and TxA_2 are normally formed and released together with norepine-phrine in response to adrenergic stimulation and that PGI_2 and TxA_2 work as a mechanism for local control of vascular response to sympathetic activation. In IHD patients this mechanism is impaired. When adrenergic stimulation, performed by cold application, was carried out a significantly higher increase of TxA_2 and significantly lower PGI_2-like activity production could be seen in IHD patients than in controls. IHD patients with coronary angiographic lesions showed significantly higher levels of TxB_2 in coronary sinus blood in comparison to patients unaffected by IHD. Moreover, in patients suffering from frequent anginal attacks, i.e. with active IHD, this modulating mechanism of the vascular response is further impaired. In these patients the PGI_2 production was even lower and TxA_2 formation was even higher than in patients free from anginal attacks.

The consequence is that forearm vascular resistence after adrenergic stimulation is significantly higher in comparison to that found in controls and in patients free from anginal attacks. Thus, the imbalance in vessel wall production of thromboxane and prostacyclin results in the impairment of the intravascular modulating mechanism of the vascular response and, as a consequence, in the inappropriate contraction of the vascular wall to adrenergic stimulation. From the pathophysiological point of view, the abnormalities of the haemostatic system found especially in patients with anginal attacks, result in a facilitation to thrombus formation and to coronary vasospasm. Three therapeutical implications come from these abnormalities of the haemostatic system: (1) Control of blood clotting activation; (2) caution in using conventional antiaggregating agents; and, (3) correction of abnormal TxA_2 formation by the vessel wall. The occurrence of a hypercoagulable state in IHD patients suggests the use of anticoagulant therapy, especially in patients with active disease.

Obviously, we should remember that hypercoagulability is only one of the mechanisms responsible for thrombus formation, and, therefore, anticoagulant therapy does not necessarily prevent the occurrence of thrombosis. However it is worth remembering that a well done anticoagulant therapy seems to lower reinfarction rate (Sixty Plus Study, 1980).

Moreover i.v. heparin has been reported to be able to significantly decrease the incidence of myocardial infarction in patients with intermediate syndrome (Telford and Wilson, 1981). In our department subcutaneous calcium heparin in dosage of 12500 U/day effectively counteracted hypercoagulability as shown by the significant lowering of FPA plasma levels in IHD patients. The perplexity in using antiaggregating agents comes from the awareness that they are not always able to inhibit platelet aggregation (for instance that one induced by thrombin or collagen) and when used in non-appropriate schedule they can worsen the equilibrium between TxA_2 and PGI_2 production, so facilitating the vasoconstrictor response of the vascular wall. Probably the use of selective inhibitor of thromboxane–synthetase or stable prostacyclin analogues or drugs able to stimulate prostacyclin synthesis, as dipyridamole (Neri Serneri, 1981d) will prove to be more useful.

Finally, we could try to correct the abnormalities of the arachidonic acid metabolism in platelets and in vessel wall by controlled diets rich in eicosapentaenoic acid. Eicosapentaenoic acid is a fatty acid with five-double-bonds, instead of four-double-bonds as in arachidonic acid. The metabolism of eicosapentaenoic acid results in the formation of TxA_3 and PGI_3 which are metabolites with three-double-bonds in the side chain, instead of two-double-bonds as in TxA_2 and in PGI_2. Thromboxane A_3 has been reported to be devoid of any aggregating activity, whereas prostaglandin I_3 possesses antiaggregating activity like that of prostacyclin. Moreover eicosapentaenoic acid inhibits arachidonate conversion into thromboxane A_2 by competing at the level of cyclooxygenase. The first results in efforts to manipulate the availability of arachidonic acid have been encouraging. When a controlled diet, largely composed of coldwater fish rich in EPA, approximating the diet of Greenland Eskimos, was fed to some volunteers, platelet aggregation and TxA$_2$ production were reduced (Siess *et al.*, 1980). Let's hope that these results will open a new way for the control of the abnormalities in the haemostatic system.

Acknowledgements

This investigation has been supported by grant n° 82·02255·56 (CNR, Rome, Italy).

References

Hoffman, V. and Straub, P. W. (1977). *Thromb. Res.* **11**, 171.
Neri Serneri, G. G. (1979). *In* "Myocardial infarction" (Mason, D. T., Neri Serneri, G. G. and Oliver, M. F. Eds), p. 299. Excerpta Medica, Amsterdam.
Neri Serneri, G. G., Gensini, G. F., Abbate, R., Mugnaini, C., Favilla, S., Brunelli, C., Chierchia, S. and Parodi, O. (1981a). *Am. Heart J.* **101**, 185.
Neri Serneri, G. G., Masotti, G., Gensini, G. F., Abbate, R., Poggesi, L., Galanti, G. and Favilla, S. (1981b). *Atherosclerosis Reviews* **8**, 139.
Neri Serneri, G. G., Masotti, G., Gensini, G. F., Poggesi, L., Abbate, R. and Mannelli, M. (1981c). *Cardiovasc. Res.* **15**, 287.
Neri Serneri, G. G., Masotti, G., Poggesi, L., Galanti, G. and Morettini, A. (1981d). *Eur. J. clin. Pharmacol.* **21**, 9.
Siess, W., Scherer, B., Böhling, B., Roth, P., Kürzmann, J. and Weber, P. C. (1980). *Lancet* **i**, 441.
Sixty Plus Reinfarction Study Research Group. (1980). *Lancet* **ii**, 899.
Telford, A. M. and Wilson, C. (1981). *Lancet* **i**, 1225.

IV. Perspectives in Heart Surgery and Extracorporeal Assistance

Surgery For the Coronary Patient: When, Which (Venous Arterial or Artificial Grafts) and/or Plexectomy?

G. SOOTS

Department of Cardiovascular Surgery A,
Regional and University Hospital Centre of
Lille, Lille, France

The increasing number of aorto-coronary bypass (ACBP) operations has been the most evident fact in cardiac surgery in the seventies. This has been due to the success on relief of angina as well as low mortality and morbidity rates (Griffiths *et al.*, 1979; Miller *et al.*, 1981).

Important progress has also been accomplished in the field of physio-pathology of angina at rest, showing the importance of coronary spasm (Gensini, 1975); cardiac denervation procedures have been proposed (Clark *et al.*, 1977; Grondin and Limet, 1977; Warembourg *et al.*, 1977). We may now ask ourselves whether is it possible to further improve results of ACBP and if denervation procedures may prevent recurrence of coronary artery spasm?

The first question "When?" concerns indications for coronary arterio-graphy. Schematically symptomatic patients with angina on effort are selected by exercise stress tests; those with angina at rest are studied by continuous EKG recording. Asymptomatic patients, who experienced a recent myocardial infarction are explored by arteriography; in others, exercise test helps to select those who need coronary arteriography. This may show fixed organic narrowings and also coronary artery spasm, which if not spontaneous has to be demonstrated with ergot alkaloid provocation test. Coronary arteriography is also of value in assessing left ventricular function.

When To Recommend Surgery?

Surgery For Fixed Narrowings

The answer depends on actually established results. Early criteria for surgery were proximal and severe narrowing over 70%; good run-off; and ejection fraction over 35%. The results of surgery have been assessed on following criteria: operative mortality; peri-operative infarction; relief of angina; long-term survival; and grafts patency.

Operative mortality

This decreased to low figures in recent years and is actually 2% in most centres (Kennedy et al., 1980). The number of vessels involved does not affect mortality, but the degree of loss of ventricular function is important, resulting in 5% mortality or more when ejection fraction is less than 25%. Operative risk remains high in presence of congestive heart failure which is considered as a contra-indication by many authors.

Peri-operative myocardial infarction

The rate has been diversely appreciated, with extremes from 2% to 25% (Cachera and Bourassa, 1980). This depends largely on adopted criteria: EKG modifications and clinical manifestations (low cardiac output or severe ventricular arrythmia) or CKMB serial determinations. Recent studies (CASS) seem to consider a rate of 5% in most centres (Kennedy et al., 1980).

Myocardial infarction (MI) is only in 25% to 35% of cases related to acute occlusion of a graft. Twenty-five per cent do occur in a non-grafted area. The majority of MIs do occur in a territory which is revascularized by a patent graft.

Despite definite progress due to use of cardioplegia, myocardial protection is not yet perfect, especially in coronary surgery, since cardioplegic solutions are introduced via stenotic arteries, and some additional protection such as topical hypothermia is necessary (Landymore 1981). Topical hypothermia is also not perfect especially when the ventricles have to be lifted for the exposure of circumflex arteries.

As observed by Videcocq et al. (1981) 75% of perioperative MI are clinically silent and only 25% are accompanied by low cardiac output or severe rythm disturbances. Those with low cardiac output are susceptible to a high rate of recurrent MI during the first year as well as higher late mortality. Improvement in protective measures against reperfusion myocardial damage is still necessary.

Relief of angina

Relief of angina following ACBP is now recognized as being superior to any other form of treatment, with 80% asymptomatic patients at one year.

Long-term survival

Long-term survival as well as low rate of late MI is the main objective of coronary artery surgery. This point is still controversial (Hurst *et al.*, 1978). Data concerning natural history of the disease often do not consider progress which has been accomplished in medical treatment during recent years. Criteria for ACBP have been progressively modified and technical progress has resulted from increased surgical experience. Only randomized trials could answer the question of choice between medical and surgical treatment.

However there are now sufficient data (Hurst *et al.*, 1978) to consider long-term survival rates in favour of surgery for left main coronary artery as well as for triple-vessel disease (Table 1).

Data shown in Table 1 concerning two vessel disease and single vessel disease have been criticized. Data concerning "surgical candidates" in the

Table I *Late survival after ACBP*

	Vessels involved	Follow-up	% Survival	
			Surgical candidates	Surgery
Left	CLC	6 years	52	88
Main	VA	3 years	61	83
	CLC	5 years	56	82·6
3 vessel	VA	54 months	76	85
disease	UAH	46 months	53	83
2 vessel	CLC	5 years	69	85·4
disease	UAH	24 months	73	93·8
1 vessel	CLC	5 years	90	91·5
disease	UAH	5 years	94	96

CLC = Cleveland clinic (Proudfite *et al.*, 1982, Sheldon and Loop, 1982). UAH = University of Alabama Hospital (Hurst *et al.*, 1978). VA = Veterans Administration Study (Hurst *et al.*, 1978).

study of Bruschke *et al.*, (1981) concern patients admitted from 1963 to 1965 and who did not benefit from modern medical therapy. The Veterans Administration randomized cooperative study carried an initial high mortality rate. Medical and surgical series from the University of Alabama Hospital (Hurst *et al.*, 1979) were not randomized but concomitant. It should be remembered that two vessel disease carries a higher risk when the left descending artery is one of the involved vessels. Also in single vessel disease prognosis of High severe stenosis of LAD is more severe than for any other single vessel disease.

This lead Hurst (1979) to conclude that the comparison favoured surgical treatment for all patients except those with single vessel obstruction.

"For a single LAD bypass, a competent surgical team should be able to achieve an operative mortality rate of less than 1%, a perioperative rate of myocardial infarction less than 4% and a patency rate of more than 90%. Provided that such a low morbidity and mortality rate can be achieved, it is logical to anticipate that surgical therapy will benefit a subgroup of symptomatic patients with an isolated proximal lesion of the LAD without collateral vessels and with normally contracting myocardium in its distribution".

Recent success from catheter dilatation may alter this opinion in future. Long-term survival is also affected by pre-operative left ventricular impairment.

A study by Vliestra *et al.* (1977) has demonstrated that left ventricular function alteration with ejection fractions between 25% and 49% result in a survival rate of 89% at four years for operated cases in comparison with 68% in "surgical candidates" medically treated.

Correlation between results and graft patency: (which?)

It has been demonstrated that relief of angina does parallel graft patency. At one year, 85% of patients with complete revascularization are asymptomatic (Cachera and Bourassa, 1980).

Early graft occlusion, occurring during the first year is due to indication or technical factors which have been progressively recognized; late graft occlusions are mainly due to progression of the disease, either in the distal artery or in the graft. Recurrence of angina may also be due to progression of the disease in a non-grafted artery.

An aggressive attitude has been advocated (Johnson and Lepley, 1970) toward extensive revascularization but one has to consider what is the real benefit, taking into account the additional risk of longer aortic clamping and extracorporeal circulation times (Ulyott, 1980). Moreover extensive revascularization is only justified if grafts have a high rate of patency. The problem is what is "Optimal revascularization"? (Weisel *et al.*, 1981). Patency rate depends on artery diameter, being 89% when superior to 2 mm (Ulyott, 1980) and decreasing to 51% when below 1·5 mm (Liddle, 1981).

Internal mammary artery (IMA) anastomosis proposed by Green (1977) is certainly excellent with more than a 95% early rate of patency and over 90% at five years.

But its use is restricted to the LDA or diagonal branches of LDA; IMA is not available in all cases, due to its diameter or arteriosclerotic changes in proximal subclavian artery. Operative technique is more difficult and requires a "learning time". Tector *et al.*, (1976) have shown some advantages in using IMA to revascularize LDA with narrow lumen or distal arteriosclerotic alterations.

Is it possible to improve patency rate with venous grafts? Diameter discrepancy between graft and artery has been discussed and use of the lesser saphenous vein recommended by Crosby and Craver (1975).

Bartley *et al.* (1972) and Sewell (1974) introduced the use of "sequential" grafting where several arteries are anastomosed to the same venous graft, resulting in a higher output and augmented velocity in the graft. This concept was extended by Grondin *et al.* (1978) to "circular" grafts with up to five or six anastomoses to a single graft. Despite some criticism, risk of proximal stenosis or occlusion, results show a high rate of early patency and good late results (Grondin *et al.*, 1978; Knaepen, 1982).

Thrombo-endarteriectomy may be the only way to revascularize otherwise non-graftable arteries. It is not recommended as a sole procedure, but in addition to grafts in a more "attractive artery". Rates of patency have been only slightly inferior to ACBP (Yaccoub, 1982).

Other grafts?

PTFE (Gore-tex) grafts have been occasionally used (Cohn, 1978) and also Dacron (Sauvage *et al.*, 1976). Homologous saphenous vein has shown poor results (Bical *et al.*, 1980) and experience with human umbilical artery is not yet well established. The use of radial artery has been abandoned. Progress may be expected to be slow, since, ethically, use of these materials may not be extensive, considering excellent results with vein or IMA. Progression of the disease will be of more and more concern since results of reoperations are now better known. By repeating coronary arteriography in non-operated "surgical candidates", Bruschke *et al.* (1982) have shown at one year progression of the disease in 46% of cases, and at 5 years in 87%. After 37 months, 27% of patients should have had more grafts than at that time of the first arteriography and 16·6% experienced alteration of the left ventricle.

Should we operate narrowings inferior to 50%? Cosgrove and Loop (1981) have shown that patency rates were identical in arteries with > 50% or < 50% narrowings when they were grafted. But they found more progression of the disease in the native artery proximal to the graft when narrowing is < 50%. Grafting of arteries with less than 50% narrowing should only be undertaken when other more stenotic arteries have to be grafted or in the presence of high-risk factors such as dyslipidemia.

Reoperations are expected to be more and more frequent. Loop *et al.* (1981) have shown better results of reoperation for "graft failure" (early graft occlusions) than for those due to progression of the disease. Results however are good with 2·6% death, 2·7% MI, and patency rates of 79% at 19 months. At 5 years 87% of grafts are still open but 31% of the patients have some alteration of left ventricular function.

Should we Operate on Asymptomatic Patients?

Asymptomatic patients are those who have been studied by arteriography after MI or positive exercise test. Grondin *et al.* (1979) obtained disappointing results in a series of 55 operated cases, with no deaths, 4% MIs and 20% occluded grafts as control. These results have been attributed to "failure to differentiate between anatomical coronary artery disease (CAD) and ischaemic heart disease" (Anderson and Arentzen, 1979). In such patients, it is necessary to assess ischaemic disease by appropriate measures showing reduction of blood flow to the myocardium. From this part of our study, it seems that we may expect to improve the results of ACBP surgery in patients with fixed narrowings by appropriate application of different methods of grafting. Post-operative mortality and peri-operative MI may be lowered by further improvements in myocardial protection.

Possibilities of Surgery on Coronary Artery Spasm?

Mechanism of angina at rest

As demonstrated by Maseri *et al.* (1976), mechanism of attacks of angina is different in angina at rest than in other forms of the disease. Maseri demonstrated that attacks of Prinzmetal variant angina (PVA) do occur without augmentation of myocardial demand but on the contrary are due to a sudden decrease in transmural blood flow to the myocardium concomitant to coronary artery spasm. Coronary artery spasm occurs either spontaneously during arteriography or may be induced by ergotrate or methergine provocation test. Spasm is frequently demonstrated in angina at rest and almost in all cases of Prinzmetal variant angina (Maseri *et al.*, 1975; Bertrand *et al.*, 1980). Various anatomic narrowings are found in addition to spasm in PVA and there is no parallel between degree of fixed narrowings and severity of the disease.

Results of ACBP in PVA have been less satisfactory than in other forms of

CAD (Grondin and Limet, 1977). Failures despite patent grafts (Betriu *et al.*, 1974) have been related to the recurrence of spasm soon after operation (Pichard *et al.*, 1980) or late (Zeff *et al.*, 1982) either in a grafted artery distal to patent graft or in another artery. Different mechanisms may result in coronary artery spasm, neurogenic or humoral.

Yasue *et al.* (1974) advanced the hypothesis "that enhanced activity of the parasympathetic nervous system does stimulate the sympathetic nerves and possibly induces coronary artery spasm by way of activating alpha receptors (vasoconstrictors) present in large coronary arteries.

Cardiac denervation

This leads us to think that a denervation procedure should be added to ACBP for fixed lesions in PVA (Warembourg *et al.*, 1977; Bertrand *et al.*, 1980).

Attempts to denervate the heart are not new but, due to the absence of coronary arteriography, indications and results were not appreciated with objective tests and these procedures were abandoned.

Arnulf's technique described in 1939 seemed to us the most logical. From anatomical and physiological studies, Arnulf (1939) did demonstrate that nervous fibres, both from parasympathetic and sympathetic origin are concentrated in the pre- and sub-aortic area before they reach the coronaries. The only difficulty in this procedure is to make sure that cellular tissue removal is large enough to realize complete denervation. As the sternal approach for ACBP affords a large exposure of the aortic arch, we described an enlarged procedure (Plexectomy) (Warembourg *et al.*, 1977) which we have used since 1973 in PVA cases.

Results of plexectomy

Two groups of patients have been studied.

In the first group (n = 50) all had severe narrowings and had plexectomy in addition to ACBP.

Spasm was demonstrated in 38 cases (13 spontaneous and 25 provoked among 26 attempts). (No provocation test was done in 11 most severe cases.) There were two early deaths. One was due to MI from kinking of a graft. The other death occured during dissection, from intractable PVA attack despite ACBP. In another patient the same problem was encountered but spasm was immediatly controlled by local anaesthetic infiltration. This was done routinely as a preventive measure in all other cases. Two non-lethal MIs were observed; one of them occurred during sternotomy. At late evaluation (from 1 to 65 months), 46 patients were studied. Forty-four are asymptomatic and have no medication (88%); two have symptoms suggesting PVA reccurrence. In all successful cases, post-operative tachycardia was observed (instead of bradycardia in failures). Pathologic examination did not show nervous tissue in one of the two failures (and was not done in the

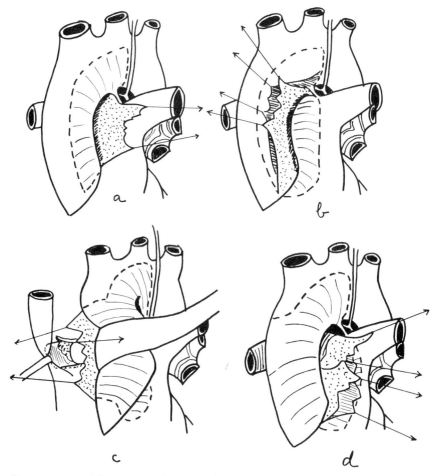

Figure 1. (a) Adventitia is dissected from left anterior wall of ascending aorta, nervous fibres from vagus nerve to the right are cut. (b) adventitia dissected from right half of anterior wall of main pulmonary artery. (c) adventitia dissected free all around ascending and horizontal aorta. Aorta pulled to the left using a retractor; adventitia dissected on anterior wall of the right pulmonary artery, starting from superior vena cava. (d) All dissected tissue pulled to the left below aortic arch. Dissection of the Wrisberg area is conducted deeply until contact with carina. Arterial ligament is completely dissected, taking care of left laryngeal nerve.

other). No spasm was provoked in successful cases by methergine; one of the two failures accepted recatheterization and methergine did provoke a spasm distal to a patent graft.

Group II (n = 8) exhibited less satisfactory results, those patients had no significant organic stenosis. In all eight cases spasm was demonstrated; all patients being resistant to long-lasting medical treatment including nitrates, amiodarone and calcium inhibitors. Follow-up in this group was 3 to 27 months. One asymptomatic patient died suddenly; five are free of pain and MI without any medication. The methergine test was negative in 3 among 3 successful cases and positive in two failures.

In another patient (Bertrand *et al.*, 1981) who had extremely severe PVA with no angiographically demonstrable narrowing but with spasm, a plexectomy was done in another institution without any result (pathologic examination of removed specimen did not show nervous tissue). PVA attacks were as frequent as 7 to 15 episodes/day. No result was obtained despite three more months of intensive medication (nifedipine – 60 mg/day, verapamil – 360 mg/day, propranolol – 120 mg/day, amiodarone – 1600 mg orally and 600 mg i.v.). In this patient we performed an auto-transplantation by transecting both atria as well as aorta and pulmonary artery and resuturing in the same manner as homotransplantation. The patient was improved by described atypical pain. After 10 months a new angiography was performed with the methergine test showing coronary artery spasm with S–T segment elevation but no chest pain. After 33 months he was hospitalized in another centre where during an episode of pain at rest S–T segment elevation was recorded (Bertrand *et al.*, 1981).

Questions concerning mechanisms of coronary spasm

The first question arising from these facts is whether a complete denervation of the coronaries is obtained by plexectomy? We found in successful patients, heart rate diagrams very similar to those of transplanted patients. But more investigations are necessary to assess the completeness of denervation. Secondly, the results were excellent in Group I patients having plexectomy and ACBP; failure to reproduce spasm by ergot alkaloid test leads us to think that relief of angina is not only the result of the interruption of sensitive pathways.

Results however were less satisfactory in patients without demonstrable narrowings. Stimulation test was positive in cases with clinical failure. At least one recurrent episode has been proved in the patient who had auto-transplantation and methergine test was positive.

Studies made by the group at Stanford (Buda *et al.*, 1981) did not show heart reinnervation in transplanted patients, but they observed a patient who experienced, 20 months after transplantation, chest pain at rest, S–T segment elevation, and ergonovine maleate provocation test was positive showing spasm in the RCA, pain and EKG changes.

It has to be mentioned that there is a difference in patient selection between Group I, Group II and the autotransplanted case. Group I patients were operated on primarily because they were symptomatic and had severe coronary narrowings and long-term medical treatment was not attempted. In Group II plexectomy was done after the failure of long-lasting medical treatment including calcium inhibitors; autotransplantation was decided only after the failure of medical treatment and previous plexectomy.

Different degrees of severity of the disease seem to exist and may involve several different mechanisms simultaneously, explaining good results of plexectomy in less severe cases where nervous mechanism could be predominant. These findings should stimulate further investigations concerning coronary artery spasm and its role in coronary artery disease.

References

Anderson, R. W. and Arentzen, C. E. (1979). *Ann. thorac. Surg.* **31**, 97–99.

Arnulf, G. (1939). *Press. Med.* **47**, 1635.

Bartley, T. D., Bigelow, J. C. and Scott Page, U. (1972). *Archs Surg.* **105**, 915–917.

Bertrand, M. E. Lablanche, J. M., Rousseau, M. E. Warembourg, H. H. Jr, Stankowiak, C. and Soots, G. (1980). *Circulation* **61**, 877–882.

Bertrand, M. E., Lablanche, J. M., Tilmant, P. Y., Ducloux, G., Warembourg, H. Jr and Soots, G. (1981). *Am. J. Cardiol.* **47**, 1375–1378.

Betriu, A. Solignac, A. and Bourassa, M. G. (1974). *Am. Heart J.* **87**, 272–278.

Bical O., Bachet, J., Laurian, C., Camilleri, J. P., Goudot, B., Menu, P. and Guilmet D. (1980). *Ann. thorac. Surg.* **30**, 550.

Bruschke, A. V. G., Visser, R. F., Plokker, H. W. M., Wijers, Th. S. and Kolsters, W. (1981). *In* "Coronary Artery Disease Today" (A. V. G. Bruschke, G. van Herpen and F. E. E. Vermeulen, eds) *Exerpta Medica Int. Congress Series* **557**, pp. 4–50. Utrecht.

Buda, A. J., Fowles, R. E., Schroeder, J. S., Hunt, S. A., Cipriano, R., Stinson, E. B. and Harrison, D. C. (1981). *Am. J. Med.* **70**, 1144–1149.

Cachera, J. P. and Bourassa, M. (1980). "La maladie coronarienne". Flammarion Ed., Presse de l'Université de Montreal C.P. 6128 Succ. "A" Montreal QUE CANADA H 3 C 3 J 7.

Cipriano, P. R., Guthaner, D. F., Orlick, A. E., Ricci, D. R., Wexler, L. and Silverman, J. F. *Circulation* **59**, 82–88.

Clark, D. A., Quint, R. A., Mitchell, R. L. and Angell, W. W. (1977). *J. thorac. cardiovasc. Surg.* **73**, 332–339.

Cohn, L. H. (1978). *In* "Vascular Grafts" (Sawyer, Ph. and Kaplitt, M. J., Eds), 398–430. Appleton Century Crofts, New York.

Cosgrove, D. M., Loop, F. D., Saunders, C. L., Lytle, B. W. and Kramer, J. R. (1981). *J. thorac. cardiovasc. surg.* **82**, 520–531.

Crosby, I. and Craver, J. M. (1975). *Ann. thorac. Surg.* **20**, 703.

Gensini, G. C. (1975). *Chest* **68**, 709–713.

Green, G. E. (1972). *Ann. thorac. Surg.* **14**, 260.

Griffiths, S. P., Zazula, B. M., Courtney, D., Spencer, F. C., Malm, J. R. (1979). *Am. J. Cardiol.* **44**, 3, 555–562.

Grondin, C. M. and Limet, R. (1977). *Ann. thorac. Surg.* **23**, 111–117.

Grondin, C. M., Vouhe, P., Bourassa, M. G., Lesperance, J., Bouvier, M. and Campeau, L. (1978). *J. thorac. cardiovasc. Surg.* **75**, 161–167.

Grondin, C. M., Kretz, J. G., Vouhe, P., Tubau, J. F., Campeau, L. and Bourassa, M. G. (1979). *Ann. thorac. Surg.* **31**, 113–118.

Hurst, J. W., King, S. B., Logue, R. B., Hatcher, C. R., Jones, E. L., Craver, J. M., Douglas, J. S., Franch, R. H., Dorney, E. R., Cobbs, B. W., Robinson, P. H.,

Clements, S. D., Kaplan, J. A. and Bradford, J. M. (1978). *Am. J. Cardiol.* **42**, 308–329.

Johnson, W. D. and Lepley Jr D. (1970). *J. thorac. cardiovasc. Surg.* **59**, 128–138.

Kennedy, J. W., Kaiser, G. C., Fisher, L. D., Maynard, C., Fritz, J. K., Myers, W., Mudd, J. G., Ryan, T. J. and Coggin, J. (1980). *J. thorac. cardiovasc. Surg.* **80**, 876–887.

Knaepen, P., Geldorp, Th. V., Dekker, F., Alfieri, O., De Geest, R., Vermeulen, F. (1981). *In* "Coronary artery disease today" (A. V. G. Bruschke, G. van Herpen and F. E. E. Vermeulen, eds) *Exerpta Medica Int. Congress Series).*

Landymore, R. W., Tice, D., Trehan, N. and Spencer, F. C. (1982). *J. thorac. cardiovasc Surg.* **82**, 832–837.

Liddle, H. V. (1981). *J. thorac. cardiovasc. Surg.* **81**, 1–10.

Loop, F. D., Cosgrove, D. M., Kramer, J. R., Lytle, B. W., Taylor, P. C., Golding, L. A. R. and Groves, L. K. (1981). *J. thorac. cardiovasc. Surg.* **81**, 675–685.

Maseri, A., Mimmo, R., Chierchia, S., Marchesi, C., Pesola, A. and L'Abbate, A. (1975). *Chest* **68**, 625–632.

Maseri, A., Parodi, O., Severi, S. and Pesola, A. (1976). *Circulation* **54**, 2, 280–288.

Miller Jr, D. W., Ivey, T. D., Bailey, W. W., Johnson, D. D. and Hessel, E. A. (1981). *J. thorac. cardiovasc. Surg.* **81**, 423–427.

Pichard, A. D., Ambrose, J., Mindich, B., Midwall, J., Gorlin, R., Litwak, R. S. and Herman, M. V. (1980). *J. thorac. cardiovasc. Surg.* **80**, 149–154.

Proudfit, W. L., Bruschke, A. V. G., Sones, F. M. Jr. (1982). *In* "Coronary Artery Disease Today" (A. V. G. Bruschke, G. van Herpen and F. E. E. Vermeulen, Eds), *Exerpta Medica Int. Congress Series* **557**, pp. 120–125. Utrecht.

Sauvage, L. R., Schloemer, R., Wood, S. J. and Logan, G. (1976). *J. thorac. cardiovasc. Surg.* **72**, 418–421.

Sewell, W. H. (1974). *Ann. thorac. Surg.* **17**, 538.

Sheldon, W. C. and Loop, F. D. (1982). *In* "Coronary Artery Disease Today" (A. V. G. Bruschke, G. van Herpen and F. E. E. Vermeulen eds), *Exerpta Medica Int. Congress Series* **557**, pp. 120–125. Utrecht.

Tector, A. J., Davis, L., Gabriel, R., Gale, H., Singh, H. and Flemma, R. (1976). *Ann. thorac. Surg.* **22**, 515–519.

Ulyott, D. S. (1980). *Ann. thorac. Surg.* **30**, 192–203.

Videcocq, M., Maille, J. G., Dupras, G., Kretz, G., Du Cailar, C., Delva, E. and Bourassa, M. G. (1981). *Coeur*, **XII**, 275–287.

Vliestra, R. E., Assad Morell, J. L., Elveback, L. R., Connolly, D. C., Ritman, E. L., Pluth, J. R., Barnhorst, D. A., Danielson, G. K. and Wallace, R. B. (1977). *Mayo Clinic Proceedings* **52**, 85.

Warembourg, Jr H., Bertrand, M. E. and Soots, G. (1977). *Nouv. Press. Med.* **6**, 2521.

Weisel, R. D., Goldman, B. S., Baird, R. J., Scully, H. E., Schwartz, L., McLoughlin, M. J., Teoh, K. H., McLaughlin, P. R. and Aldridge, H. E. (1981). *J. thorac. cardiovasc. Surg.* **81**, 376.

Yaccoub, M. *In* "Coronary Artery Disease Today", (A. V. G. Bruschke, G. van Herpen and F. E. E. Vermeulen, eds) *Exerpta Medica Int. Congress Series* **557**, pp. 4–50. Utrecht.

Yasue, H., Touyama, M., Shimamoto, M., Kato, H., Tanaka, S. and Akiyama, F. *Circulation* **50**, 415–646.

Zeff, R. H. *et al.* (1982). *Ann. thorac. Surg.* **34**, 196.

A Future for Heart Transplantation

T. A. H. ENGLISH

Cardiac Surgical Unit, Papworth
Hospital, Papworth Everard,
Cambridge, UK

It is now almost fourteen years since Christiaan Barnard (1967) performed the first human heart transplant. This was followed by a spate of transplants by surgical teams in many different countries. Most of them were failures and within two years the procedure was abandoned in all but a few centres. Chief of these was Stanford University in California, where Dr Shumway and his colleagues continued with a careful programme of evaluation and where over 200 patients have now received orthotopic heart transplants.

During the last few years there has been a general renewal of interest in the possibility of treating terminal heart disease by transplantation. This has partly been due to the improved results from Stanford, where the chances of surviving 5 years after a transplant is now nearly 50% (Jamieson *et al.*, 1979). Another reason is the relatively large number of patients with severely damaged left ventricles secondary to ischaemic heart disease, who fail to obtain a satisfactory result from conventional operations in the form of coronary artery bypass grafting with or without resectional surgery of the left ventricle and for whom heart replacement may provide a more logical therapeutic modality. The possibility of the development of more effective immunosuppressive agents is also an important factor.

Frontiers Cardiol. for the 80s.
0-12-220680-0

Selection of Recipients

Patients being considered for transplantation should be in severe congestive cardiac failure despite full medical therapy and have a poor prognosis for surviving the next six months. They should be aged between 15 and 50 years and come from a stable social background in order that they can comply with long-term immunosuppressive therapy and a programme of rehabilitation after transplantation. A recent complete cardiac catheterization is always necessary and the pulmonary vascular resistance should be less than 8 Wood units. There should be no active infection or insulin-dependent diabetes. Recent pulmonary infarction is a relative contraindication. ABO blood group compatibility between recipient and donor is necessary, as is a negative lymphocyte cross match. Tissue typing is performed on all recipients and donors, but the importance of HLA compatibility remains uncertain (Stinson *et al.*, 1971).

Donor Heart Acquisition

Advances in the preservation of donor hearts (English *et al.*, 1979) means that it is now possible to accept donor organs from hospitals within at least a 500 mile radius of the transplant centre. Donors should be less than 35 years of age because of the prevalence of undetected coronary disease in the general population and because the Stanford group has recently shown that accelerated graft atherosclerosis tends to develop more rapidly in recipients with hearts from donors older than that (Bieber *et al.*, 1981).

The usual cause of brain damage is cerebral trauma due to road traffic accidents. Intracranial haemorrhage and primary brain tumour account for a smaller proportion. The diagnosis of brain death is made according to defined criteria by doctors entirely independent of the transplant team (Conference of the Medical Royal Colleges and their Faculties in the United Kingdom, *Br. med. J.*, 1976).

Coordination of Donor and Recipient Operations

The donor operation is timed to commence in accordance with the preparation of the recipient after his admission to hospital. Close communication by telephone is maintained from the time the donor is taken to the operating room. The donor heart is excised during venous inflow occlusion and cold cardioplegic arrest. It is then cooled further by serial passage through bowls of cold saline and stored in cardioplegic solution at 4°C within a Coolbox.

Only after the heart has been removed without complication is instruction given to start the recipient operation.

Once on cardiopulmonary bypass the recipient's heart is removed, dividing the aorta and pulmonary artery distal to the semilunar valves and leaving the posterior walls of the left and right atria with their venous connections. The donor heart is removed from the Coolbox and trimmed of excess tissue. The right atrium is opened by a curved incision from the inferior vena caval orifice to the base of the right atrial appendage, thereby protecting the region of the donor sinu-atrial node. The donor atria are then sutured to corresponding structures in the recipient and the pulmonary arterial and aortic anastomoses completed. After revascularization of the donor heart, supportive bypass is continued for 20 min to allow recovery from the ischaemic period. Two temporary pacemaker wires are placed on the donor right atrium. These are of value for the diagnosis of atrial dysrhythmias and the early detection of rejection episodes.

Postoperative Management and Immunosuppression

Immunosuppressive therapy is most intense during the first four weeks after transplantation. During this period the patient is nursed in as sterile an environment as possible in a specially prepared transplant cubicle in the Intensive Care Unit. After completing the primary course of antithymocyte globulin, he is transferred to a single room fitted with an electrostatic clean air unit. Thereafter masks are worn only by those entering the room or by the patient when he is in other parts of the hospital. Rehabilitation is commenced with daily sessions in the physiotherapy gymnasium and the patient is taught how to take his own drugs and instructed in their potential side-effects. A close surveillance is kept for any signs of infection, which usually start in the respiratory tract. Daily chest radiographs are taken and any new radiographic opacities investigated immediately.

Immunosuppression starts before operation with loading doses of azathioprine and i.v. methylprednisolone and antithymocyte globulin. After operation oral prednisolone is started at 1 mg/kg body weight, reducing to 0·5 mg/kg by one month and 0·3 mg/kg by three months. Azathioprine is administered at a dose of up to 2·5 mg/kg with the purpose of keeping the white cell count in the region of 5000 per cu.mm. Equine antithymocyte globulin (Upjohn) is given by daily i.v. injection for the first four weeks and is regarded as an important part of the primary immunosuppressive regimen. The dose is adjusted to suppress the T-cell fraction of the circulating lymphocytes to less than 50 cells per cu.mm., which is equivalent to about 5% of their preoperative value. This is usually in the range of 10–15 mg/kg body weight.

Rejection tends to be episodic and of most help in its detection are changes in the daily electrocardiogram and endomyocardial biopsy. It is most frequent during the first three months after transplantation, when the average incidence is one per 22 patient days. Thereafter it becomes much less frequent, declining to one episode per 325 patient-days after the first year. Clinical evidence of graft rejection, which includes fluid retention, a diastolic gallop rhythm, and signs of a low cardiac output are late phenomena and every effort is made to detect rejection before it has progressed this far. A drop of the summated QRS voltages in leads I, II, III, V1 and V6 of more than 20%, or a similar fall in voltage of the atrial electromyogram, suggests impending rejection and is an indication for cardiac biopsy, which is otherwise undertaken at intervals of about ten days. Atrial dysrhythmias may also be an early sign of rejection.

The treatment of rejection episodes depends on their timing and severity. Most respond to a temporary increase in oral prednisolone, with or without three or four daily doses of 1 g methylprednisolone and a further short course of antithymocyte globulin.

Patients are maintained on a low-cholesterol, low-sodium diet and encouraged to exercise daily. After leaving hospital they are seen in the outpatient clinic once a week for the first three months, and then about twice a month until the end of the first year. Continuing potential complications in the years after transplantation include infection (Remington et al., 1972), accelerated coronary atherosclerosis in the transplanted heart (Griepp et al., 1977), and malignant neoplasms, usually of the lymphomatous type (Krikorian et al., 1978). Complications arising from long-term steroid therapy are also important. Every year patients are admitted to hospital for a complete review, which includes exercise testing, coronary arteriography, left ventriculography and cardiac biopsy.

Results

Twenty-two patients received heart transplants at Papworth Hospital from January 1979 to August 1981. Their ages ranged from 16 to 52 (mean 37) years and all but one were men. Ten patients had cardiomyopathies and 12 ischaemic heart disease. During this period 220 patients were referred for consideration of transplantation, 98 of whom were admitted to hospital for further evaluation. Forty-eight patients were accepted for transplantation, of whom 19 died while awaiting operation.

The ages of the donors ranged from 16 to 35 (mean 21) years. Seven were women and 15 men. Donor hearts were brought to Papworth by road in six cases and by a combination of road and air transport in sixteen cases. The total donor heart ischaemic time varied from 108–205 min (mean 160 min). Early function of the transplanted heart was excellent in all cases. Postoperative cardiac output was measured by an electromagnetic flow probe placed around the aorta in 18 of the 22 cases and in these the mean measured cardiac output before closing the chest was 6·9 l/min.

At the end of August 1981 14 of the 22 patients were alive. During the 18-month period January 1979 to July 1980 12 patients were transplanted and of these six are now alive between one and two years after transplantation. During the next year between August 1980 and July 1981 ten patients were transplanted, of whom eight are alive seven weeks to 11 months after operation. Six patients have been investigated one year after transplantation and shown angiographically to have normal left ventricular function and normal coronary arteriograms. On exercise there is a delayed increase in heart rate and an abnormal rise in left ventricular filling pressure, illustrating the denervated transplanted heart's dependence on the Frank-Starling mechanism for increasing cardiac output.

Of the eight deaths, five have been from rejection (at 51, 59, 76, 223 and 252 days), one from a dysrhythmia (at 131 days) and two from infection secondary to brain damage (at 17 and 64 days). No grafts have been lost to rejection during the first six weeks after transplantation and major infectious complications have been relatively uncommon.

The quality of life of the 13 survivors who have been discharged from hospital has been greatly improved and most are delighted with the degree of rehabilitation attained.

Conclusions

For the patient with terminal heart failure as a result of irreversible left ventricular damage, replacement of the heart by either a mechanical device or a transplant becomes the only conceivable solution. Some patients will prefer to let life take its course and decline either option. Others, however, and particularly those with young families, may seize the opportunity of a return to a more normal existence, even if the duration of rehabilitation cannot be accurately predicted. Only the future will decide which of these two methods of heart substitution will be the most successful. In the meantime, it would seem reasonable that both avenues should be explored.

Considerable progress has been made with the development of left ventricular assist devices during the past decade. However, the ultimate goal of a totally implantable artificial heart still seems a long way off. Here, perhaps the two most difficult problems relate to the power source and to bio-incompatibility of the constituent materials.

So far as orthotopic heart transplantation is concerned, we have confirmed that the actual operative procedure can be accomplished at a low risk, despite the fact that the patient may be critically ill at the time of transplantation. Here, it is the provision of a normal cardiac output immediately after the operation which is of crucial importance and which allows for the rapid recovery of other organ systems previously compromised by chronic congestive cardiac failure.

However, having survived the operation, it would seem correct to conclude from the Stanford data and our own early experience that, with current methods of immunosuppression, about a third of those transplanted will die from rejection, or infection secondary to immunosuppressive therapy, during the first year after operation. Most of these deaths occur during the first six months. For those patients who are alive and well and on a moderate immunosuppressive regime one year after transplantation the future becomes brighter, as the mortality for this group is approximately 10% per annum, giving an overall 5-year patient survival rate at Stanford of about 45% (Jamieson *et al.*, 1979). It is also evident that, despite chronic immunosuppressive therapy and its attendant complications, the quality of life for the majority of these patients is reasonably good (Hunt *et al.*, 1976).

We conclude, therefore, that heart replacement does indeed have a future and that the immediate tasks now lie with the biomedical engineers and the immunologists. We believe that, even with existing immunosuppressive agents, cardiac transplantation offers a reasonable therapeutic option to certain patients with terminal heart disease. Furthermore, the scope of its application would be broadened and the whole cost-benefit equation improved by the development of more effective and less toxic methods of immunosuppression.

References

Barnard, C. N. (1967) *S. Afr. J. Med.* **41**, 1271–4.
Bieber, C. P., Hunt, S. A., Schwinn, D. A., Jamieson, S. A., Reitz, B. A., Oyer, P. E., Shumway, N. E. and Stinson, E. B. (1981). *Trans. Proc.* **3**, 207–11.
Conference of the Medical Royal Colleges and their Faculties in the United Kingdom (1976). *Br. med. J.* **2**, 1187–8.
English, T. A. H., Cooper, D. K. C., Medd, R., Walton, R. and Wheeldon, D. (1979). *Proceedings of European Society for Artificial Organs* **6**, 340–4.
Griepp, R. B., Stinson, E. B., Bieber, C. P., Reitz, B. A., Copeland, J. G., Oyer, P. E. and Shumway, N. E. (1977). *Surgery* **81**, 262–9.
Hunt, S. A., Rider, A. K., Stinson, E. B., Griepp, R. B. Schroeder, J. S., Harrison, D. C. and Shumway, N. E. (1976). *Circulation* **54**, Suppl. 3, 56–60.
Jamieson, S. W., Reitz, B. A., Oyer, P. E., Bieber, C. P., Stinson, E. B. and Shumway, N. E. (1979). *Br. Heart J.* **42**, 703–8.
Krikorian, J. G., Anderson, J. L., Bieber, C. P., Penn, I. and Stinson, E. B. (1978). *JAMA* **240**, 639–43.
Remington, J. S., Gaines, J. D., Griepp, R. B. and Shumway, N. E. (1972). *Trans. Proc.* **4**, 699–705.
Stinson, E. B., Payne, R., Griepp, R. B., Dong, E. Jr and Shumway, N. E. (1971). *Lancet* **2**, 459–60.

Perspectives of Infant Cardiac Surgery

Ch.-H. CHALANT

Department of Cardiovascular Surgery,
University Clinic St. Luc, UCL Brussels,
Belgium

Futurology always remains a challenging problem for everyone concerned. Past experience in the field of cardiology taught us that the predictions on the development of the techniques were often wrongly evaluated. Nevertheless we remain convinced that the effort to predict the future is an absolute necessity to improve the quality of our medicine. This is the best way to progress from a pure handicraft period to a more sophisticated and a more effective surgery. It is the same for other fields, for instance: in the field of artificial hearts, surgery may admit a "chair to bed" mode of life provided that a more normal mode of life can already be hopefully foreseen (Fig. 1). An overall realistic and perhaps optimist view on cardiac congenital malformations makes us divide them into three main groups:

The first group includes favourable malformations giving a normal quality of life and life expectancy after a well codified surgical correction at low risk, for example: patent ductus arteriosus, atrial septal defect, ventricular septal defect, coarctation, favourable forms of tetralogy of Fallot . . .

The second group includes malformations giving submormal quality of life and life expectancy after a more sophisticated therapy; f.i. palliative valvulotomy requiring subsequent valvular replacement, simple transposition of the great arteries . . .

The third group gathers complex or associated malformations requiring difficult corrections and sometimes the use of foreign material with an

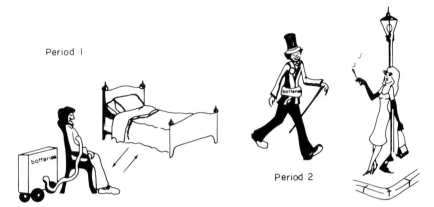

Figure 1. The artificial heart. Period 1 – Experimental devices. Period 2 – Sophisticated devices.

unknown future evolution: f.i. tricuspid atresia or pulmonary atresia, truncus arteriosus, univentricular heart, complex transposition. Life expectancy and the quality of life of this last group are not comparable with those of the other two groups. Fortunately this group concerns a small number of patients and therefore should be more reserved to very specialized teams. Nevertheless, this group is very useful to improve the knowledge of the other more simple malformations and the management of the diagnosis and the treatment of all congenital cardiac diseases. This specific sector is for cardiac surgery what Cape Canaveral has been for spatial research.

We would not focus our discussion on this last group but on the more numerous and more curable population of young patients of the first two groups. Nobody will discuss the fact that some phenomena are nocious in themselves: hypoxaemia, ventricular overloading, pulmonary and systemic hypertension are such phenomena. If the disease will not spontaneously heal, surgical decision is absolutely indicated.

For psychological and physiological reasons we estimated that the procedure has to be performed before the school-age; in other words, long before the age of professional and family responsabilities. The main purpose of our future policy must be the prevention of cardiac malformations in elderly patients. In the future we hope never to see such malformations: prenuptial patient ductus, soldier's aortic coarctation, atrial septal defect of the coronary patient, unoperable ventricular septal defect. This attitude supposes a precise and early diagnosis, a constant reevaluation of the status of the patient in time, and a low risk surgery. In this prospect if the disease is well tolerated the child will be operated on, at the ideal age of 3 or 5 years; if not, it should be corrected as soon as possible, sometimes during the first days of life. We must keep in mind that some anatomically simple malformations, may have a disastrous and fatal spontaneous evolution.

Experience in our university hospital for the last 10 years has taught us that the number of infants operated upon under the age of 1 year is increasing every year. Following examples clearly illustrate this point of view.

Patent Ductus Arteriosus in Premature Infants

Failure of the ductus to close after birth results in well known conditions which may lead to difficulties in infants with an otherwise normal heart.

In premature infants, the patency of the ductus may either aggravate cardiorespiratory difficulties associated with a hyaline membrane syndrome or lead to cardiac failure. In our experience, twelve threatened premature infants ranging in age from 24 to 37 weeks (mean age: 31 weeks) and in weight from 600 g to 3600 g (mean weight 1·4 kg) underwent surgical closure of patent ductus arteriosus. All these newborns were refractory supported; the ratio of left atrial to aortic diameter demonstrated by echocardiography was always greater than 1·3. Eight months to 3 years after procedure, six children are in excellent condition; meanwhile six others, operated upon too late, died from cardiac failure, pulmonary complications or necrotizing enterocolitis.

Presently, according to the advice of Nadas (1981), we "don't rush to the drugstore to get indomethacin", and we consider that surgical ligation is virtually without risk if performed before impairing the patient. This surgery can easily be realized in an intensive care unit and the results are lasting.

Coarctation in Infancy

Infants with coarctation of the aorta who are in cardiac failure and not responsive to medical treatment should be considered for surgical management. "The primary objective of the surgical management of these infants is to relieve the coarctation to close the ductus and to perform any other simple manoeuvre that is necessary to bring the infant out of cardiac failure" (Hamilton, 1981).

The secondary objective is to reconstruct the pathological aortic segment in order to enable it's growing in the future. The left subclavian artery onlay flap technique described by Waldhausen and Nahrwold (1966) may help for the reconstruction of some difficult types of coarctation of the aorta in infancy.

In our institution, 21 infants underwent this type of correction; 16 of them were less than two months old, five were between two and six months old. Indication for surgery was: refractory cardiac failure in 16, systemic hypertension in four and both in one patient. Postoperative course evaluated two months to three years after surgery was excellent in 18 infants. Three late deaths were related to associated malformations. In some surviving cases, evidence of growth of the aortic reconstruction was proved by angiography.

Ventricular Septal Defect (VSD)

The natural history of large isolated VSD with high pulmonary flow and intractable heart failure in infancy is poor. Primary surgical closure should be done early, keeping in mind that residual abnormalities in left heart function seem to be reversible if the defect is closed in younger patients, less than 2 years of age (Cordell *et al.*, 1976).

Primary repair in our experience was always performed under deep hypothermia and circulatory arrest, it concerns 30 infants less than one year old, (mean weight: 4·6 kg); all were in congestive heart failure. The Q_p/Q_s ratio was ranged from 2·5 to 4. There were no hospital deaths. A six months to six years follow-up period showed one late death, 22 excellent and seven good clinical results; in one of these patients a small residual shunt was detected.

Tetralogy of Fallot

All children with tetralogy of Fallot will require surgical treatment, and delay may not be desirable and can even be a danger to life. In infants, less than one year old, cyanosis is almost invariable reason for admission. As the spontaneous course in many of these infants leads to a higher incidence of hypoxic spells, treatment will be indicated sometimes in emergency. The problem of primary correction vs palliative shunt and subsequent correction still remains unsolved. Nevertheless primary intracardiac repair remains an ideal objective in symptomatic infants with favourable anatomy of the pulmonary arterial tree (Sunderland *et al.*, 1980). In a long-term prospective view we hope to become able to prove that functional results will be better in patients operated on at an earlier age. In a more immediate prospective point of view, we continue to favour primary repair as the operation of choice for symptomatic infants with favourable anatomical conditions.

Our experience concerns 15 infants operated upon before one year of age and weighing from 3·5 to 8 kg. Surgical indication was based on the following data: an increasing cyanosis, life-threatening hypoxic spells and well-developed pulmonary arteries (Fig. 2). Two patients died after surgery for low cardiac output. Nine infants could be considered as excellent and four as good results with a follow up from six months to six years.

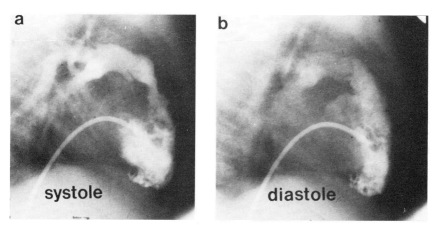

a

systole

b

diastole

Figure 2. Preoperative right angiogram of a favourable form of tetralogy of Fallot.
Well developped pulmonary artery tree with predominant infundibular stenosis.

Transposition of Great Arteries

Simple transposition of the great arteries has a disastrous spontaneous evolution in infancy. Senning's technique (1975) seemed to us to be especially well-adapted to correct a heart of a very small size by preventing postoperative obstruction of systemic or pulmonary venous return. From July 1977, 24 infants less than three months of age underwent Senning's operation. They ranged in age from one day to three months (mean age 57 days) and weighed from 2·5 to 5·5 kg (mean weight: 3·8 kg). The operation was performed by choice in 15 and urgently required in nine because of severe hypoxia or congestive heart failure. Postoperative evaluation of 19 survivors was recently performed with a mean follow up of 23 months (6 months–4 years). There were no late deaths. All the children were normal with respect to growth, physical activity and ability for exertion.

Clinically all infants are in good condition, without cyanosis, any signs of congestive heart failure or clinical evidence of caval or pulmonary venous obstruction. Postoperative cine-angiography has been performed in 14 patients: six months to three years after surgery. Atrial and ventricular contractions were efficient in all cases. Tricuspid insufficiency was never detected. We observed a mild superior vena cava stenosis in only one asymptomatic patient.

Concerning rhythm and conduction, repeated standard ECG confirm sinus rhythm in all patients. Fourteen patients were submitted to a 24-h Holter monitoring: all these patients were in sinus rhythm with significant atrial extrasystoles in two and ventricular extrasystoles in one.

From the haemodynamic and electrocardiographic point of view, we have shown that the Senning's method is technically possible and efficient even in the first days of life.

We can conclude that our attention should mainly focus in future on the following points:

(1) An improvement in our surgical technology to correct complex malformations that still constitue a group of operations at high risk. A better quality of foreign material which can be used in this kind of procedure is also desirable.
(2) A more precise knowledge of the malformations and of their evolutions imposes the use of more and more sophisticated invasive and non-invasive diagnostic techniques that will allow the cardiologist to perform a constant reevaluation of the patient's status.
(3) Thanks to the improvement of the techniques, we will see the possibility of earlier correction before irreversible lesions have definitely handicapped the future of the child. This aggressive attitude will be more and more justified. In this way we hope to allow the children to lead a relatively normal way of life as soon as possible.

What should we expect from the future? Nothing extraordinary. The only way to tackle any particular problem is to form a team with a wide knowledge of the different fields of science. In any kind of research, the purpose is not to discover a new technique but to form a team able to deal with any problem. Personal experience shows that it is difficult to have total agreement between all members of a group. Therefore one could say that it's easier to create an artificial heart than to work in a team.

References

Cordell, D., Graham, T. P. Jr, Atwood, G. F., Boerth, R. C., Boucek, R. J. and Bender, M. W. (1976) *Circulation* **54** 394–298.
Hamilton, D. I. (1981). *In* "Congenital Heart Disease in the First 3 Months of Life" (L. Parenzan, G. Crupi and G. Graham, Eds), pp. 328–339. Patron, Bologna.
Nadas, A. S. (1981). *N. Engl. J. Med.* **305**, 97–98.
Senning, A., (1975). *Ann. Surg.* **182**, 287–292.
Sunderland, C., Nichols, M., Feucht, K., Ho, L., Menashe, V., Starr, A. and Lees, M. (1980). World Congress Paediatric Cardiology, London, 2–6 June 1980, Abstract 37.
Waldhausen, J. A. and Nahrwold, D. L., (1966). *J. thorac. cardiovasc. Surg.* **51**, 582.

Surgery for Arrhythmias

H. H. BENTALL

Royal Postgraduate Medical School,
University of London, Cardiothoracic Unit,
Department of Surgery, Hammersmith
Hospital, London, UK

The Wolff–Parkinson–White (WPW) syndrome may be associated with life-threatening rhythm disturbances which are still refractory to management by modern drugs. Wolff *et al.* (1930) originally described healthy, young people prone to paroxysmal tachycardia who showed bundle branch block with short PR interval in the electro-cardiogram, in 1930. The possible mechanisms for this were discussed by Holzmann and Scherf in 1932 and Wolferth and Wood in 1933, and a hypothesis made that an accessory pathway of atrioventricular conducting tissue was present. Ten years later, Wood *et al.* (1943) demonstrated that this hypothesis was correct and that there was firm histological evidence of such a connection. It was not, however, until the late 1960s and the early 1970s that electrophysiological studies had progressed far enough to be able to predict with confidence the anatomical location of this accessory conduction pathway and thus render it amenable to surgery. The pioneer work in this field was largely that of Sealy, Gallagher and their colleagues at Duke University, Durham, North Carolina (Cobb *et al.*, 1968; Sealy and Wallace, 1974; Sealy and Gallagher, 1981a, b), and it was the same group that first suggested the use of cryothermic techniques for the ablation of accessory atrioventricular connection in 1977 (Gallagher *et al.*, 1977). Two patients were successfully cured by this method and three further patients were subsequently added. Since that time, however, patients have been almost exclusively treated by surgical incision rather than cryothermic methods. We therefore decided to investigate further the use of cryosurgical methods in the treatment of our patients with a number of tachycardia syndromes. We were fortunate in having a very

Frontiers Cardiol. for the 80s.
0-12-220680-0

sophisticated and satisfactory apparatus manufactured in England, which uses the rapid expansion of nitrous oxide under controlled conditions to cool the end of a probe, which we have specially designed for use in cardiac surgery. After about 1 min, the tissues within a few millimetres of the probe have cooled to about 0°C, and cardiac conduction in the vicinity ceases. If the foot-switch is raised at this moment, rapid re-warming of the probe occurs and conduction will return. This re-warming is achieved automatically by the machine by reversing the flow of gas as the foot-switch is released and the probe rapidly detaches itself from the tissues to which it has become adherent. Should a destructive freeze be required, the foot-switch is left depressed for 5 min, when the temperature in a ball of myocardium approximately 1 cm in diameter, falls to around −60°C, and this is destructive of the conducting tissue. The Duke University Group have recently shown (Milcat et al., 1977) that direct application of the cryothermic probe to the epicardium over a coronary artery will produce changes in the arterial wall in dogs, and it is, therefore, obviously important that the position of the coronary arteries is kept clearly in mind when making use of this instrument. At Hammersmith Hospital, we have used cryothermic ablation to deal with three groups of conditions.

(1) Re-entrant arrhythmias of the Wolff–Parkinson–White type (ablation of Kent bundles).
(2) Intractable atrial tachycardias, for example atrial flutter with one-to-one conduction (ablation of A–V node and insertion of demand pacemaker).
(3) Recurrent ventricular tachycardias of a focal type.

Wolff–Parkinson–White Syndrome

In this syndrome persistent specialized conduction tissue is present between the atrium and ventricle in addition to the bundle of His. This tissue is arranged in fasciculi known as bundles of Kent. There may be one or more such fasciculi and they may be either between right atrium and right ventricle or left atrium and left ventricle. They may conduct upwards (retrograde) and/or downwards (anterograde). The latter produces the characteristic delta wave of pre-excitation.

We have now operated on eleven patients with the WPW syndrome. In three, the abnormal conducting bundles were on the right side (Type B) and eight were on the left side (Type A). The results are shown in Table 1.

Intractable Atrial Tachycardias

Two patients with almost continuous tachycardias unrelieved by drugs were treated by cryoablation of the A–V node followed by insertion of a permanent pacemaker with complete symptomatic relief.

Table 1 *WPW accessory pathways*

			Type	Age	Arrhythmia	Duration (years)	Follow-up (years)	
1.	I.H.	♀	'B'	27	RT(2), PA Fl	9	3	Asymptomatic – no therapy
2.	A.M.	♂	conc 'A'	46	RT, PAF	20	3	Asymptomatic – no therapy
3.	S.D.	♂	'B'	21	RT	5	3	Mild recurrence
4.	M.D.	♂	'B'	36	RT	15	2/12	Asymptomatic – no therapy
5.	M.J.	♀	'A'	40	RT, PAF	10	2	Asymptomatic (amiodarone)
6.	A.T.	♀	'A'	47	RT, PAF	3	2	Asymptomatic – no therapy
7.	M.G.	♀	conc 'A'	59	RT	40	2	Asymptomatic (quinidine)
8.	J.M.	♀	conc 'A'	48	RT	25	1/12	Asymptomatic – no therapy
9.	T.K.	♀	'A'	49	RT	33	–	Cerebral Haem'ge (haemangioma)
10.	O.M.	♀	'A'	49	RT, PAF, VT	21	4/12	Asymptomatic – no therapy
11.	M.P.	♂	'A'	35	RT, PAF	?	2/12	Asymptomatic – no therapy

Recurrent Ventricular Tachycardias of a Focal Type

One patient, a male aged 21, gave a history of being kicked in the chest by a horse at the age of 6 years. He suffered repeated ventricular tachycardias requiring hospital treatment during the last 3 years. He was found to have a small ventricular aneurysm (3 cm in diameter), in the territory of the first diagonal branch of the left anterior descending coronary artery. Epicardial mapping showed the origin of the ventricular tachycardia to be situated about 1·5 cm below the visible extent of the aneurysm. This region was cryoablated and the ventricular tachycardia could not be reinvoked and has not recurred during the years since the operation. The aneurysm itself was electrically silent and was obliterated with two sutures.

The surgical treatment of multifocal ventricular tachycardias in patients with ischaemic heart disease, particularly those with ventricular aneurysm, is a rather different problem, well studied by Guiraudon, Fontaine and Frank in Paris (Guiraudon *et al.*, 1974, 1978; Fontaine *et al.*, 1977); it is excellently reviewed by Harken, Horowitz and Josephson (1980), and will not be discussed here.

The Effects of Cryothermia on the Heart: an Experimental Study

These early results with cryosurgery stimulated us to undertake a long-term experimental study in animals. We used the sheep and applied the cryothermic probe in exactly the same manner as in patients, both to the epicardium in 15 animals, and, imitating the situation when treating WPW, to the artrioventricular ring in a further 15 animals, in the latter group using cardiopulmonary bypass. The animals were then killed at 1, 3, 5, 7 and 14 days, and at 1, 2, 3, 6, 12 and 18 months.

Cryothermia always produced a zone of muscle necrosis radiating from the site of application of a 5 mm probe for about 6 mm. Necrotic muscle was sharply demarcated from unaffected tissue. Necrosis occurred after 1 minute's cooling but extended into myocardium for only 3 mm. After 7 days, fibrous tissue began to replace the necrotic muscle, but little cellular infiltrate was evident at any time. By 1 month, healing (fibrosis) was complete. Blood vessels were little affected: minor damage to the adventitia immediately adjacent to the probe was noted, but permanent damage had not occurred up to 18 months after operation.

In summary, therefore, there are many ways in which surgery can help patients with intractable, disabling or life-threatening arrhythmias. The precise technique chosen depends upon the individual case, but there is now a wide variety of safe and accurate techniques available. The closest collaboration with one's electrophysiological colleagues is, of course, mandatory. This is not the kind of surgery which can be successfully carried out by a cardiac surgeon working in isolation. In a well-equipped cardiac centre with experienced electrophysiological help available in the operating theatre, the results are safe and predictable and at times spectacular.

References

Cobb, F. R., Blumenschein, S. D., Sealy, W. C., Boineau, J. P., Wagner, G. S. and Wallace, A. G. (1968). *Circulation* **38**, 1018.

Fontaine, G., Guiraudon, G. and Frank, R. (1977). *In* Kulibertus, H. E. (Ed.) "Re-entrant Arrhythmias", p. 334. MTP Press, Lancaster, England.

Gallagher, J. J., Sealy, W. C., Anderson, R. W., Kasell, J., Millar, R., Campbell, R. W. F., Harrison, L., Pritchett, E. L. C. and Wallace, A. G. (1977). *Circulation* **55**, 471.

Guiraudon, G., Frank, R. and Fontaine, G. (1974). *Nouv. Press Med.* **3**, 321.

Guiraudon, G., Fontaine, G., Frank, R. *et al.* (1978). *Ann. thorac. Surg.* **26**, 438.

Harken, A. H., Horowitz, L. N. and Josephson, M. E. (1980). *Ann. thorac. Surg.* **30**, 499.

Holzmann, M. and Scherf, D. (1932). *Z. Klin. Med.* **121**, 404.

Mikat, E. M., Hackel, D. B., Harrison, L., Gallagher, J. J. and Wallace, A. G. (1977). *Lab. Invest.* **37**, 632.

Sealy, W. C. and Gallagher, J. J. (1981a). *J. thorac. cardiovasc. Surg.* **81**, 698.

Sealy, W. C. and Gallagher, J. J. (1981b). *J. thorac. cardiovasc. Surg.* **81**, 707.

Sealy, W. C. and Wallace, A. G. (1974). *J. thorac. cardiovasc. Surg.* **68**, 757.

Wolferth, C. C. and Wood, F. C. (1933). *Am. Heart J.* **8**, 297.

Wolff, L., Parkinson, J. and White, P. D. (1930). *Am. Heart J.* **5**, 685.

Wood, F. C., Wolferth, C. C. and Geckeler, G. D. (1943). *Am. Heart J.* **25**, 454.

Circulatory Assistance in Acute Potentially Reversible Syndromes: Cost/Benefit Perspectives

F. UNGER

1st Surgical Clinic, University of Innsbruck,
Innsbruck, Austria

Despite the encouraging results in modern cardiac surgery, in replacing valves, repairing congenital defects and revascularing the coronary arteries it is still a challenge to replace a non-functioning myocardium. The heart transplantation tends to become a standardized technique in certain defined indications (Oyer *et al.*, 1979): however lack of donor hearts available, especially at the spot, when a heart definitely fails after an open-heart operation, has led to the development of several mechanical assist devices which are now in clinical use: intra-aortic balloon pump (IABP); left ventricular assist devices (LVAD); and artificial hearts to be implanted in orthotopic position (Cooley *et al.*, 1969; Cooley, 1981), driven pneumatically.

The IABP (Bregman, 1974) is very well established in cardiac surgery. In approximately 10% of open-heart cases weaning off from the cardio-pulmonary bypass presents some kind of complications. Of these patients 80% can be treated conservatively, but 20% need the help of the IABP.

* With the support of the Austrian Research Council, (Project N°3829, F. Unger principal investigator) the Austrian National Bank (Jubiläumsfond, Project N° 1785) and the Austrian Research Society (Project N° 06/0069).

Costs of this treatment are contained: an approximate total of 200 US dollars for the patient back in good condition.

Still there are patients, who do not respond to the IABP: in this desperate situation after a cardiac operation, left ventricular assistance is required. After the first clinical trial of De Bakey in 1962 (De Bakey, 1971), 71 patients have been implanted already with pneumatic assist devices since 1975. The indication of LVAD is at present limited to patients with cardiac failure after an open-heart operation: not in all cases the desired beneficial effects are obtained, the following situation may occur: (a) direct response to the LVAD and subsequent wean off; (b) direct response, but the patient remains dependent from the LVAD; (c) no response to the LVAD. In the first group there are mainly patients whose heart failed after an aortic valve replacement. The metabolism of the heart muscle, brought out of steady state due to cardiopulmonary bypass, can be reestablished with a strong supporting system.

In the second group there are mainly patients whose heart failed after

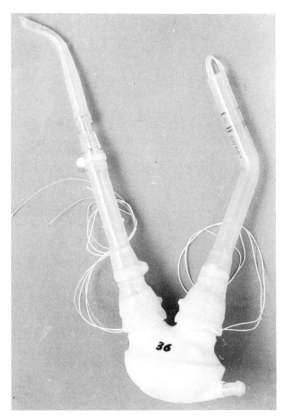

Figure 1. Ellipsoid left ventricular assist device (E-LVAD).

coronary revascularization. The patients show isolated left ventricular failure, with good initial response to the LVAD, but finally an additional right heart failure syndrome takes place and makes the LVAD ineffective.

The third group is characterized by the presence of left ventricular power failure, or right ventricular power failure due to general myocardial insufficiency or to a high pulmonary vascular resistance. In these cases the LVAD is ineffective. These cases are an indication for a biventricular assist device (BVAD) or for an artificial heart (TAH) (Unger, 1979).

In cases with good response pneumatical driven LVAD (Fig. 1) results in

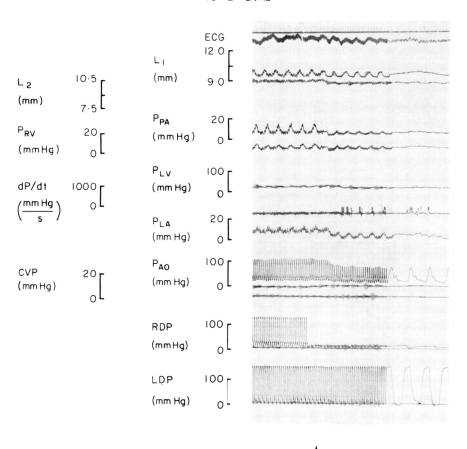

Figure 2. *Haemodynamic of the E-RVAD in a failing heart (P_{PA} = pulmonary artery pressure; P_{LV} = left ventricular pressure; P_{LA} = left atrial pressure; P_{AO} = aortic pressure; R_{DP} = right driving pressure; L_{DP} = left driving pressure; CVP = central venous pressure; P_{RV} = right ventricular pressure).*

full maintaining of the circulation, partially or totally, even for relatively long periods of time and during ventricular fibrillation: left ventricle end-diastolic pressure goes down, aortic pressure, cardiac output and cardiac index increase. In certain cases the myocardium state improves within 24 h, with narrowing of the QRS complexes.

The most beneficial effect can be expected in patients with isolated left ventricular power failure due to unbalance in the steady state of the myocardial metabolism resulting from aortic valve replacement.

In order to treat biventricular power failure, a biventricular assist device must be available: this device acts as a functional artificial heart since the circulation can be maintained fully independently of the state of the myocardium (Fig. 2). The driving management, however, is quite difficult, and also the high output of the artificial heart chambers is diminished due to the hindrance of the cannulas.

From the hydraulic point of view, driving a total artificial heart is much easier (Fig. 3), since without the cannulas the system is more responsive to changes in the venous return in the sense of the Starling's law (Fig. 4).

The indication for circulatory assistance by means of left ventricular assist device or biventricular assist devices is restricted to patients with cardiac failure after heart operations with inadequate response to drugs alone or in combination with intra-aortic balloon pumping. To implant a total artificial mechanical heart is a definitive step in the operating theatre and might be

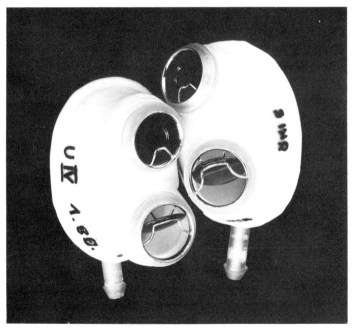

Figure 3. Ellipsoid heart for total artificial heart replacement.

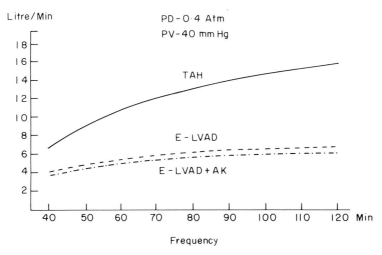

Figure 4. Haemodynamic of an artificial heart.

considered in subjects whose heart would never recover and should hence be replaced because of extensive myocardial failure due to massive lesions of the coronary system. Currently, different artificial hearts are being evaluated (in Salt Lake City, Berlin, Cleveland, Hershey, Vienna, Houston, Brno, Innsbruck) to act as temporary support in view of heart transplantation.

Besides the surgical indications, cardiomyopathies might also be considered as a possible indication for mechanical circulatory support. The worldwide incidence is 60 000 per year, and possibly 30 000 patients might become candidates for heart transplantation. Carefully designed but complex clinical trials with left ventricular assist devices will show if the failing heart can recover during resting. A total artificial heart might help in subjects in the terminal stage to overcome the time-lag for finding an acceptable donor heart.

The implantation of these devices should be performed by a skilled surgeon, with experience in cardiac assistance of artificial hearts. This requires the establishment of experimental units: the cost of such a "training unit" is US $ 200 000/year without personnel costs, and the activity should be of 10–15 experiments per year.

In desperate situations like cardiac failure after open-heart surgery, the artificial heart and the LVAD are at present the extreme resources.

The costs for intra-aortic balloon pumping are acceptable and we feel that they are adequately paid out with a discharged patient. The costs in left ventricular assistance and artificial hearts are at present very high. Taking into account the required research input, the cost of an implantation is probably of the order of 100 000 US dollars. These costs will drop down rapidly, as soon as there will be more implantations and positive results. In any case, it is too early to assess a cost/benefit ratio, but no effort should be spared in the attempt to bring man back to work (Pope John Paul II: "man has right to work", from the encyclica "Laborem exercens").

References

Bregman, D. (1979). *In* "Assisted Circulation" (Ed., F. Unger), p. 31. Springer, Berlin, Heidelberg and New York.

Cooley, D. A., (1981). *Bulletin of the Texas Heart Institute* **8**, 305.

Cooley, D. A., Liotta, D., Hallman, G. L., Bloodwell, R. D., Leachman, R. D. and Milam, D. (1969). *Trans. Am. Soc. artif. intern. Organs* **15**, 252.

DeBakey, M. E. (1971). *Am. J. Cardiol.* **27**, 3.

Oyer, P. E., Stinson, E. B. and Shumway, N. E. (1979). *In* "Assisted Circulation" (Ed., F. Unger), p. 406. Springer, Berlin, Heidelberg and New York.

Unger, F. (1979). "Assisted Circulation". Springer, Berlin, Heidelberg and New York.

Perspectives in Extracorporeal Oxygenation and Blood Substitution

A. AGOSTONI

Institute of Clinica Medica VII, University of
Milan, San Paolo Hospital, Milan, Italy

Five different topics will be discussed in this presentation: (1) the control of anticoagulant treatment in extracorporeal circulation; (2) the use of prostacyclin in extracorporeal circulation (ECC); (3) the use of blood substitutes in extracorporeal circulation (namely Hb solution and fluorocarbon); (4) possibility of stimulate anaerobic glycolysis with infusion of fructose-1, 6 diphosphate (FDP) solution; and (5) perspectives of CO_2 removal by means of carbonic anhydrase immobilized on artificial lung in chronic hypercapnic patients.

During cardiopulmonary bypass blood is subjected to mechanical trauma and exposed to artificial surfaces as plastic tubing and bubble or membrane oxygenator. This produces activation of clotting factors, platelet aggregation, alteration in endothelial prostaglandin synthesis, protein consumption and neutropenia. Complement activation may be central to these complications, including pulmonary dysfunction (post-perfusion lung).

The use of heparin inhibits the appearance of thrombotic phoenomena, but does not eliminate the other problems. Great attention has been paid by our group in studying changes of haemostasis parameters and in monitoring the anticoagulant therapy in 11 patients with acute respiratory insufficiency treated for several days (2–13 days) with a particular extracorporeal

Frontiers Cardiol. for the 80s.
0-12-220680-0

approach indicated as "low frequency positive pressure ventilation with extracorporeal CO_2 removal" (LFPPV–$ECCO_2R$). Strictly after the onset of bypass striking modifications in the coagulation parameters occur: namely a fall in platelet number accompanied by a great PF4 release. The remaining circulating platelets show an impaired function tested by aggregation capacity. As a consequence of fibrinogen deposition on artificial surfaces a fibrinolytic reaction produces a rise in FDP level, that are not an expression of disseminate intravascular coagulation (DIC) and are quickly cleared from circulation. White blood cells show a dramatic fall due exclusively to PMN fraction.

For heparinization monitoring we have introduced a modified activated clotting time: citrated blood is thermostatized in a bath and activated through kaolin before the registration of the clotting time. The advantages of this test, which has been called RACT, are the following: the start of the measurement and the temperature could be standardized, the influence of physiological anticoagulants could be eliminated allowing a good correlation with heparin levels. After the equilibration period, RACT was kept around two times the basal value and corresponded to a quite low and stable heparin dosage (around 0·2 mg/kg/h).

Considering the fundamental role played by platelets in haemostasis impairment during ECC we decided the use of prostacyclin (PGI_2), which inhibits platelet aggregation and release. For its properties PGI_2 has successfully been used in man for charcoal haemoperfusion, for dialysis and also for cardiovascular surgery. We studied coagulation and haemodynamic in 8-h experiments of extracorporeal circulation with a membrane lung in sheep, treated with PGI_2 plus a minimal dose of heparin compared with a control group treated with a standard dose of heparin only. Platelet count is preserved by PGI_2 infusion until administration is stopped (Fig. 1). Platelet aggregation capacity is completely inhibited during all infusion periods and this effect is reversed in about 20s after PGI_2 stoppage. Similarly PF4 release is greatly limited by PGI_2 infusion. Activated clotting time is much lower in the PGI_2 group because of the small amount (1/4) of heparin, required only to avoid activation of the intrinsic clotting mechanism. No significant changes in fibrinogen and haematocrit could be detected, while the PMN fall could not be preserved.

The main haemodynamic effect was a decrease both in diastolic and mean arterial pressure, while systolic pressure remained unchanged. We can conclude that PGI_2, compared to other antiaggregant drugs previously tested like sulphinpyrazone or dipyridamole seems to have reached the task of ameliorating the blood compatibility paralyzing platelets.

Haemodilution has become a widely used method during surgery due to the claimed advantages of blood saving and improving haemorrheology. Clinical experience has now documented that if maximum blood conservation with haemodilution is practised, it is possible to operate upon as many as 70% of patients requiring cardiopulmonary bypass without the use of homologous blood. However, with the large number of

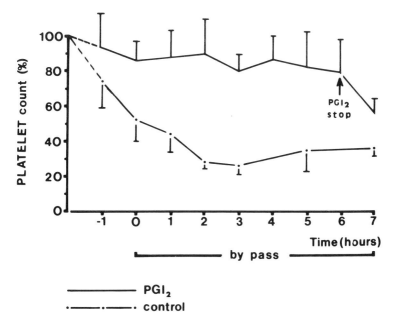

Figure 1. Effect of PGI₂ infusion on platelet number during long-term ECC with membrane lung in sheep. Each value is a mean of six experiments. Comparison with a control group.

cardiopulmonary bypass procedures being performed today blood procurement is still a problem. In extending haemodilution limits, the use of a cell-free oxygen-carrying blood substitute could be of obvious benefit: (a) no more problems in homologous blood procurement, (b) no more risk of viral infection, (c) possibility of bypass surgery in Jehovah's witnesses. Moreover, meeting the oxygen requirements of the tissue with a further reduction in the haematocrit level during cardiopulmonary bypass may allow for an extension of the benefits of haemodilution, such as (d) decreased viscosity, (e) improved tissue perfusion.

Two different types of artificial blood have been proposed: (1) stroma-free haemoglobin solution and (2) fluorocarbon emulsion. Stroma-free haemoglobin (SFH) solution in addition to its oxygen-transporting characteristic has many beneficial effects: it is a naturally occuring protein, it does not need typing and crossmatching, it has low viscosity, it has oncotic activity, it does not produce microaggregate, it does not produce allergic reactions, it has a good solubility, it can be stored without degradation. However, with SFH some problems have to be faced: (1) stromal lipid contamination, as a source of possible altered renal function; (2) short intravascular persistence of haemoglobin, (3) high oxygen affinity of the haemoglobin solution (P50 = 12 mmHg). Indeed initial *in vivo* assessment in baboons using an exchange transfusion model showed that all the control animals treated with dextran died at haematocrit of 5%, while all SFH animals survived for 3 h at zero haematocrit and at a haemoglobin level of 6 g%.

Several methods have been described to improve the half-life of haemoglobin solutions. One technique is polymerization of the haemoglobin molecule by adding glutaraldehyde to the solution. Good results have been obtained using SFH bound to Dextran 20 000 in a 1/1 molar ratio. Preliminary experiments done by our group have shown that the oxygen dissociation curves of haemoglobin bound to dextran have an hyperbolic pattern, thus indicating the absence of structural interactions between the four subunits. The problem of high oxygen affinity of SFH which is presumably due to the loss of 2,3 DPG and other organic phosphate ligands could be faced using pyridoxal phoshate (a compound which has analogous effects to 2,3 DPG on the oxygen affinity, but it is more stable). The final issue concerns a difference between haemoglobin in solution and that present in the red blood cells. Following exchange transfusion with SFH, in contrast to acute normovolemic anaemia, cardiac output does not change, thus indicating a fundamental difference in cardiac response between haemoglobin solution and erythrocytic haemoglobin. Thus, the physiology of O_2 transport with haemoglobin solution appears to be different from that of erythrocytic haemoglobin. Indeed, it has been recently shown that in experimental myocardial infarction a procedure of haemodilution with SFH resulted in improvement in myocardial tissue pO_2 and reduction in the presumptive infarct volume when compared to that seen following haemodilution with dextran or reinfusion of whole blood. In fact, haemodilution with SFH was shown not only to reduce the blood viscosity in proportion to the reduction in hematocrit, but also to produce a blocking effect on the viscosity increase and erythrocyte aggregation accompanying acute myocardial ischaemia.

Further work is necessary to explore the possibility that the oxygen dissociation curve might have a different role with SFH, with other factors becoming increasingly important. In recent years great interest has been focused on the evaluation of oxygen-carrying capacity of fluorocarbon emulsion. The best preparation is an emulsion of perfluordecalin and perfluortripropylamine which is isotonic, isoosmotic, stable, and it does not produce aggregates. It has been called Fluosol-DA. Good results have been obtained using Fluosol-DA as a priming solution in extracorporeal circulation in different animals. The capacity of Fluosol-DA to deliver oxygen to the tissue is good enough even the animal is depleted of blood and perfused for 1 or 2 h with Fluosol-DA. In Japan 75 patients have been treated with Fluosol-DA in different clinical situations: including severe haemorrhages, surgical procedures with high O_2 consumption, Jehovah's witnesses, etc. However, the use of Fluosol-Da has not been approved till now by the American FDA and by the European authorities. In fact information on the toxic effect at long term are now lacking.

It has recently been claimed that the infusion of an organic phosphate fructose-1,6 diphosphate, is able to activate intracellular glycolysis. Indeed, FDP is a very important factor in regulating glycolysis enhancing both phosphofructokinase activity, which is the glycolysis limiting factor due to its high sensitivity to pH variations, and pyruvatekinase activity. Benefits of FDP infusion were reported during cardiopulmonary bypass in normo-thermic cardiac arrest. The reported *in vivo* results prompted us to study *in vitro* FDP effects on some erythrocytic metabolic aspects. The results indicate that incubation of blood with FDP produces an intraerythrocytic alkalosis. In Fig. 2 the extra-intracellular pH differences were plotted against plasmatic pH in presence of FDP, fructose and inorganic phosphate. It is possible that a relative intracellular alkalosis could stimulate anaerobic glycolysis removing the acidotic inhibiting effect due to hypoxia. Thus, enhancing phosphofructokinase activity intracellular levels of FDP could increase without needing a transmembrane transfer of FDP into the cell, and the infusion of FDP solution seems to be theoretically warranted in extra-corporeal circulation.

A large quantity of CO_2 is stored in a normal body particularly in the tissue. However, we do not know how much these stores increase in hyper-capnic patients, but it seems logical to try to assist patients with severe lung insufficiency by an artificial and practical support as it is now done by an artificial kidney in uremic patients. The requirements for an extracorporeal CO_2 removing system in chronic hypercapnic patients are:

(1) Possibility of periodical application.
(2) Low flow.
(3) V–V shunt.
(4) Easy vascular access.
(5) Membrane with high capability of CO_2 removal.
(6) Avoidance of ion unbalance.

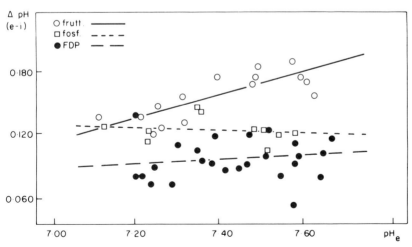

Figure 2. Erythrocytic extra-intracellular pH differences plotted against different plasmatic pH values.

Studies on isolated bloodless lung preparation perfused with bicarbonate solutions suggest that lung carbonic anhydrase (CA) accelerates the conversion cf H_2CO_3 to CO_2 and enhances CO_2 elimination as perfusate passes through the pulmonary capillaries, and that the enzyme may be present on the capillary endothelial surface. The demonstration that CA is indeed located at the alveolar–capillary barrier in the rat and monkey lung could agree with a role for it in the exchange of CO_2 over this barrier. Thus, two pathways exist at the pulmonary levels for CO_2 elimination, as indicated in Fig. 3.

Now what happens to the endothelial CA activity in chronic lung disease with hypercapnia? We do not know, but it is quite reasonable to hypothesize that CA activity in endothelial tissue could be involved in chronic lung disease. If this is the case, why do we not try to reintroduce this activity on an artificial membrane?

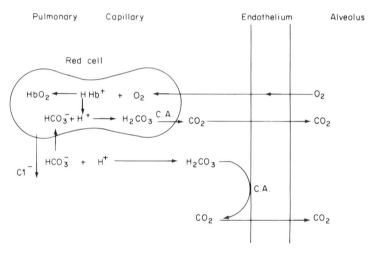

Figure 3. Schematic diagram of reaction and diffusion processes that occur within blood during exchanges of CO_2 and O_2 in a pulmonary capillary.

References

Biro, G. P. and Beresford-Kroeger, D. (1980). *Am. Heart. J.* **99**, 64.

Blumenstein, J., Tam, S. C., Chang, J. E. and Wong, G. T. F. (1978). *In* "Blood substitutes and plasma expanders" (Jamieson, G. A. and Greenwalt, T. J., Eds), p. 205. Allan R. Liss Inc., New York.

Costrini, R., Candiani, A., Cifra, E., Battocchio, G., Panico, S., Simonetti, N. and Gasparetto, A. (1980). *IRCS Med. Sci.* **8**, 257.

Crandall, E. D. and O'Brasky, J. E. (1978). *J. clin. Invest.* **62**, 618.

Effros, R. M., Chang, R. S. Y. and Silverman, P. (1978). *Science* **199**, 427.

Effros, R. M., Shapiro, L., Silverman, P. and Lieber, M. (1980). *In* "Biophysics and physiology of carbon dioxide" (Baner, C., Gros, G. and Bartels, H., Eds), p. 339. Springer-Verlag, Berlin.

Feola, M., Azar, D. and Wiener, L. (1979). *Chest* **75**, 369.

Gattinoni, L., Agostoni, A., Pesenti, A., Pelizzola, A., Rossi, G., Langer, M., Vesconi, S., Uziel, L., Fox, U., Longoni, F. and Damia, G. (1980). *Lancet* **ii**, 292.

Gonzalez, E. R. (1980). *JAMA* **243**, 719.

Gould, S. A., Rosen, A., Sehgal, L., Noud, G., Sehgal, H., De Woskin, R., Levine, H., Kerstein, M., Rice, C. and Moss, G. S. (1980a). *J. Surg. Res.* **28**, 46.

Gould, S. A., Rosen, L., Sehgal, L., Sehgal, H., Rice, C. L. and Moss, G. S. (1980b). *Trans. Am. Soc. artif. intern. Organs* **26**, 350.

Jones, J. W., Markov, A. K. *et al.* (1983). *Surg. Forum* (in press).

Lonnerholm, G. (1980). *Acta Physiol. scand.* **108**, 197.

Moores, W. Y., De Venuto, F., Heydorn, W. H., Weiskopf, R. B., Baysinger, M., Gerson Greenburg, A. and Utley, J. R. (1981). *J. thorac. cardiovasc. Surg.* **81**, 155.

Moss, G. S., De Woskin, R., Rosen, A. L., Levine, H. and Palani, C. (1976). *Surgery Gynec. Obstet.* **142**, 357.

Synder, G. K. (1977). *Science* **195**, 412.

Uziel, L., Agostoni, A., Pirovano, E., Pesenti, A., Pelizzola, A., Gattinoni, L. and Galmarini, D. (1981). *Internat. J. artif. Organs* **4**, 142.

Perspectives of Long-Term Respiratory Extracorporeal Assist Devices

L. GATTINONI

Institute of Anaesthesia and Reanimation,
University of Milan, Polyclinic Hospital, Milan,
Italy

Since the first application of Membrane Lungs for long-term support of Acute Respiratory Failure (ARF) several investigators used this new technique for assisting the failing lungs.

Gille and Bagniewski (1976), in 1974, rewieved a world-wide experience on 243 patients treated with Extracorporeal Membrane Lung Oxygenation (ECMO), reporting a survival rate of approximately 10%.

At this time, the US National Heart and Lung Institutes implemented a multicentre controlled study comparing the conventional treatment (continuous positive pressure mechanical ventilation: CPPV) with CPPV associated with ECMO.

This study failed to show any improvement in the survival of the treated group compared with control group (Zapol et al., 1979). The mortality rate, as in Gille's report, was about 90%.

The ECMO patient underwent venous–arterial high flow bypass, (with proportional decrease in pulmonary blood flow), while the diseased underperfused lungs were ventilated with CPPV. This can cause barotrauma and local alkalosis, with consequent lung infarction (Kolobow et al., 1981).

The ECMO study emphasized the technical capabilities of the extracorporeal support: good blood gas tensions were obtained easily in the arterial side; however, no basic changes in the management of the lung

Frontiers Cardiol. for the 80s.
0-12-220680-0

disease were introduced: and lung function did not improve. The ultimate goals of any form of respiratory assistance can be summarized as follows:

(1) providing adequate oxygenation; (2) providing adequate CO_2 removal; (3) avoiding pulmonary or systemic complications (e.g. barotrauma, haemodynamic or renal failure) due to the respiratory treatment; and (4) providing an "optimal" environment for lungs healing.

ECMO satisfied the first two objectives, but, in our opinion, did not modify, and possibly worsened, the last two: local and systemic complication of CPPV were not prevented, being CPPV associated with ECMO, new complications due to high flow bypass, as surgical stress, bleeding etc., were added, and the background for lungs healing was probably deteriorated, due to local pH changes and pulmonary under perfusion (Kolobow *et al.*, 1981).

We thus decided a different approach to satisfy an "ideal" respiratory assistance. This consists, basically, in dissociating the two main respiratory function, i.e. oxygenation and CO_2 removal, by using the Membrane Lungs to clear the CO_2 production and the natural lungs to oxygenate the blood.

The oxygenation is impaired during ARF by three mechanisms: (1) possible decrease of diffusion; (2) true right to left shunt; (3) ventilation/perfusion mismatching.

The hypoxaemia due to the first two components, after use of high F_1O_2 and optimal positive end-expiratory pressure, can be solved only by the parallel resolution of the basic pathology of the lungs (i.e., reversal of microatelectasis, decrease of interstitial oedema etc.), while hypoxaemia due to the VA/Q mismatching (functional) is strongly related to the mode of ventilation and to the haemodynamic pattern.

The ideal form of ventilation to overcome the problems of low VA/Q units, with different time constants, would require slow inflation and long end inspiratory plateau, to satisfy the different time constant, low pressures would also be better to prevent the blood flow diversion from relatively healthy zones, where the pressure is better transmitted, to low compliance, hypoventilated zones, already hyperperfused. However this kind of ventilation is impossible in stiff lungs because of $PaCO_2$ rise. In fact, during ARF, the total pulmonary ventilation needs to be increased to two or three times the normal values to maintain a normal $PaCO_2$. High ventilation dictates high pressures: and barotrauma, renal and haemodynamics derangements are pressure-linked complications.

We used low flow venous–venous bypass (1.5 litres/min) to clear CO_2 production while preserving the pulmonary blood flow. The extracorporeal CO_2 removal ($ECCO_2R$) cancels the need of pulmonary ventilation allowing a free choice of the kind of management most appropriate for oxygenation through the diseased lung. Apneic oxygenation, overcomes the problems due to VA/Q mismatching: the gas distribution is, by definition, ideal during static inflation of the lungs and more even blood flow distribution can be reasonably expected in this condition. We thus chose to keep the lung motionless with apneic oxygenation, while 2/3 beats/min (low frequency positive pressure ventilation with extracorporeal CO_2 removal – LFPPV) were provided to preserve lung mechanics and functional residual capacity, as we showed experimentally. CO_2 removal is accomplished at low blood-flow, and the technical problems are far less for $ECCO_2R$ than in ECMO.

The use of LFPPV–$ECCO_2R$ while providing good oxygenation and adequate CO_2 clearance avoids the complications of CPPV. We showed a great improvement of haemodynamics and renal function when comparing this technique with conventional ventilation in animal experiments (Gattinoni *et al.*, 1980).

It is also possible that the lung "rest" enhances the healing process compared to the lung "stress" of mechanical high-volume and pressure ventilation.

We applied, in 1980, LFPPV–$ECCO_2R$ in 11 patients with adult respiratory distress syndrome of various origin (the details of the technique and the clinical results have been reported elsewhere) (Pesenti *et al.*, 1981; Gattinoni *et ai.*, 1981).

The patients met ECMO entry criteria (90% mortality rate), i.e. F_IO_2 0·6, PaO_2 < 50 mmHg for 12 h after 48 h of maximal conventional therapy. We add another criterion, i.e. total static compliance (TSLC) lower than 30 ml/cm H_2O when measured at volume of 7/8 ml/kg by static inflation. The stiffness of the lung is such, in these conditions, that no form of ventilation can approach the "ideal" for oxygenation. The mean duration of the CPPV treatment was 8·6 days before the LFPPV–$ECCO_2R$ while the mean per-fusion time was 6·5 days.

Seven out of 11 patients fully recovered from ARF (spontaneous breathing with excellent blood gases without any form of respiratory assistance), two patients improved lung function (X-ray clearing and TLSC improvement) but died of sepsis and two did not improve.

During LFPPV–$ECCO_2R$ three phases can be detected:

(1) Early "functional" phase (in hours), which is probably due to gas/flow distribution improvement into the lungs. The PaO_2 rapidly rises, and right to left shunt decreases. However, no changes in underlying pathology occurs, as TSLC and X-ray film do not usually change. Blood gases are not considered signs of improvement.

(2) Healing phase (days). While excellent blood gases are maintained TSLC and X-ray improve; the mechanical improvement reflects, in our opinion, the resolution of the disease process.

(3) Weaning phase. We start to wean the patient when TSLC is greater than 30 ml/cmH_2O, which is, in our experience, appropriate to sustain spontaneous breathing in continuous positive airway pressure (CPAP).

The LFPPV–$ECCO_2R$ is a safe technique. No perfusion was interrupted because of technical problems. Blood requirement for replacing blood losses and sampling is about one-quarter of that reported for ECMO.

Our goal is to optimize the extracorporeal system to reduce the extracorporeal blood flow. Two-hundred ml CO_2/min can be theoretically cleared from $0\cdot5$ litres/min of blood flow, which approximates the blood flow requirements for renal dialysis. Promising approaches, in this sense, have recently been published (Fleming *et al.*, 1981).

References

Fleming, J. S., Becket, J., Markey, A. W. *tt al.* (1981). *Proc. Europ. artif. Organs* **8**, 296.

Gattinoni, L., Agostoni, A., Damia, G. *et al.* (1980). *Int. Care Med.* **6**, 155.

Gattinoni, L., Pesenti, A., Pelizzola, A. *et al.* (1981). *Trans. Am. Soc. artif. intern. Organs.* **27**, 289.

Gille, J. P. and Bagniewski, M. (1976). *Trans. Am. Soc. artif. intern. Organs.* **22**, 102.

Kolobow, T., Spragg, R. G. and Pierce, J. E. (1981). *Int. J. artif. Org.* **4**, 76.

Pesenti, A., Pelizzola, A., Mascheroni D. *et al.* (1981). *Trans. Am. Soc. artif. intern. Organs.* **27**, 263.

Zapol, W., Snider, M., Hill, J. D., Snider, M. T., Hill, J. O., Fallat, R. J. Bartlett, R. H., Edmunds, L. H., Morris, A. H., Peirce II, E. C., Thomas, A. N., Proctor, H. J., Drinker, P. A., Pratt, P. C., Bagniewski, A. and Miller, Jr., R. G. (1979). *JAMA* **242**, 2193.

V. The Clinical Perspectives of New Technologies

A New Look at Electro- and Magnetocardiography

B. TACCARDI

Institute of General Physiology and "Centro Simes", University of Parma, Parma, Italy

Clinical electrocardiology is expanding rapidly in many directions. To list only a few of the most important areas, we may mention: dynamic electrocardiography; intracardiac recordings, including His bundle electrograms and monophasic action potentials; exercise electrocardiography; cardiac pacing and automatic defibrillation; external His bundle recordings; automated analysis of ECG, and the mapping of cardiac fields. Recently, it has become possible to measure the magnetic activity of the heart, not only in shielded rooms, but also in ordinary hospital surroundings. Magneto-cardiography is a new, fast-developing branch of electrocardiology. In this report I shall confine myself to discussing the mapping of cardiac fields, with a few words on magnetocardiography.

It is the purpose of clinical electrocardiography to provide information on the location and time-course of the intracardiac electrical events throughout the heartbeat. Let us now consider the potential field in the heart and body tissues during ventricular excitation. The overall potential distribution is actually a mixture of several superimposed potential fields. These are generated by the following events, all of which occur during the same time interval: (a) atrial recovery; (b) one or more separate, anisotropic excitation wavefronts, spreading through the ventricular walls and the septum, (c) initial repolarization of those ventricular areas that have been reached by the excitatory process during the previous stages of activation, (d) in case of acute ischaemia, additional electrical sources must be taken into consideration, which arise at the boundary between normal and injured areas.

Frontiers Cardiol. for the 80s.
0-12-220680-0

Clearly, a realistic representation of such a complicated distribution cannot be obtained by recording a few electrocardiograms from the surface of the body. This procedure involves a definite risk of overlooking both physical and diagnostic information contained in unexplored areas. At present, the automated recording of the total body-surface information is possible by using automated, digital instruments working "on line" (Taccardi and Macchi, 1980). A mobile instrument is now commercially available as a result of a cooperative effort sponsored by the Italian National Research Council. Similar instruments are being developed in several countries (Yamada, 1981); they enable equipotential contour maps to be recorded from the surface of the body and also from the epicardial surface, during heart surgery. Maps have provided significant diagnostic information in the following heart conditions: acute and old myocardial infarction (detection of infarction in patients with normal ECG; monitoring of infarct size before and after drug administration); coronary insufficiency (exercise maps); right and left ventricular hypertrophy (congenital heart disease); left bundle branch block complicated by myocardial infarction or hypertrophy; Wolff–Parkinson–White syndrome; intractable arrhythmias, (see for reference: Taccardi and De Ambroggi, 1975, 1982; Taccardi *et al.*, 1976; Yamada, 1981).

Recent developments suggest that the mapping of cardiac fields can be of clinical use in patients at high risk of ventricular fibrillation. Irregularities in the recovery sequence, which are liable to provoke arrhythmias, can be evidenced by means of "iso-area" mappings, according to Urie *et al.* (1978). On the other hand epicardial mapping at surgery has proven indispensable to locate pre-excited areas or abnormal excitation pathways in re-entrant arrhythmias. A further improvement of the diagnostic power of body surface maps may be expected from the 'inverse' procedures, which enable the epicardial potentials to be calculated from surface electrocardiograms (Barr and Spach, 1977; Colli Franzone *et al.*, 1979).

Magnetocardiography

A magnetic field is always associated to the cardiac electric field. It is generated by a portion of the cardiac currents. Theoretically, only the so-called "impressed currents" can elicit a magnetic field, i.e., those currents that originate where chemical energy is transformed into electric energy (Williamson and Kaufman, 1981). These are the transmembrane ionic currents. The remaining currents that flow "passively" through the body tissues would not give rise to a magnetic field, if the body tissues behaved like an infinite, homogenous conducting medium.

Practically, due to the inhomogeneity and finiteness of the body tissues, the "volume" currents do participate in the generation of the cardiac magnetic field, whose strength is about 10^6 times weaker than the earth's steady field.

Magnetic maps, portraying the distribution of the sagittal component of the field on the anterior chest surface, have been recorded by Karp *et al.* (1978). The "diastolic" and "systolic" injury fields have been measured by Cohen and Kaufman (1975) in experimental animals. More recently, minute magnetic signals occurring during the P–Q interval have been detected by means of averaging procedures (Fenici *et al.*, 1980). Interpretative work, still in progress, performed by means of mathematical models simulating His bundle activity indicates that the small signals are probably the expression of His bundle activity.

In conclusion, the mapping of cardiac fields is at present the only means of achieving an accurate representation of the electrical activity of the heart. It provides basic knowledge on the time course of excitation and recovery in the heart, and also yields a considerable amount of clinical information that cannot be obtained from the conventional electrocardiogram.

References

Barr, R. C. and Spach, M. S. (1977). *Circ. Res.* **42**, 661–675.
Cohen, D. and Kaufman, A. L. (1975). *Circ. Res.* **36**, 414–424.
Colli Franzone, P., Guerri, L., Taccardi, B. and Viganotti, C. (1979). Publication n. 222 of the Institute of Numerical Analysis, University of Pavia, pp. 1–82.
Fenici, R., Romani, G. L., Barbanera, S., Zeppilli, P., Carelli, P. and Modena, I. (1980). *G. ital. Cardiol.* **10**, 1366–1370.
Karp, P. J., Katila, T. E., Saarinen, M., Siltanen, P. and Varpula, T. T. (1978). *Ann. Cardiol. Angéiol.* **27**, 65 (quoted by Williamson and Kaufmann).
Taccardi, B. and De Ambroggi, L. (1975). *In* "Cardiologia d'Oggi" (A. Beretta Anguissola and V. Puddu, Eds), Vol. II, pp. 361–381. Second edition in press (1982).Edizioni Medico Scientifiche, Torino.
Taccardi, B., De Ambroggi, L. and Viganotti, C. (1976). *In* "The theoretical basis of Electrocardiology" (C. V. Nelson and D. B. Geselowitz, Eds), pp. 436–466. Clarendon Press, Oxford.
Taccardi, B. and Macchi, E. (1980). *Rev. Latina Cardiol.* **1**, 30–36.
Urie, P. M., Burgess, M. J., Lux, R. L., Wyatt, R. F. and Abildskov, J. A. (1978). *Circ. Res.* **42**, 350–358.
Williamson, S. J. and Kaufman, L. (1981). *I. Magn. Mag. Mater.* **22**, 129–202.
Yamada, K. (1981). *Jap. Circ. J.* **45**, 1–14.

Future Trends in Implantable Devices for the Treatment of Bradycardia and Tachycardia

M. B. KNUDSON
and J. E. SHAPLAND, II

Cardiac Pacemakers Inc., St Paul,
Minnesota, USA

The current trend in implantable devices is to approximate as closely as possible normal physiology. This paper will focus on future trends in implantable devices for physiologic pacing. During the 1980s these will, in a large part, be implanted pacemakers for the treatment of bradycardia and tachycardia.

Problems associated with the treatment of tachycardia can be divided into four specific areas: (1) the treatment of atrial tachycardia, (2) the treatment of ventricular tachycardia, (3) the use of implantable defibrillators and (4) an important new trend in the 1980s – early recognition of the precursors of arrhythmias. The haemodynamic and physiologic effects of paroxysmal supraventricular tachycardia may be accompanied by dramatic falls in arterial pressure and may be life-threatening; but what non-pharmacological options are available? For atrial tachycardias, the use of orthorhythmic pacing with atrial burst pacers is currently one widely used method of conversion. Haft *et al.* (1967) published an early paper demonstrating the use of burst pacing in the treatment of tachycardias. Other methods include AV sequential or DVI pacemakers with either a normal or very short PR interval to treat atrioventricular reentry tachycardias. A more complex problem in treatment, however, is ventricular tachycardia, where orthorhythmic pacing, underdrive and overdrive pacing systems and the newer methods of scanning pacing will find application (Foster and Zipes, 1979). The scanning pacemaker, also known as an autodecremental pacemaker, is able to decrement or increment the interval between the last sensed ventricular contraction and the pacing spike using either single or paired spikes to interrupt a reentry rhythm. The use of implantable devices for the treatment of automatic tachycardias is mostly ineffective.

Another important step in the 1980s will be the development of automatic implantable defibrillators. The three major hurdles facing the use of the automatic implantable defibrillator are, first, sufficient energy from an implantable battery. (The lithium iodide cell, with its high internal impedance, is quickly exhausted by use in an implantable defibrillator.) Second, fail-safe recognition of fibrillation. Third, prevention of myocardial damage by the defibrillatory shock. One of the exciting advances is characterized by recent work from Simson (1981) on recognition of patients at risk for development of tachycardias. In the early phases of the QRS complex, there is little difference between control patients and patients who have a high risk of developing ventricular tachycardia. However, during the later phases of the QRS, there is a significantly lower frequency component in those patients who will develop ventricular tachycardia. The future of tachycardia recognition is bright and in the 1980s, we should see a tremendous growth in the use of the implantable tachyconverter with advanced detection schemes.

One of the most active aspects of physiologic pacing in the 80s will be pacemakers which are responsive to body needs for varying cardiac output. The two variables which determine cardiac output are stroke volume and heart rate. Many pacemakers function mostly to maintain AV relationships. Samet (1966, 1968) studied the effect of AV synchrony in man and found that cardiac index can be increased by approximately 20% by AV synchrony at standard rates and other studies demonstrated the differential effect with changing heart rate as well as AV synchrony. Ogowa et al. (1978) conducted similar studies in dogs. None of the subjects of these studies had significant myocardial dysfunction. An important question raised by these studies relates to the effect of left and right ventricular filling pressure on atrial contribution. Greenberg et al. (1979) commented, "When LVEDP is in the normal range, the left ventricular function curve is steepest and atrial synchrony should increase stroke volume maximally. When left ventricular end diastolic pressure is elevated, the flat portion of the ventricular function curve is approached and further increments in pressure would be expected to have progressively less effect." Further extending this work, Greenberg et al. (1979) demonstrated that there is significant inverse relationship between increasing pulmonary capillary wedge pressure and decreasing atrial contribution to stroke volume. The intercept for the line of those patients with coronary artery disease is 22 mmHg. Greenberg et al. (1979) conclude, "Atrial contribution tends to be less effective in augmenting cardiac output when filling pressure is already elevated, particularly in patients with impaired left ventricular function." This means that the less competent the ventricle, the less effective AV synchrony and atrial kick is, but the more important some method of augmenting performance becomes.

The other option, is heart rate. Koyoma, *et al.* (1976) performed a very interesting study of fixed rate ventricular pacing at the onset of strenuous exercise. In five patients aged 50–64, they found that the ability to increase cardiac output was dependent on stroke volume and that it was limited to a 66% increase in cardiac ouptut. Snell *et al.* (1980) and Knudson *et al.* (1981) extended these studies to look at the effect of fixed rate pacing on physical performance in individuals with rate programmable pacemakers. These studies showed that cardiac output at rates of 65–75 ppm is limited to a very low value (10–12 litres/min), whereas at a rate of 100, cardiac output can approach the normal range, approximately 18 litres/min. These studies further show the limitation to cardiac output is stroke volume; this stroke volume limitation applies regardless of what heart rate (in the range of 90–120 ppm) is so long as maximal exercise is reached. The costs, however, of exercising at low fixed rate are very high in terms of central pressures and volumes and potential damage to the myocardium. Figure 1 shows pulmonary capillary wedge pressures at various rates during progressively increased severity of exercise. Obviously, a rate of 100 is much more tolerable to the cardiovascular system. Ultimately, fixed ventricular rate limits cardiac out-

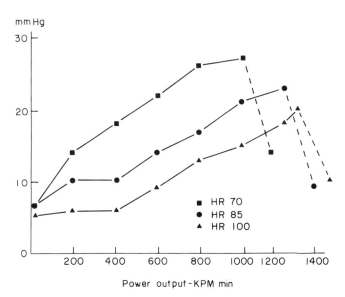

Power output - KPM min

Figure 1. Pulmonary Capillary Wedge Pressure measured at rest and during supine bicycle exercise at the exercise intensities shown. Three set heart rates were used in one subject with complete heart block and a programmable pacemaker.

put by limiting cardiac reserve to stroke volume increase alone and results in over-stretching of the ventricles, which can sharply increase pulmonary capillary wedge pressure. The question then arises: What are the relative contributions of AV synchrony and rate? Karlof (1974) performed an important study of fixed rate pacing vs P-triggered pacing during rest and exercise. Fixed rate pacing was adjusted to the maximum P-synchronous rate achieved during exercise and then exercise at 120 ppm was performed in both P-triggered and asynchronous pacing. There was no significant difference in cardiac output and function between fixed rate pacing and P-triggered pacing at the same rate and the same exercise intensity.

We have conducted a similar study with a physiologic pacemaker which responds to changes in atrial rate by increasing ventricular rate (Fig. 2). This pacemaker, called the RS4,* was clinically evaluated and the data obtained were segmented into four groups: (1) those patients paced at 65 ppm, (2) a group of patients paced at 75 ppm, (3) the same patients in group 2 in the rate responsive (RS4) mode and again tested and (4) a group who reverted to 1:1 conduction during exercise. There is an increase in exercise tolerance, expressed in METS, with increasing heart rate from a mean of 4·4 at 65 to a mean of 10·07 at 151. Figure 3 shows oxygen uptake as a function of rate for

Exercise Tolerance (METS)

		Mean ± SEM	Heart Rate	N
1	VVI (65 ppm)	4.4 ± .617	65.0 ± .43	N = 9
2	VVI (75 ppm)	6.13 ± .69	75.3 ± .27	N = 10
3	RS4	8.1 ± .712	91.0 ± 3.8	N = 9
4	1:1 Conduction	10.07 ± 1.21	151.43 ± 8.534	N = 7

Exercise Tolerance (METS)

		Mean ± SEM	Comparison	P Value
1	VVI (65 ppm)	4.3 ± .617	1 to 2	P < .01
2	VVI (75 ppm)	6.13 ± .69	1 to 3	P < .005
3	RS4	8.1 ± .712	1 to 4	P < .05
4	1:1 Conduction	10.07 ± 1.21	3 to 4	P > .05 (NS)

Figure 2.   Comparison of the four groups; three ventricular paced (VVI, 65 ppm, VVI, 75 ppm and RS) and a group exhibiting 1:1 atrial–ventricular conduction during exercise. Values are group means for maximum exercise tolerance and peak ventricular rate, N is number of patients in each group (upper). Groups with different letters are significantly different (anova and Student's t-test) (lower).

* RS-4®Pacemaker/SRT®Pacing lead, Cardiac Pacemakers, Inc., St. Paul, Minnesota.

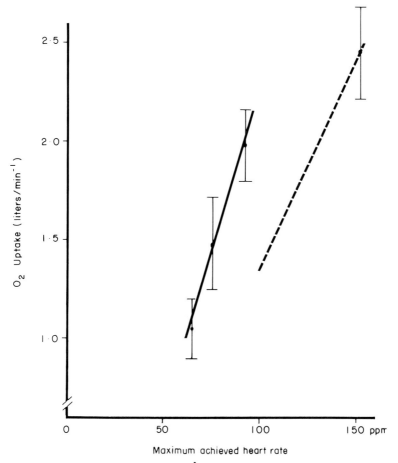

Figure 3. Maximum oxygen uptake ($\dot{V}O_2$ max.), for all groups, calculated from METS (O_2 uptake = METS × 3·5 × 70Kg) and/or measured directly.

the groups. The 1 : 1 conduction group has a similar slope to that of the paced group, although in the paced group the line is shifted slightly to the left. This may be the result of adaptation by chronic increase in stroke volume.

Figure 4 demonstrates that patients confined to very low exercise levels at 65 to 75 ppm can exercise in the normal range when in the RS4 mode; in fact, they have an exercise tolerance not significantly different from the 1 : 1 conduction group. Only one patient failed to exceed the commonly accepted normal value of six METS; even though at VVI rate of 65 and 75 ppm, in the same group of individuals, there are seven patients who did not achieve six METS. Therefore, in the same group of individuals, only one of seven was

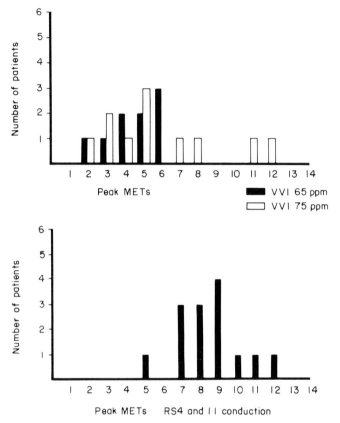

Figure 4. Distribution of maximum exercise tolerance (METS) achieved by individual patients at a fixed, paced ventricular rate of 65 ppm (upper); RS4 and 1:1 conduction group (lower).

still below normal with rate responsive pacing and that person increased from a peak of two METS to a peak of five METS, an important increase in terms of quality of life.

The current generation devices which are under test and should be out in the 1980s to deal with both sides of the cardiac output equation are the rate responsive pacemakers such as the VDD which sense in the atrium and pace in the ventricle and the dual chamber automatic pacers, the DDD pacers which pace the atrium and pace the ventricle. However, there is one significant and growing group of patients who are not treated by either of these pacemakers. These are patients who have chronotopic dysfunction and constitute one of the important challenges for the 80s. Abbott et al. (1977) demonstrated that correction of resting heart rate to normal does not treat exercise intolerance. Currently, in the USA, the sick sinus syndrome constitutes one of the major indications for pacemaker implants. Sagawa (1980) recently stated, "The current problem is how to deal more effectively with patients with so-called sick sinus syndrome in which the sinus node fails to respond to the efferent automatic nervous signals." Abbott *et al.* (1977) showed that patients with sick sinus syndrome vs control patients have considerably reduced oxygen uptake and exercise heart rate response via their sinus nodes. This means that even with a pacemaker which senses atrial activity and responds accordingly, patients with sick sinus syndrome are still limited in their exercise response. One of the new trends in pacing is the development of automatic pacemakers capable of automatic sensor controlled rate change. This will be accomplished by replacing SA node control with sensors for control. The 80s will then be the decade of implantable devices for physiologic pacing to (1) optimize myocardial performance and cardiac output through control of heart rate in the treatment not only of conduction disturbances but disturbances of impulse generation in the sinoatrial node, (2) the control of atrial ventricular synchrony optimizing PR interval (since in those patients who need AV synchrony, the AV interval is all important), and (3) the control of tachyarrhythmias.

References

Abbott, J. A., Hirschfeld, D. S., Kankel, F. W., Scheinman, M. M. and Modin, G. (1977). *Am. J. Med.* **62**, 330.

Foster, P. R. and Zipes, D. (1979). *In* "Cardiac Pacing" (P. Varriale and E. A. Naclerio, Eds), pp. 215–228. LeaFebiger, Philadelphia.

Greenberg, B., Chatterjee, K., Parmley, W. W., Werner, J. A. and Holly, A. N. (1979). *Am. Heart J.* **98**, 742.

Haft, J. J., Kosowsky, B. N., Lan, S. E., Stein, E. and Damato, A. N. (1967). *Am. J. Cardiol.* **20**, 237.

Karlof, I. (1974). *Acta med. scand.* **196**, 7.

Knudson, M. B. (1980). *Cardiostim* **80**, J. Mugica, Ed.

Knudson, M. B. *et al* (1981). *Pace* **4**, A-53.

Koyoma, T., Nakajima, S. and Horimoto, M. (1976). *Am. Heart J.* **91**, 457.

Ogowa, S. *et al* (1978). *Pace* **1**.

Sagawa, K. (1980). *Annals of Bio. Med. Eng.* **8**, 415.

Samet, P. (1966). *Am. Heart J.* **72**, 725.

Samet, P. (1968). *Am. J. Cardiol.* **21**, 207.

Simson, M. B. (1981). *Circulation* **64**, 235.

Snell, P. *et al* (1980). *Med. Sci., Sport and Ex.* **12**, 123.

Cardiovascular Physical Measurements by Means of Fibre Optic and Piezoelectric Polymer Transducers

D. DE ROSSI and P. DARIO

Institute of Clinical Physiology CNR and
"E. Piaggio" Centre, Faculty of Engineering,
University of Pisa, Pisa, Italy

Introduction

Stronger impact on the quality of health care will be probably exerted in the next decade by a better interpretation of presently available clinical measurements and by the definition of more precise correlations between measured variables and patient clinical status; nevertheless the continuous advancement of sensor technology will offer potentially valuable tools for new, more precise and more reliable biomedical measurements.

Fibre optic sensors and piezoelectric polymer sensors are now attracting considerable interest for measurements of physical quantities such as temperature, pressure, sound, ultrasound, blood velocity and blood flow.

This paper reviews these classes of sensors and outlines new configurations and possible advantages for their use in cardiovascular physical measurements.

Fibre Optic Sensors

Signal transmission through fibre optics is particularly attractive in cardio-vascular measurements mainly because of the minimal interference between the optical signal and lower frequency noise usually present in the biological environment and because of absence of any risk of lethal electric shock (Christensen, 1980). Several measuring techniques using fibre optics have been proposed and some of them appear to be promising in the field of cardiovascular physical measurements.

Most of fibre optic sensors make use of the fibres just as light conductors to have access to the measuring site, while the sensing mechanism is provided by some other detector located at the tip of the transmitting and receiving fibre optic bundle and capable of converting the quantity to be measured into optical information.

For another class of detectors (Bucaro and Cole, 1979) the optical fibre itself provides the mechanism of transduction of the sensed physical quantity into an optical signal. Light travelling through the fibre is intensity modulated or phase shifted in response to external stimuli and such variations can be detected by a simple photodetector in the former case, while interferometric techniques must be used in the second one.

Temperature Measurements

Several classes of materials change their optical properties in response to temperature variations. Liquid crystals, gallium arsenide and rare earth phosphors have been used for the construction of temperature sensor located at the tip of fibre optic bundles. Small dimensions, fast response and accuracy in the range of physiological temperatures are distinctive features of these transducers.

Liquid crystals, or more appropriately mesomorphic substances, belong to a thermodynamically stable state, intermediate between amorphous liquids and crystalline solids. The combination of strongly anisotropic material constants, a characteristic feature of solid crystalline state, with liquid-like rheological properties, allow liquid crystals to exhibit relevant molecular structure reorganizations in response to external stimuli, (Carrol, 1973). Liquid crystal mixtures can be formulated to perform temperature measurements in different ranges. An accuracy of $0\cdot1°C$ is generally obtained in the range of physiological temperatures with liquid crystal-fibre optic probes (Johnson and Rozzell, 1975).

The temperature dependence of light absorption in gallium arsenide due to changes in the energy gap between the valence band and the conduction band, has been used to construct a temperature probe having an accuracy of $0\cdot1°C$ and resolution of $0\cdot01°C$ in the range 20–50°C with a sensor tip diameter as small as 240 microns (Christensen, 1977).

The measurement principle of recently developed rare earth phosphor temperature sensors is based on the temperature dependence of the intensity of selected spectral lines emitted by certain rare earth phosphors excited by ultraviolet light transmitted through plastic fibre optics. Temperature reading can be obtained from the intensity ratio of two selected spectral lines, making the measurement immune to eventual fluctuations of the light source brightness.

Temperature dependence of optical path of the light travelling through a fibre optic has been recently proposed as a possible mechanism for temperature sensing (Bucaro *et al.*, 1977). The proposed instrumental configuration is based on a interferometric detection system. The light emitted by a monochromatic, coherent light source is conveyed into the reference and a measuring fibre optic arm. Some length of the measuring arm, acting as the sensing element, is exposed to the temperature field. The phase shift between luminous signals travelling through the two optical fibres can be converted into temperature reading.

Pressure and Sound Measurements

Catheter-tip transducers have been designed in which the small displacement of a diaphragm exposed to intravascular pressure is detected by measuring the intensity of the light reflected back in the receiving fibres of a fibre optic bundle and correlated with the differential pressure across the diaphragm itself (Lindstrom, 1970).

Pressure-induced light scattering in a temperature-insensitive cholesteric–nematic liquid crystal mixture has been investigated in the range of physiological blood pressure and a fibre optic catheter for intravascular blood pressure measurements has been proposed (Jeudy and Robillard, 1976).

Several other fibre optic devices presently under evaluation as highly sensitive underwater hydrophones can be considered for pressure and sound measurement in the cardiovascular field.

Optical losses induced by bending an optical fibre under the action of pressure and sound result in light intensity modulation which can be measured and correlated with the acting pressure (Fields *et al.*, 1979).

Another relatively simple configuration is used for the movable grating sensor (Tietjen, 1981). A fine grid grating, moving with a diaphragm with respect to a similar stationary grating, under the action of pressure, intercepts the light from a transmitting to a receiving optical fibre. A light intensity modulation is obtained, proportional to diaphragm deformation and, in a certain range, to pressure variations.

The most sensitive fibre optic devices employ an interferometric detection scheme where the optical phase shift induced in the sensing fibre by pressure stimulated photoelastic effect is compared with the optical phase shift in a shielded reference arm (Cole *et al.*, 1977). Extremely high sensitivity, far beyond the requirements for biomedical measurements, is expected using interferometric techniques, but at the expense of additional complexity in the detection probably confining this class of sensors to very specialized measurements.

Blood Velocity and Blood Flow Measurements

Blood velocity measurements have been performed by means of an intra-vascular fibre optic catheter using Doppler frequency shift effect (Tanaka and Benedek, 1975). Light emitted by a He–Ne laser is transmitted into a vein by an optical fibre which also collects the light scattered back from moving erythrocytes. Optical mixing spectroscopy has been used to measure the spectrum of Doppler shift between the light scattered from the erythro-cytes and the reference light reflected back from the exit of the fibre optic catheter. Velocity distribution of moving erythrocytes proportional to the spectrum of Doppler shift in the scattered light has been measured in the range from $0 \cdot 01$ cm/s up to 100 cm/s. Although this technique allows very accurate measurements, blood flow more than blood velocity is a physical quantity of high diagnostic value.

Indicator dilution techniques are commonly used for blood flow measure-ment. Fibre optic catheters are used to record dye dilution curves to calculate cardiac output. Densitometric measurements of dye concentration are performed by recording the ratio of the intensity of the light back-scattered by the blood–dye mixture at two different wavelengths (Hugenholtz *et al.*, 1965).

Blood flow measurement by thermodilution is widely used in clinical practice because of its accuracy, easy repeatability and harmlessness.

A liquid crystal–fibre optic catheter for simultaneous measurements of blood flow by thermodilution and oxygen saturation by reflection spectro-photometry in the coronary sinus has been developed and tested *in vitro* and *in vivo* (De Rossi *et al.*, 1980). In Fig. 1 the recordings of an animal experiment performed using this catheter are reported.

Piezo- and Pyroelectric Polymer Sensors

The unique properties of piezo- and pyroelectric polymers (Broadhurst and Davis, 1980) – low density, good mechanical impedance match to human soft tissue, flexibility, non-toxicity and ease of fabrication of complex pattern and array–make them ideally suited to biomedical transducers and artificial organ technology.

The strongest piezo- and pyroelectric activity among different polymers has presently been found in polyvinylidene fluoride (PVDF or PVF_2 in the literature). External sensors, catheter-tip sensors and sensor arrays can be designed and they are under preliminary tests to monitor cardiovascular and

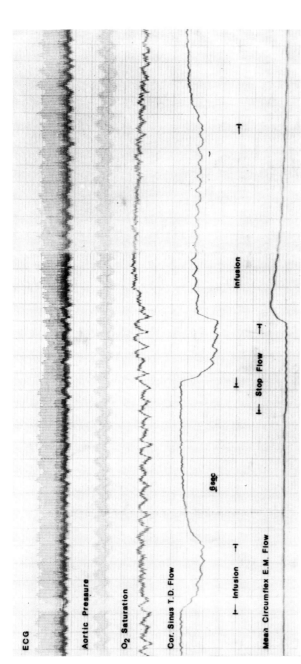

Figure 1. In vivo experiment recording on anaesthetized dog. Thermodilution (TD) curve obtained with the infusion of saline at room temperature at a rate of 10 cm³/min is shown during steady-state flow (left) and during reactive hyperaemia following transient occlusion of the circumflex artery (CF) (centre portion). In the latter instance, infusion of saline starts during the stop flow and continues 70s after the CF has been released. Blood temperature as well as O_2 saturation change in accordance with the CF flow. In the recording of the thermodilution curve, starting blood temperature is 37·2°C and vertical grid scaling 0·6°C per mesh spacing. O_2 saturation curve shows an initial value of about 75% and falls to 50% during reactive hyperaemia. (Reproduced from De Rossi, D. et al., 1980, by permission of the publishers, I.P.C. Business Press Ltd.[c])

respiratory phenomena over a wide frequency range of signals of mechanical origin taking advantage of the inherent large bandwidth and flat frequency response of piezoelectric plastics. Piezoelectric polymer transducers have been applied to monitor peripheral pulse (Shuford *et al.*, 1976), to record simultaneously ECG and carotid pulse to calculate systolic time intervals (De Rossi *et al.*, 1981), to monitor uterine contractions and foetal heart

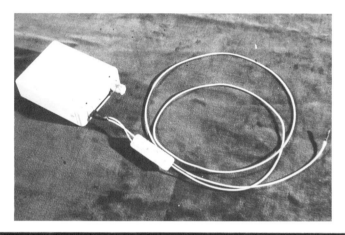

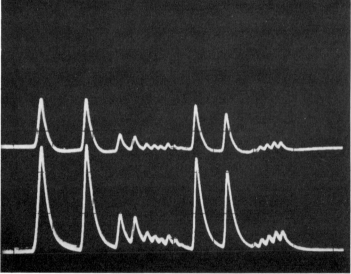

Figure 2. Top: French 5 catheter tip PVF$_2$ sensor, connected to the battery operated electronic unit. Bottom: Simultaneous in vitro *recording of pressure tracings for the PVF$_2$ sensor (lower trace) and a National LXI60ID semiconductor pressure transducer.*

sounds (Kobayashi and Yasuda, 1981). Intravascular catheter-tip sensors for simultaneous dynamic pressure and sound measurements have been developed and preliminarily evaluated (Dario *et al.*, 1980).

In Fig. 2 a French 5 catheter with tip mounted PVF_2 sensor is shown, together with results of *in vitro* tests.

The robustness, high voltage sensitivity, large bandwidth and potential low cost of such a device suggest the possibility of developing a truly disposable catheter-tip dynamic pressure and sound transducer.

The flexibility and low mass of piezoelectric polymers allow also to conceive longitudinal arrays of sensor to be located along the course of peripheral vessels to locate eventual stenoses. They can also be incorporated into artificial organs to detect organ movements or changes in the compliance of distensible components.

Vascular prostheses, artificial assist devices and artificial hearts with built-in sensor capabilities are conceivable and under preliminary evaluation.

Low acoustic impedance, very close to human soft tissue, allows piezoelectric polymers to provide outstanding match with the human body.

This property, together with the characteristic low-Q resonant behaviour of this class of materials, implies that broad bandwidth and a very short impulse response improving axial resolution and angular response are achievable in echo imaging with piezoelectric polymer ultrasonic receivers (Callerame *et al.*, 1978). Here again, the ability of polymers to conform to irregular shapes and the relatively easy preparation of high density bidimensional arrays (Swartz and Plummer, 1979) open new avenues for research in ultrasonic instrumentation for diagnostic use.

References

Broadhurst, M. G. and Davis, G. T. (1980). *In* "Electrects" (G. M. Sessler, Ed.), Topics in Applied Physics, Vol. 33, pp. 285–319. Springer Verlag, Heidelberg.

Bucaro, J. A. and Cole, J. H. (1979). EASCON'79 Record, pp. 572–580.

Bucaro, J. A., Dardy, H. D. and Crome, E. F. (1977). *Appl. Optics* 16, 1761–1766.

Callerame, J., Tancrell, R. H. and Wilson, D. T. (1978). *In* "IEEE Ultrasonic Symposium Proceedings", IEEE Cat. N°78, Ch 1344 ISU, pp. 117–121.

Carrol, P. L. (1973). "Cholesteric liquid crystals". Ovum Ltd, London.

Christensen, D. A. (1977). *J. Bioeng.* 1, 541.

Christensen, D. A. (1980). *In* "Physical sensors for Biomedical Applications" (M. R. Neuman, D. G. Flemming, W. H. Ko and P. W. Chung, Eds), pp. 67–81. CRC Press Inc., Boca Raton.

Cole, J. H., Johnson, R. L. and Bhuta, P. G. (1977). *J. acoust. Soc. Am.* 62, 1136.

Dario, P., Bedini, R. and De Rossi D. (1980). Digest of papers "Biomed 80" pp. 229–330, Marseille.

De Rossi, D., Benassi, A., L'Abbate, A. and Dario, P. (1980). *J. biomed. Eng.* 2, 257–264.

De Rossi, D., Dario, P., Marchesi, C., Trivella, M. G., Pedrini, F., Contini, C., De Reggi, A. S., Edelman, S. and Roth, S. (1981). Proc. IEEE Computers in Cardiology 1981, pp. 111–114, ISSN Nº 0276–6574.

Fields, J. N., Smith, C. P., Asawa, U.K., Morrison, R. J., Ramer, O. G., Tangonana, G. L. and Barnosky, M. K. (1979). Presented at the Optical Fiber Comm. Meeting, Washington D.C.

Hugenholtz, P. G., Gamble, W. S., Monroe, R. G. and Polanyi, M. (1965). *Circulation* **31**, 344–355.

Jeudy, M. J. and Robillard, J. J. (1976). *Optics and Laser Technology* 117–119.

Johnson, C. C. and Rozzell, T. C. (1975). *Microwave J.* **18**, 55–57.

Kobayashi, K. and Yasuda, T. (1981). *Ferroelectrics* **32**, 181–184.

Lindstrom, L. H. (1970). *IEEE Trans. biomed. Eng.* BME-**17**, 207–219.

Shuford, R. J., Wilde, A. F., Ricca, J. J. and Thomas, G. R. (1976). Proceedings 1976 Army Science Conference, Vol. 3.

Swartz, R. G. and Plummer, J. D. (1979). *IEEE Trans. Elect. Dev.* ED 26–12, 1921–1932.

Tanaka, T. and Benedek, G. B. (1975). *Appl. Opt.* **14**, 189–196.

Tietjen, W. B. (1981). *J. acoust. Soc. Am.* **69** (4), 993–997.

Computer-assisted Multivariate Analysis in Cardiovascular Measurements

A. K. REAM

Department of Anesthesia, Institute
of Engineering Design in Medicine,
Stanford University Medical Center,
Stanford, California, USA

Introduction

Because of the limitations of time and space, this paper must concentrate on concepts. They are illustrated by examples, as time permits, and references are provided. Remember: these are difficult, but useful ideas. The use of examples and applications is essential to full understanding (Ream, 1978).

Measurement Needs

The use of measurements in clinical care may be divided into four parts: (1) assure the quality of measurements (techniques), (2) make the measurements (application), (3) derive results (data reduction), and (4) formulate interpretation (analysis). Any device used to assist the clinician, as the computer, must meet these needs.

The value of the computer is usually thought to be threefold: (1) It is faster (the fastest category is "on line": the user does not wait for results). (2) It is more reliable (there are fewer errors). (3) It is more consistent (it has better repeatability and accuracy). But initial applications of the computer, to make more and better measurements, caused users to be overwhelmed with data. A fourth attribute is the most important, and leads to the solution to this problem: (4) The computer significantly enhances the ability to perform multivariate analysis.

Multivariate Analysis

Multivariate analysis refers not only to the act of making simultaneous measurements of several variables, but to the consideration of the information contained "between" them. Sometimes the information "between" is a small but significant part of the total information. An example is the measurement of filling pressure (or peak systolic wall stress) vs ejection fraction, which enhances the definition of normal values (Strauer, 1979, (Fig. 1)). And sometimes the desired information is completely represented

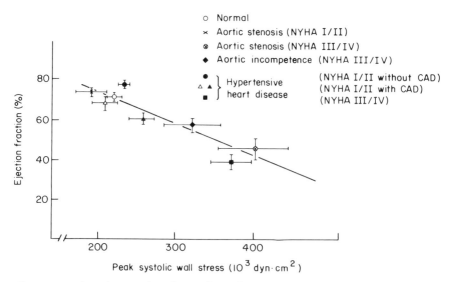

Figure 1.   The relation of peak systolic wall stress and ejection fraction. Note that the ejection fraction, which is used for clinical assessment of the adequacy of cardiac performance, is sensitive to wall stress. In clinical practice, when the ejection fraction is reported, it is implied that the patient has been titrated to the appropriate portion of the Starling Curve, i.e. that the wall stress has been adjusted to the physiologically most efficient value (Strauer, 1979).

between the measurements. This is demonstrated below in a non-clinical example, since most clinical situations are not so clear cut:

Imagine a set of coins, black on one side and silver on the other. Half are arbitrarily marked "A" and the other half "B". If we define the "head" side of "A" coins as black and the "head" side of "B" coins as silver, then if we desire to know if the "head" side is up, we must measure both attributes. A moment's reflection indicates that knowing "A" or "B" alone, or black-side-up or silver-side-up is not enough. All of the useful information in this example is contained in the *combination* of data (Fig. 2). (See Ream 1980 for further discussion.)

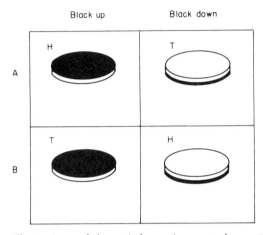

Figure 2. An illustration of how information can be entirely contained "between" measurements. A set of coins is created which are black on one side and silver on the other. Half are arbitrarily marked "A" and the other half "B". If we define the head side of A coins as black, and the head side of B coins as silver, then if we desire to know if the head side is up, we must measure both attributes. A moment's reflection indicates that knowing A or B alone, or black-side-up or silver-side-up is not sufficient. All of the useful information in this example is contained in the combination of data.

A clinical example is the assessment of cardiac (pump) failure. The measurement of small isolated changes in central venous pressure (CVP), heart rate (HR) and mean systemic arterial pressure (MAP) may be impossible to interpret. However, a small simultaneous decrease in MAP and HR with an increase in CVP is a virtually certain indicator of pump failure.

Optimization Techniques

It is clear from these simple examples that, while the concept of multivariate analysis is powerful, it is also difficult and intimidating. Let's examine some of the "tricks" which make the concept practical and useful. There are four general areas where specifics are helpful: (1) timing, (2) selection of measured variables, (3) indirect measurements, and (4) assistance to human thought. We examine each in turn.

Timing

In order for multivariate measurements to be maximally useful, they must be simultaneous. If they are changing, which is the usual situation of interest, then non-simultaneous measurements reduce their correlation, and hence their information. Similarly, measurements must be made often enough to demonstrate any changes. Sampling too slowly can lead to missed (and even false) results!

Timing effects lead to three major measurement categories:

(1) *Diagnostic* devices are expensive, measure slowly, and are often used only once in a given situation. An example in cardiac catheterization.
(2) *Observation* devices are simpler, less expensive, and used more than once. An example is bedside measurement of cardiac output.
(3) *Monitoring* devices are used for continuous measurement, and therapeutic interaction. An example is the continous measurement of systemic arterial and pulmonary artery pressures.

Note the increase in utility as the problems of timing and simultaneity are reduced; and cost, quality, and reliability improve.

Selection of Measured Variables

Much can be said on this subject: we here attempt to state the most important concepts in a practical way. Further reading is strongly recommended.

Maximize the statistical independence of measurements

This is another way of saying that each measurement must add *new* information. Each variable which adds *new* information, and is correlated with the result of interest, increases our confidence in the calculated result (Harman, 1967).

Limit the number of measurements used for deriving any result

This is an extraordinarily important and subtle concept. If we make excess measurements, new uncertainty is added to the result without adding an equivalent amount of new information. This degrades the result. This is shown in Fig. 3 reproduced from Hall (1977). As the number of independent

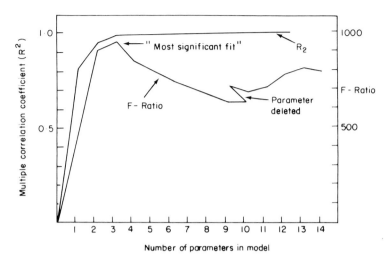

Figure 3. Multiple correlation coefficient (r squared) and F-ratio variation as parameters are added to the model. (Hall, 1977). See text. (In effect, the F-ratio is correlated with the probability of predicting the result correctly.)

measured variables increases, the F ratio reaches a maximum, then once more decreases. Note that the correlation coefficient is not sensitive to this phenomenon. In other words: quality is more important than quantity of variables when talking about the number of variables measured. Another way of looking at this concept is to note that even when many variables are measured, using only a few of them in subsequent calculations gives the most accurate result (e.g. Schneider *et al.*, 1979; Shoemaker and Czer, 1979).

Minimize loss of results with loss of any measurement

This is illustrated by an example from our artificial heart laboratory (Fig. 4; Robinson *et al.*, 1977). The diagram shows variables measured along the top, and variables calculated from them along the left side. Entries in the table show the measurements required for each calculation. The general scatter in these entries is good: it means that the loss of a single measurement minimizes the impact on the results. An important exception is the dependence of almost every measurement on the ECG; this is done to facilitate extra accuracy in calculation. The undesirable result is that adequate monitoring is extraordinarily dependent on the availability of the ECG signal. This concept may be referred to as the "belt and suspenders approach". If one measurement fails, then another will provide support.

Indirect Measurements

(1) Indirect measurements increase convenience because they are less

CALCULATED VARIABLES

	ECG	LAP	LVP	PIP	AP	PAF	POF	IPV	DVDT	POP	DPP	CVP	ARF	RAP	PAP	CAF	CVPI	DP	PTHR	SVMN
1. SV(V)								X	X										X	
2. F(F)	A					X		B	B										B	
3. F(V)								X	X										X	1,28
4. RSV	A				A			X	X											1,2,28
5. POP	X											X								
6. Q–E	X							X	X										X	
7. E–F	X							X	X										X	
8. HR	X																			
9. PAF	X					X														
10. LAP	X	X																		
11. LVPMX	X		X																	
12. APMX	X			X																
13. APMN	X			X																
14. AP	X			X																
15. AF–E	X					X	A	B	B										B	9,3,2
16. LVSVE	X					X	A	B	B										B	15,8
17. DD/P100	X		X									X								
18. LVMW	X		X	X		A		B	B					X				X	B	29, 30
19. R	X		X	X	X								B				A			14,9
20. EFR	X							X	X										X	
21. EER								X	X										X	
22. LVSWP	X		X	X		A		B	B									A	B	30,8
23. LVMWE	X		X	A	X													A	B	9
24. LVSW	X		X	X		A		B	B									X	B	18,8
25. QESD	X							X	X										X	
26. EFSD								X	X										X	
27. E																				TIME
28. PR								X	X										X	
29. LVMWA	X		X											X			X			
30. LVMWP	X		A			A		B	B									A	B	
31. DATE																				Keyboard
32. TIME																				Keyboard
33. TTI	X		X															X		
34. DP/PO	X		X									X								
35. DTI	X		X	X														X		
36. ARF	X												X							
37. CALF																				Keyboard
38. PMW					X			X	X											
39. PTI	X		X	X																
40. S–DP/P	X		X									X								
41. CAF	X															X				
42. LVPED	X		X									X								

A – pump off
B – pump on

Figure 4. A source diagram for calculation of physiologic variables. Measured variables are shown along the top and calculated variables along the left side. Entries in the table show the measured variables necessary to calculate a given calculated variable. This table represents the calculation routines in use in the Stanford Artificial Heart Laboratory, using a computer assisted monitoring system.

invasive, and therefore often reduce skill requirements and patient risk.

(2) Indirect measurements tend to increase error, because physical distance from the measurement site reduces the opportunity to make multiple simultaneous independent measurements (see above), and increases the opportunity for noise to enter the path between the object of interest and the site of measurement. Reducing noise in the pathway can improve monitoring. An example is that the use of a conductive catheter for cardiac catheterization permits less stringent constraints on leakage current for ECG monitors, thereby permitting reduction of the noise sensitivity of the ECG monitor (Lipton *et al.*,1978).

(3) Indirect measurements are usually more complex, because of the need to overcome the problems just cited.

(4) Indirect measurements usually represent a continuum from direct to remote, permitting some choice in the tradeoffs involved. Two examples: (1) intracranial pressure can be measured from the ventricle, subdurally, epidurally, and through a fontanelle (Ream *et al.*, 1979); and (2) Left Atrial pressure can be measured directly, or estimated from pulmonary artery wedge pressure or pulmonary artery diastolic pressure (Yelderman, 1979).

(5) A special problem is the relative value of *objective* vs *subjective* measurements. Subjective measurements are those where the patient or clinician must estimate values, as exercise tolerance. (An objective measure might be a treadmill test.) Furthermore, where diagnostic computer programs have been written which perform better than individual clinicians, the addition of subjective data often degrades their performance (Warner, *et al.*, 1961 (congenital heart disease) and Leaper *et al.*, 1972 (abdominal pain)).

Some of this error may be due to differences between observers (when lumped together in the input to the computer program), but it also appears evident that out ability to subjectively evaluate such information has limited utility.

Assistance to Human Thought

Analytic vs sequential analysis

The human approach to analyzing problems requires two steps. First, all of the data are reviewed (history and physical examination) and an overall (tentative) picture is developed (the presumptive diagnosis), then a sequential plan is implemented for confirming the diagnosis and optimizing therapy.

Computer-implemented approaches have tended to emphasize the analytical, or overall view. There are several frequently applied techniques, at least squared error, clustering or Bayes' rule (Shortliffe *et al.*, 1979). An example of a researcher using this approach is the controlled study. Data gathering is global, and partial analysis is discouraged.

Yet the most promising approach to computer-assisted data evaluation appears to be the sequential approach, just now beginning to be widely applied. An example of a researcher using this example is the *play the winner rule*, which acquires and evaluates data sequentially. Each subsequent trial uses the previous technique if the previous result was the one desired. It is much faster than the controlled study when differences are clinically significant (a very practical point!) (Zelen, 1969).

Advantages of the sequential approach include: there is little to remember at each step, it is easier to see when the decision rules don't make sense, and it is easier to stop with diminishing returns.

I believe that this is one reason personal computer application among physicians presently is so heavily oriented to word processing: the attraction is not just the savings in time, but also the ability to *piecewise* refine a difficult text. The savings in time and mental anguish can be truly enormous!

Specific benefits

(1) Fewer measurements are required, reducing cost and effort.
(2) Measurements are more likely to be independent, increasing information.
(3) The implementation of a hierarchy for substituting measurements when the most desired are not available increases monitoring reliability.
(4) Measurements are more likely to be nearly optimized over the range of interest, because formal analysis is more likely to reveal (and emphasize) gaps in knowledge.
(5) It is possible to formally minimize loss of information with loss of any given measurement parameter. Ordinarily, the complexity of measurement leads to significant deficiencies with reference to this problem.
(6) The clinician is less likely to be misled by the inappropriate use of mathematical trnasformations which do not enhance information (as the Fourier transform or frequency analysis), since the results can be made more evident.
(7) Progress toward a widely accepted definition of *normal* vs *abnormal* will be accelerated; a practical consideration, since all therapy must be conditioned on definition of a point of reference.
(8) The optimal sequence of therapy will be made more evident. An example is the treatment of a failing heart in the order: arrhythmias, preload, afterload and contractility (ignoring short-term measures). Convergence on this approach has become widespread, despite much contrary advice in the literature.

Also Kirklin and Osborn have reported that performance of nursing personnel is significantly enhanced after a period of work with a computer monitoring system, presumably on the basis of consistent reinforcement of the use of proven clinical algorithms.

Summary

We can summarize these ideas:

(1) Originally, the computer was used to obtain more data, faster. Now, we emphasize better analysis of data, and the implementation of alternatives based on measurements.

(2) The progression from diagnostic measurement, to observation, to monitoring is a natural sequence, and to be desired. As our analysis grows more complex, multivariate analysis is an essential part of this progression.

(3) Multivariate analysis simplifies clinical evaluation, letting the user concentrate on the difficult and unresolved aspects.

(4) Multivariate analysis increases the rate of learning by making thought processes more explicit, and offering the possibility of both a simulator (as the "LINK" trainer for pilots), and assisted clinical management.

I agree with Komaroff:

> We see little benefit in the continuing freedom to collect and analyze medical data in a way which is generally ill-defined, variable, inaccurate and unmonitored. We agree with Francis Bacon: It is easier to evolve the truth from error than from confusion.
>
> A. L. Komaroff, September 1979

References

Hall, W. E. (1977). *Naval Research Reviews* **30**(4), 1–20, (p. 10).

Harman, H. H. (1967). "Modern Factor Analysis", University of Chicago Press, Chicago.

Komaroff, A. L. (1979). *Proc IEEE* **67**(9), 1196–1206.

Leaper, D. J., Horrocks, J. C., Staniland, J. R. and de Dombal, F. T. (1972). *Br. med. J.* **4**, 350–354.

Lipton, M. J., Ream, A. K. and Hyndman, B. H. *Circulation* **58**, 1190–1195.

Ream, A. K. (1978). *Science* **200**, 959–964.

Ream, A. K. (1980). *In* "Essential Noninvasive Monitoring in Anesthesia", (Gravenstein, J. S., Newbower, R. J., Ream, A. K. and Smith, N. T., Eds) pp. 53–74. Grune and Stratton, New York.

Ream, A. K., Silverberg, G. T., Corbin, S. D. *et al.* (1979). *Neurosurgery* **5**, 36–43.

Robinson, D. J., Ream, A. K., Corbin, S. D *et al.* (1977). *Proc. San Diego Biomed. Symp.* **16**, 233–242.

Schneider, A. J. L., Knoke, J. D. and Zollinger, R. M. *et al.* (1979). *Anesthesiology* **51**, 4–10.

Shoemaker, W. C. and Czer, L. S. (1979). *Crit. Care Med.* **7**, 424–429.

Shortliffe, E. H., Buchanon, B. G. and Feigenbaum, E. A. (1979). *Proc. IEEE* **67**(9), 1207–1224.

Strauer, B. E. (1979). *Am. J. Cardiol.* **44**, 730–740.

Warner, H. R., Toronto, A. F., Veasey, L. G. and Stephenson, R. (1961). *JAMA* **177**(3), 177–183.

Yelderman, M. L. and New, W. (1979). *Anesthesiology* **51**(3S), S210.

Zelen, M. (1969). *Am. Statistical Assoc. J.* **64**, 131–146.

Functional Monitoring: A Review of the Main Questions, Seen Through the Example of Electrocardiographic Ambulatory Monitoring

C. MARCHESI

Institute of Clinical Physiology, CNR, Pisa, Italy

Foreword

Long-term monitoring of vital signs, through biological signal instrument-based analysis, put analogous questions in all the fields of its clinical applications. However the specialized care units for continuous monitoring are much more characterized by the level of the required care and by the level of instability of the patient's condition, than by the particular pathology.

From a methodological point of view, the peculiar characteristic of this diagnostic tool is the possibility of obtaining dynamic information about the patient's condition. This goal determines the design choices as far as methods and techniques are concerned. In this short analysis the main questions arising from patient monitoring will be reviewed from the point of view of ECG ambulatory monitoring.

Ambulatory Monitoring Systems

State of the Art

The main operations involved in the ambulatory monitoring systems are shown in Fig. 1. For introduction and review see: Holter, 1961; Cox et al., 1972; Kennedy and Caralis, 1977; Stott, 1977; Thomas et al., 1979; Feldman, 1981; Wenger et al., 1981.

ECG sensing

The problem of a stable, noise-free, skin-electrode contact allowing reliable long-term monitoring (24–72 h) is still open. The solutions adopted are along the following lines: disposable adhesive electrode; active electrode; differential electrode (SMART); and aesophageal electrode.

The last two solutions are intended to improve the artifact immunity, but they require an extra channel on the portable recorder (McFee and Baule, 1972; Liberghien et al., 1976; Feldman et al., 1979; Collins et al., 1979; Wenger et al., 1981).

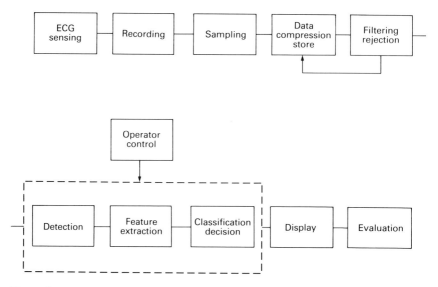

Figure 1.

Recorder

At the present time a number of recorders of acceptable quality are available, most of them of the cassette type. Still there is a lack of standardization of the specifications and requirements. One of the critical parameters, bandwidth, particularly important for ST-interval analysis, ranges from $0 \cdot 4$–$20\,$Hz to $0 \cdot 04$–$100\,$Hz (Feldman, 1981; Wenger, 1981).

Filtering and sampling

All the modern systems are built to process digital signals. This is because digital electronic techniques are becoming less and less expensive and a crucial problem of the older systems, the real time presentation of the signal, is made possible by the inexpensive present day digital memories (Lynn, 1971; Pryor, 1971; Berson *et al.*, 1977).

Data compression

When permanent storage of the 24-h sampled ECG is required, namely in computer-based systems, the capacity neeeded (10 to 40 Millions of Computer Words depending on sampling rate and number of channels) is still very expensive. Storage on the mag tape memory is a possible solution, but it does not allow the necessary fast access. Thus the use of fast access memories (disc units) requires the reversible compression of the original sampled signal, through encoding techniques. It is thus possible to reduce storage by a factor of three at the expenses of computer time (Ripley and Cox, 1976; Ruttimann and Pipberger, 1979; Pahlm *et al.*, 1979).

Operator control

This procedure is necessary to tailor the analysis procedures to the characteristics of the single patient. This operation is useful not only for limiting the effect of the inter-patient variability, but also to allow the flexibility necessary to obtain particular answers about the patient conditions. The method of interaction is strictly dependent on the particular system.

Detection of the QRS

Cited inter-patient variability, but also the large intra-patient variability during long-term observation, are still a challenge to the solution to this basic problem. A reliable QRS detector is an essential prerequisite to the subsequent analysis. The most successful solutions seem to derive from the adoption of algorithms able to self adjust to the patient's changing characteristics (McClelland and Arnold, 1976; Murthy and Rangaraj, 1979; Okada, 1979; Fraden and Neuman, 1980).

Feature extraction

The methods used to achieve a simplified description of the ECG cycle are grouped in three categories: empirical selection of traditional parameters (RR, QRS width, etc.); stylization of morphology (slopes and flat signal portions); and integral parameters, extracted through signal transforms.

The last method is the most promising because of its accuracy in the morphology description. This characteristic is particularly important when the system includes both rhythm and ST analysis (Cox *et al.*, 1969; Nygards *et al.*, 1975; Hamba and Tachibana, 1976; Temel and Linkens, 1978; Marchesi *et al.*, 1980a; Udupa and Murthy, 1980; Meffert *et al.*, 1980; Marvell and Kirk, 1980b).

Classification

Most procedures used fall into one of the following types: a priori (predetermined decision), and a posteriori (decision after classification).

The first group assumes a knowledge of the characteristics of the abnormal cycles. Thus whenever a cycle fits one predetermined class, it is labelled with that type of abnormality. The class attribution is made through logical functions or through a fixed template matching. The second group include methods of clustering the extracted features in "families" of abnormality, or using a self-learning template matching scheme. In both cases it is the observer's responsibility to label the determined class. As an alternative approach statistical modelling has been proposed, to assess rhythm diagnosis (Sibson, 1972; Swenne *et al.*, 1977; Gustafson *et al.*, 1978a; Hubelbank and Feldman, 1978; Udupa and Murthy, 1980; Marchesi *et al.*, 1980b).

Display

A convenient data presentation technique is a key concept in this long-term analysis. Infact, in spite of the reasonable accuracy of the state of the art systems, very often a visual validation is required during the analysis process or at the end (depending on the system characteristics).

Solutions adopted can be grouped:

(a) Hard copy
Very compact beat by beat presentation of all the 24-h ECG, or of part of it.
Very compact presentation of the main features of the ECG (histograms, time plots).
(b) CRT (cathode ray tube) screen
In place, synchronized presentation of running beats.
Page mode display of many cardiac cycles.

Dynamic – perspective – contour mode (Likoff and Pennock, 1972; Tyler, 1973; Cashman, 1977; Tyler and Mitchell, 1977; Biagini *et al.*, 1981; Mancini, *et al.*, 1981).

Evaluation

It is still a fundamental problem waiting for a convenient solution. The usual man–machine comparison can no longer be applied to the evaluation of the classification of about 100 000 beats per patient per day. Even the solution of the so-called annotated data base, while very accurate, is still far from a general practical solution because of a total lack of standardization in all the processes so far illustrated. Let us consider the controversies surrounding the opportunity of including ST analysis among system performances, to pick up only one question out of many others. Thus the trade off is now that many "reference institutes" are developing their own data base (Romhilt *et al.*, 1973; Ripley and Arthur, 1975; Frost, *et al.*, 1977; Schang and Pepine, 1977; Various Authors, 1977; Lustig *et al.*, 1978; Schoenberg *et al.*, 1979; Balasubramanian *et al.*, 1980; Jain *et al.*, 1980; Marvell, 1980a; Willems, 1980, Wenger *et al.*, 1981.)

Cost/benefit

The usual considerations are applicable. The difficulty, also in ambulatory monitoring, in defining the goals of health technology, is a limiting factor to define cost/benefit analysis procedures. A very interesting review on this matter is reported in Jurado *et al.*, 1977.

Available Systems

They can be grouped into three broad classes: hard wired, computer-based, dedicated, and computer-based, general purpose.

The claimed lack of standardization and the complexity of the operations required, make it clear that a synthesis about the various solutions adopted is very difficult. A possible unitary view point is the level of interaction required by the operator, which is an important practical limiting factor.

A list is presented, certainly not complete, grouping some of the available systems according to the interaction level required.

Level 1 – Totally operator dependent, through:
– hard copy   : EDWARDS (ELIMINATOR)
                                  AVIONICS (VIS-U SCAN)
                                 : IMC (QUICK SCAN)
– CRT, page   : AVIONICS (HEART SCREEN)
– CRT, dynamic contour   : REMCO (ETA LONG)

To this level belong also small portable units for recording on sampled basis (like CIRCADIAN from Reynolds).

Level 2 – Interaction in combination with automatic procedures:

- CAMBRIDGE Inst. (CAMSCAN)
- REYNOLDS (PATHFINDER)
- OXFORD Med. Sys. (MEDILOG 2)
- ICR (SCAN MASTER)
- AVIONICS (TREND SETTER)

Level 3 – Computer-based:

- Washington University System
- Stanford University System
- Cardio Data
- Dynagram
- CNR Clinical Physiology System
  (Nolle *et al.*, 1974; Lopes *et al.*, 1975; Grant *et al.*, 1976; Ripley and Cox, 1976; Sheppard and Hansmann, 1977; Hubelbank and Feldman, 1978; Biella *et al.*, 1979.)

Level 4 – Real time analysis on portable unit (development)

- MIT System
- MEDTRONIC System (announced)

Perspectives

The long-term final goal of the ambulatory monitoring technique is perhaps the real time processing of vital signs performed by the portable unit. This approach would solve all the present day complexity of the reduction of 100 000 cardiac cycles to a few episodes, made available to the cardiologist for fast final diagnosis. Moreover, transforming the simple signal registration into a true monitoring, it should be of immediate aid to the patient for early intervention. The achievement of such a goal should pass through the following steps:

- Establishment of standardized data bank to allow extensive evaluation of the analysis criteria.
- Monitoring of ECG plus other signals, because the ECG alone is not sufficient to assess reliable alarm conditions (Hill, 1976; Mark *et al.*, 1980; De Reggi *et al.*, 1981; Jirak *et al.*, 1981).

References

Balaubramanian, V., Lahiri, A., Green, H. L., Stott, F. C. and Raftery, E. B.. (1980). *Br. Heart J.* **44**, 419–425.

Berson, A. S., Ferguson, T. A., Batchlor, C. D., Dunn, R. A. and Pipberger, H. V. (1977). *Comput. Biomed. Res.* **10**, 605–616.

Biagini, A. L'Abbate, A. Carpeggiani, C. *et al.* (1981). Poor Detection Rate of Transient Electrocardiographic St-T Changes by Visual Monitoring in CCU, CNR Clinical Physiology Institute, Pisa (unpublished data).

Biella, M., Contini, C., Kraft, G., Marchesi, C., Mazzocca, G. F. and Taddei, A. (1979). *Comp. Cardiol.* IEEE Computer Society, 201–204.

Cashman, P. M. M. *J. med. Eng. Tech.* 20–28.

McClelland, K. M. and Arnold, J. M. (1976). *Comp. Cardiol.* IEEE Computer Society, 447–450.

Collins, S., Jenkins, J., Brown, D., Dean, R. and Arzbaecher, R. (1979). *Comp. Cardiol.* IEEE Computer Society, 189–192.

Cox, J. R., Fozzard, H. A., Nolle, F. M. and Oliver, G. C. (1969). "Computers in Biomedical Research", Vol. 3, (Stacy and Waxman, Eds), pp. 181–206. Academic Press, London and New York.

Cox, J. R., Nolle, F. M. and Arthur, R. M. (1972). *Proc. IEEE* **60**, 1137–1159.

De Reggi, A. S., Edelman, S., Roth, S. C., De Rossi, D., Dario, P., Marchesi, C., Trivella, M. G., Pedrini, F., Contini, C., De Reggi, A. S., Edelman, S. and Roth, S. (1981). *Comp. Cardiol. IEEE Computer Soc.*, 111–114.

McFee, R. and Baule, G. M. (1972). *Proc. IEEE*, **60**, 290–317.

Feldman, C. L. (1981). *In* "How to Evaluate a New Antiarrhythmic Drug", Martinus Nijhoff B. V., The Hague. (In press.)

Feldman, C. L., Hubelbank, M., Haffajee, C. I., Kotilainen, P. (1979). *Comp. Cardiol.* IEEE Computer Society, 285–288.

Fraden, J. and Neuman, M. R. (1980). *Med. biolog. Eng. Comp.* **18**, 125–132.

Frost, D. A., Yanowitz, F. G. and Pryor, T. A. (1977). *Am. J. Cardiol.* **39**, 538–587.

Grant, M. E., Camm, A. J. and Hanson, J. S. (1976). *J. Electrocardiol.* **9**, 351–356.

Gustafson, D. E., Willsky, A. S., Wang, J. Y., Lancaster, M. C. and Triebwasser, J. H. (1978a). *IEEE Trans biomed. Eng.* BME-**25**, 344–353.

Gustafson, D. E., Willsky, A. S., Wang, J. Y., Lancaster, M. C. and Triebwasser, J. H. (1978b). *IEEE Trans biomed. Eng.* BME-**25**, 353–361.

Hamba, S. and Tachibana, Y. (1976). *Electrical Eng. Japan* **96**, 111–117.

Hill, D. W. (1976). The development of the impedance cardiogram. A report prepared at the request of the commission of the European communities.

Holter, N. J. (1961). *Science* **134**, 1214–1220.

Hubelbank, M. and Feldman, C. L. (1978). *Med. Instr.* **12**, 324–326.

Jain, U., Rautaharju, P. M. and Horacek, B. M. (1980). *Comput. biomed. Res.* **13**, 132–141.

Jirak, T. L., Smith, R. and Benditt, D. G. (1981). A new ambulatory ECG Monitoring with pacemaker analysis capability. Presented at ISAM 81, Fourth Int. Symp. on Amb. Mon. GENT 1981 (F. D. Stett, E. Roftery, D. L. Clement, S. L. Wright, Eds), pp. 2–8.

Jurado, R. A., Fitzkee, H. L., De Alsa, R. A., Lukban, S. B., Litwak, R. S. and Osborn, J. J. (1977). *Circulation* **56**, 44–49.

Kennedy, H. L. and Caralis, D. G. (1977). *Ann. intern. Med.* **87**, 729–739.
Liberghien, J., Cornelis, J., Taevman, J., Steenhout, O. and Konreich, F. (1976). *J. biom. Eng.* 249–250.
Likoff, W. and Pennock, R. (1972). Detection and Analysis of Cardiac Dysrhythmias and Conduction Defects: Comparison of an Automated System with Visual Review of Monitor and Electromagnetic Tape. Div. of Cardiology, Hahnemann Medical College, Philadelphia. (Unpublished data, 1972.)
Lopes, M. G., Fitzgerald, J., Harrison, D. C., Fitzgerald, J., Harrison, D. C. and Scroeder, J. S. (1975). *Am. J. Cardiol.* **35**, 816–823.
Lustig, R., Cohen, S. I., Ransil, B. J. and Abelman, W. H. (1978). *Heart and Lung* **7**, 72–80.
Lynn, P. A., (1971). *Med. and biol. Eng.* **9**, 37–43.
Mancini, P., Taddei, A., Macerata, A. and Marchesi, C. (1981). *Proc. on Visual Psychophysics,* IEEE Computer Society, 1981, (in press).
Marchesi, C., Giovani, L. and Landucci, L. (1980a). *Computer applications in Medical Care,* IEEE Computer Society, 1128–1132.
Marchesi, C., Varanini, M. and Guidi, M. (1980b). *Comp. Cardiol.* IEEE Computer Society, 315–318.
Mark, R. G., Moody, G., Schulter, P., Oslon, W. and Peterson, S. (1980). Proc. on "Changes in health care instrumentation due to microprocessor technology", IFIP 1980 (in press).
Marvell, C. J. and Kirk, D. L. (1980a). *J. biomed. Eng.* **2**, 61–64.
Marvell, C. J. and Kirk, D. L. (1980b). *J. biomed. Eng.* **2**, 216–220.
Meffert, B. Schubert, D. Lazarus, T., Poll, R. and Henssge, R. (1980). New and known methods of the application of Transforms to quasi periodic Biomedical Signals. IEEE 1980, CH 1538-8/80/pp. 336–341.
Murthy, I. S. N. and Rangaraj, M. R. (1979). *IEEE Trans biomed. Eng.* BME-**26**, 409422.
Nolle, F. M., Oliver, G. C., Kleiger, R., Cox, J. R., Clark, K. W. and Ambos, H. D. (1974). *Comp. Cardiol.* IEEE Computer Society, 37–42.
Nygards, M. E., Blomqvist, P. Hulting, J., Matell, G. and Wigertz, O. (1975). *Comp. Cardiol.* IEEE Computer Society, 193–194.
Okada, M. (1979). *IEEE Trans biomed. Eng.* BME-**26**, 700–703.
Pahlm, O., Borjesson, P. O. and Werner, O. (1979). *Comp. Prog. Biomed.* 293–300.
Pryor, T. A. (1971). *Comp. biomed. Res.* **4**, 542–547.
Ripley, K. L. and Arthur, R. M. (1975). *Comp. Cardiol.* IEEE Computer Society, 27–32.
Ripley, K. L. and Cox, J. R. (1976). *Comp. Cardiol.* IEEE Computer Society, 439–445.
Romhilt, D. W., Bloomfield, S. S., Chou, T. C., Bloomfield, S. S., Chon, T. C. and Fowler, N. O. (1973). *Am. J. Cardiol.* **31**, 457–461.
Ruttimann, U. E. and Pipberger, H. V. (1979). *IEEE Trans biomed. Eng.* BME-**26**, 613–623.
Schang, S. J. and Pepine, C. J. (1977). *Am. J. Cardiol.* **39**, 396–402.
Schoenberg, A. A., Grahn, A. R. and Booth, H. E. (1979). *Comp. Cardiol.* IEEE Computer Society, 289–291.
Sheppard, J. J. and Hansmann, D. R. (1977). *Comp. Cardiol.* IEEE Computer Society, 211–219.
Sibson, R. (1972). *Comp. J.* **16**, 30–34.
Stott, F. D. (1977). *Br. J. clin. Equip.* 61–68.

Swenne, C. A., van Bemmel, J. H., Relik, F. M. and Versteeg, B. (1977). *IEEE Trans biomed. Eng.* 63–71.

Temel, Z. B. and Linkens, D. A. (1978). *Med. and biol. Eng. and Comp.* 188–194.

Thomas, L. J., Clark, K. W., Mead, C. N., Ripley, K. L., Spenner, B. F. and Oliver, G. C. (1979). *Proc. IEEE* **67**, 1322–1335.

Tyler, C. W. (1973). *J. Physiol.* **228**, 637–647.

Tyler, C. W. and Mitchell, D. E. (1977). *Vision. Res.* **17**, 83–88.

Udupa, J. K. and Murthy, I. S. N. (1980). *IEEE Trans. biomed. Eng.* BME-**27**, 370–375.

Various Authors (1977). "Optimal Electrocardiography". Tenth Bethesda Conference. *Am. J. Cardiol.* **41**, 113–193.

Wenger, N. K., Mock, M. and Ringquist, I. (Eds) (1981). Ambulatory Electrocardiographic Recording. Year Book, Medical Pub., 1981.

Willems, J. L. (1980). *Comp. and biom. Res.* **13**, 120–131.

Non-Invasive Monitoring of Normalized Cardiac Output and Left Ventricular Function by A Convenient Doppler Technique

L. H. LIGHT[1], G. CROSS[1],
E. MOSCARELLI[2], M. PAOLETTI[2],
A. DISTANTE[2] and A. MEARNS[3]

[1] Clinical Research Centre, Harrow,
Middlesex, UK; [2] Institute of Clinical
Physiology, CNR and Institute of Patologia
Medica, University of Pisa, Pisa, Italy;
[3] Royal Infirmary, Bradford 9, UK

None of the traditional haemodynamic measurements, such as blood pressure, central venous pressure or limb-core temperature difference, give unambiguous or immediate information on central blood flow, yet it is this flow which often determines a patient's chances of survival and the incidence of complications, such as venous thrombosis, pulmonary embolism and graft blockage. Unfortunately, because of the variability of individual response, measures designed to raise cardiac output can be safety employed only with flow-oriented haemodynamic monitoring. In coronary care, for example, this has hitherto confined the use of such interventions to the minority of

Frontiers Cardiol. for the 80s.
0-12-220680-0

patients who are so ill as to justify the risk, trouble and expense of catheter measurements.

A convenient non-invasive technique – Transcutaneous Aortovelography (Light and Cross, 1972) – is now available, which not only gives the information on flow required to optimize cardiac output, but also gives further data on left ventricular function by allowing the global manner of ejection to be visualized. It is a continuous wave Doppler technique (Cross and Light, 1974) developed to give trustworthy recordings of "mainstream" aortic flow velocity with some latitude in the aim of the ultrasound beam, which is directed from the supra-sternal notch towards the transverse aorta*. (The angle of intersection between beam and flow there will normally be less than 26°. For this special case, angular tolerance is high and actual velocities may be determined without knowledge of the exact angle to within ± 5% by the Doppler equation.)

The velocity recorded reflects aortic flow and is thus responsive to the many factors (including inotropic state, myocardial lesions and circulating blood volume) which determine left ventricular function as well as to valve defects. While the Transcutaneous Aortovelograph was primarily designed for ease of bedside use by relatively unskilled personnel, its applications include haemodynamic research and teaching of the pathophysiology of left ventricular function and circulatory regulation. We have summarized the results of experience gained in several machine-years of scientific and clinical trials.

Quantitative Information on Changes in Cardiac Output

Instantaneous mainstream blood velocity is quantitatively indicated by the outline of darkened complexes, which represent in grey scale the time-varying spectrum of the Doppler shifts back-scattered by the moving blood. Providing that sharp outlines are obtained (indicating that mainstream flow was indeed insonated), the measurement has proved reproducible (7% s.d.) (Fraser et al., 1976), and free of the vagaries sometimes shown by invasive indicator-dilution techniques. The area under the outline should be closely proportional to *stroke volume* in any one subject. Comparisons with invasive cardiac output measurements have shown this proportionality to be within 9–13% in serial physiological and clinical studies (Sequeira et al., 1976; Light et al., 1979; Distante et al., 1980). These trials have covered a wide range of pathology, interventions and depression/elevation of cardiac output. (Table 1). We may therefore conclude that the accuracy with which TAV measures *changes in cardiac output* is of the same order as that of invasive techniques.

* This is preferable as a measurement site to the ascending aorta for a number of reasons: ease of making the measurement, negligible sensitivity to asymmetric ejection patterns in left ventricular dyskinaesia, reduced incidence of flow disturbances and absence of discomfort for the patient.

Table 1   Quantitative studies of TAV

TRIAL	DEVIATION from exact agreement or proportionality (s.d. as % of mean)	TOTAL RANGE COVERED	TRIAL CENTRES
REPRODUCIBILITY – (4 trials) Within-observer agreement Between-observer agreement	6·6 7·3	42 subjects, aged 3–67 years 14 observers, including 8 inexperienced	Brompton Hosp./CRC Bristol Royal Infirmary Sefton Gen. Hosp. Liverpool
Proportionality against acetylene CARDIAC OUTPUT during exercise	11	CO = 7–22 litres/min (13 normal/athl. subjects)	Field Physiol. Lab. NIMR
Proportionality against intra-aortic BLOOD VELOCITY measurement	6	V_{pk} = 48 to 120 cm/s (8 myocard. isch. patients)	Northwick Park Hosp./CRC
Proportionality against green dye measurement of STROKE VOLUME	13	SV = 20 to 160 ml (20 myocard. isch. patients)	Northwick Park Hosp./CRC
Proportionality against thermodilution CARDIAC OUTPUT (reproducibility = 5% s.d.)	9.7	CO = 2·5 to 10 litres/min (14 critically ill patients)	Whipps Cross Hosp. (ITU)
Proportionality against thermodilution CARDIAC OUTPUT	12	CO = 2·7 to 9 litres/min (5 cardiomyop. patients)	Fisiol. Clinica, CNR Pisa, Italy

Optimization of Therapy

Transcutaneous Aortovelography has been used clinically to assess patients' circulatory response to a variety of interventions in coronary care, intensive therapy, pacemaker clinics and emergency admissions. The feedback obtained on percentage change in cardiac output is more immediate and sensitive than that given by less direct measurements and allows therapy to be adapted to the individual (Fig. 1). Optima in drug dosage, ventilator pressures, circulating blood volume, pacing rate (Fig. 2) and balloon pump settings can thus be found in the light of the patient's response (Hanson and Buchthal, 1977; Light et al., 1979). The need for a change in management strategy may also become evident from failure to obtain a positive response.

Biological Normalization of Aortic Velocities – Indication of Circulatory Depression

Absolute values of cardiac output are never required for clinical purposes. What is required instead, (but rarely obtainable) is the degree of circulatory depression – the ratio of the patient's present cardiac output to *his* normal resting value (Light, 1980). We have followed up clinical reports that TAV recordings of newly admitted patients seemed to give this information. Evidence was indeed found that blood velocities (particularly peak velocity) are normalized during childhood development so that the subject's normal resting cardiac output – be it large or small – is carried within the same, fairly narrow range of mainstream velocities. Thus transcutaneous measurement of blood velocity in normal children aged $\frac{1}{2}$–12 years showed no significant variation in peak velocity with age, though cardiac output must have increased by $> 200\%$. The inter-subject spreads were also relatively low ($\sim 14\%$ s.d.). We may therefore conclude that vascular cross-sectional area is sensitively and continuously regulated so as to carry resting cardiac output with constant peak velocity (Light, 1978). (Evidence has been summarized to suggest that the agent responsible for this biological normalization of blood velocity is the transient flow disturbance (Light et al., 1979) of the physiological murmur.) As this adaptive capability is lost in adult life, even chronic deviations from the individual's normal resting cardiac output are then apparent from deviations in his measured blood velocity from the normal range. The appropriate index for assessing abnormality in adults' cardiac output is time-averaged velocity, which is highly correlated with peak velocity and has a spread of $\sim 20\%$ s.d. in young adults. A gradual fall-off in normal velocities with age during adult life ($\sim 1\%$/year) must however be borne in mind when degree of flow abnormality is assessed from the abnormality of observed blood velocity. Note that Doppler velocity measurements on their own suffice for quantitation of the degree of cardiac output depression – neither aortic cross-section nor absolute cardiac output

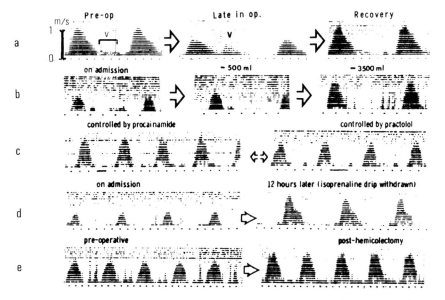

Figure 1. Serial TAV recordings of aortic blood velocity from five patients showing the response of stroke volume (area of complex) and manner of left ventricular ejection (shape of complex) to interventions. The outline of the darkened areas indicates the time-course of mainstream aortic blood velocity in m/s. The pre-operative recording in patient (a) is typical of the normal aortic velocity pattern. The vertical scale is common to all recordings. Dots along the horizontal zero-velocity axis mark 100 ms time intervals. (a) Deep (hypotensive) halothane anaesthesia: Stroke volume and early systolic acceleration are greatly depressed by the anaesthetic. Unlike acute heart failure, the "heart failure" thus induced is not accompanied by waveform evidence of sympathetic stimulation (Light, 1976). The venous signal (marked "V"), which happened to be co-recorded, is seen to change during the period of cardiac depression from the normal low-velocity, long-duration flow pattern to one peaking in early diastole. (b) Acute myocardial infarct with volume overload: Cautious successive withdrawals of fluid under TAV monitoring raised stroke volume considerably in this patient. (This example illustrates the desirability of being able to fit the treatment to the individual in the light of his response.) (c) Ventricular Tachyarrhythmia: A patient's differing response to the minimum effective dose of two anti-arrhythmic agents is evident from differences in acceleration (up-slope), peak velocity, stroke volume and heart rate. (d) Barbiturate Overdose: Initial and final recordings. The rate of isoprenaline infusion was titrated against circulatory response throughout the resuscitation period. (e) Septic shock: Haemodynamic deterioration with characteristically abnormal waveform was reversed by major surgery. Characteristic waveform abnormalities are also seen in aortic stenosis (sustained turbulence), aortic regurgitation (reverse flow assessable on a bidirectional range), non-obstructive cardiomyopathy (shift of peak towards the right), hypertrophic obstructive cardiomyopathy (dual peaks) and cardiac tamponade (pronounced respiratory modulation of stroke volume). Recordings by courtesy of Dr Gillian Hanson, ITU, Whipps Cross Hospital and Dr D. C. White, Anaesthetics Department, Northwick Park Hospital.

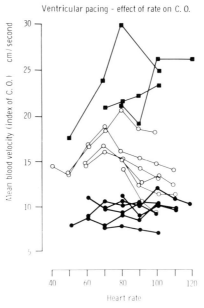

Figure 2.   Effect of pacing rate on mean blood velocity (the TAV index of cardiac output) in patients with implanted programmable pacemakers. Optimum settings can thus be found for individual patients. The unexpectedly clear separation of patients' responses into "peaked" and "flat", with all the latter having mean blood velocities < 12 cm/s, incidentally confirms that this variable provides a useful quantitative index of the degree of depression of cardiac output (which in this group of patients is due to – and reflects – the degree of left ventricular dysfunction). Recordings by Drs E. Moscarelli, M. Paoletti and C. Contini, Fisiologica Clinica, CNR and Institute of Patologia Medica, University of Pisa, Pisa, Italy.

being required for this clinical application. Velocity values also suffice to communicate results and to derive indices of peripheral resistance, etc. (Mowat *et al.*, 1983).

Waveform Information

Blood-flow velocity in the aortic arch closely reflects that of volumetric flow across the aortic valve and thus the global time-course of left ventricular ejection. As such, it is influenced by myocardial contractile ability, the coordination of myocardial contraction, stimulant and depressant effects on the myocardium and filling/load conditions. Nevertheless, the complete waveform gives so much information that interpretation has not proved difficult (Light *et al.*, 1979). Amongst the conditions with characteristic waveforms are hypovolaemia and septic shock. Figure 1 shows some waveforms encountered in intensive/coronary care and the response to interventions. While much work on the characterization of waveforms remains to be done, it is clear that instantaneous blood velocity recordings by TAV give diagnostic clues to the aetiology of shock, allow reduced myocardial capability to be recognized in spite of high sympathetic drive, and show the effect of interventions on contractile state as well as on stroke volume (Light *et al.*, 1979).

Other Clinical Applications

Good correlation ($r = 0·95$) was found between *% aortic regurgitation* and the ratio of retrograde to forward velocities (Light *et al.*, 1979). (Reverse flow is recordable on the bi-directional range on the instrument.) Quantitation is however reliable only in moderate and severe regurgitation. Blood velocity in the pulmonary artery, which in children is also measurable by TAV, was found to be raised above aortic in septal defects whenever O_2 saturation studies showed shunts to be $> 2:1$. Transcutaneous Aortovelography also provides a quick means of verifying the source of murmurs, as periods of disturbed flow are indicated by irregularities of outline (Light *et al.*, 1979).

Limitations

Transcutaneous access proved possible in 95% of a working population, but an oesophageal approach is often required in the presence of hyper-inflated lungs or surgical emphysema. Quantitation is possible only when a smooth outline over much of systole shows that flow is predominantly laminar.

For the sake of excluding artefacts etc., quantitative evaluation of the recordings is carried out off-line. A dedicated digitizer–microprocessor conveniently allows this to be done, and provides a printed summary of the haemodynamic and waveform information in a form suitable for insertion in the patient notes.

Conclusion

Central blood flow is the prime variable in the circulation, but has hitherto been measurable only by relatively demanding invasive techniques which are restricted to short-term use. In contrast, Transcutaneous Aortovelography gives the various flow-orientated items of information required in cardiology, intensive care, emergency medicine and anaesthesia in a safe and patient-acceptable manner, and is usable from the moment of admission to long-term follow-up. The manner and degree to which TAV satisfies these requirements in initial assessment and in patient management are summarized in Table 2. In particular, it allows both changes in cardiac output and its degree of depression to be quantitated in adults.

Table 2. Quantitative information of the central circulation

	Clinical requirement	Defined/indicated by	TAV indicator	Accuracy of TAV indicator
Initial assessment	Degree of circulatory depression	$\dfrac{\text{Patient's CO}}{\text{Patient's normal CO}}$	$\dfrac{\text{Patient's } V_{av}}{\text{Normal } V_{av} \text{ for patient's age}}$	Useful[a]
	Global left ventricular function	Outflow waveform	Aortic velocity waveform	Useful[a]
Patient Management	Improvement in cardiac output	$\dfrac{\text{New CO}}{\text{Previous CO}}$	$\dfrac{\text{New } V_{av}}{\text{Previous } V_{av}}$	Remarkably good
	Change in left ventricular function	Change in waveform	Change in waveform indices	Useful[a]
Specific defects	Regurgitant fraction	$\dfrac{\text{Regurgitant SV}}{\text{Ejected SV}}$	$\dfrac{\text{Area under retrograde velocity}}{\text{Area under forward velocity}}$	Accurate if >35%
	Severity of left-to-right shunt	$\dfrac{\text{Pulmonary artery flow}}{\text{Aortic flow}}$	$\dfrac{\text{Pulmonary artery } V_{av}}{\text{Aortic } V_{av}}$	Ratio > 1 in significant shunts only

[a] Useful denotes that the TAV derived information has been found of practical value by senior and less experienced clinicians alike, but that quantitative evaluation is hampered by lack of appropriate yardsticks.
(CO = cardiac output; SV = stroke volume; V_{av} = time average of recorded aortic blood velocity.)

Clinicians and para-medical staff proved capable of obtaining adequate signals on the great majority of patients after some two hours' beside tuition. The diagnostic information given neatly complements that readily gathered by echocardiography, while TAV's speed (typ. 1 min), simplicity of use and mobility fit it for routine monitoring of pump function in post-operative/coronary care and emergency resuscitation.

We conclude that Transcutaneous Aortovelography offers a convenient non-invasive tool which gives reliable and usefully accurate data on left ventricular function and cardiac output over a wide variety of circumstances. The full importance of this extension in our cardiovascular measurement capability cannot, however, be assessed yet, as virtually every imaginative study with the new tool is producing something of clinical or fundamental interest.

Acknowledgements

We thank the many clinicians who have contributed to the evaluation of Transcutaneous Aortovelography and Muirhead Medical Products, London, for further development of the instrument.

References

Cross, G. and Light, L. H. (1974). *Biomed. Eng.* **9**, 464–471.
Distante, A., Moscarelli, E., Rovai, D. and L'Abbate, A. (1980). *J. nucl. Med. all. Sci.* **24**, 171–175.
Fraser, C. B., Light, L. H., Shinebourne, E. A., Buchthal, A., Healy, M. J. R. and Beardshaw, J. A. (1976). *Eur. J. Cardiol.* **4**, 181–189.
Hanson, G. C. and Buchthal, A. (1977). *In* "Non-invasive Clinical Measurement", (D. E. M. Taylor and J. Whammond, Eds) p. 32. Pitman Medical, London.
Light, L. H. (1976). *Br. Heart J.* **38**, 434–442.
Light, L. H. (1978). *J. Physiol.* **285**, 17–18 P.
Light, L. H. (1980). *Br. J. clin. Equipm.* **5**, 240.
Light, L. H. and Cross, G. (1972). *In* "Blood Flow Measurements", (C. Roberts, Ed.), p. 60. Sector Publishing, London.
Light, L. H., Sequeira, R. F., Cross, G., Bilton, A. and Hanson, G. C. (1979). *J. nucl. Med. all. Sci.* **23**, 137–144.
Mowat, D. H. R., Haites, N. E. and Rawles, J. M. (1983). *cardiovasc. Res.* **17**, 75–80.
Sequeira, R. F., Light, L. H., Cross, G. and Raftery, E. B. (1976). *Br. Heart J.* **38**, 443–452.

Echo and Pulsed Doppler Ultrasound Applied to Carotid Artery Disease

D. J. PHILLIPS and
D. E. STRANDNESS Jr

Department of Surgery, University of
Washington, Seattle, Washington, USA

In the Department of Surgery at the University of Washington, we have been using ultrasound in a research setting for the assessment of atherosclerotic disease in the carotid arterial system. This occlusive disease tends to be localized in the carotid bifurcation and its accessability to both surgical intervention and direct diagnostic testing make this site highly important from a clinical standpoint. While diagnostic tests to date, either direct or indirect, can be used to detect disease greater than 50% diameter reduction, our goals are to detect and quantify disease states less than 50% diameter reduction; and secondly, to distinguish high grade lesions from total occlusion. Significantly, once total occlusion is reached, surgical intervention for plaque removal is no longer possible. With respect to the first goal mentioned, a retrospective study has shown that people with either transient ischaemic attacks (TIA) or strokes were just as likely to have disease in the less than 50% diameter reduction category as in the greater than 50% category (Thiele et al., 1980). It is currently believed that at least 70% of patients with TIAs or strokes have them secondary to emboli which arise from ulcerated plaques and not due to a reduction in hemispheric blood flow from high grade stenoses.

Patient risk associated with arteriography and problems associated with arteriogram interpretation (Chikos *et al.*, in press) have provided the incentive to find alternative non-invasive diagnostic methods. Ultrasound is attractive because of its strong interaction with tissues coupled with its non-invasive and non-destructive nature. Repetitive studies can be performed without patient risk. At the University of Washington we have had considerable success with an approach that combines pulse echo imagining with pulsed Doppler ultrasound (Phillips *et al.*, 1980). Basically, we use pulse echo to define the blood vessel location and anatomy and the pulsed Doppler is used to acquire blood flow velocity information at specific arterial sites. The degree of stenosis is then determined by analysis of the velocity waveform.

The combined echo–Doppler system currently used at our institution is commercially available and incorporates many of the features of earlier University research prototypes. Referring to Fig. 1, in the pulse echo mode, a real time image of anatomical structure within 4 cm of the skin surface is displayed. The real time capability permits the operator to rapidly survey vessels and establish spatial relationships of the local anatomy. Once an

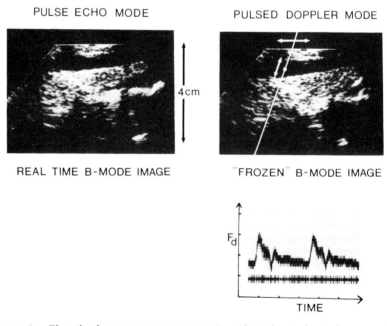

Figure 1. The duplex scanner operates in either the pulse echo or pulsed Doppler mode. The pulse echo mode provides a real time image of soft tissue interfaces within 4 cm of the skin surface. While holding the scan head still, the system switched to the pulsed Doppler mode. A stored or "frozen" image is used as an anatomical road map for sample volume placement. The pulsed Doppler signal is frequency analysed and recorded in a grey scale format for analysis and documentation.

image of a vessel of interest is acquired, the scan head is held still and the system is switched to the pulsed Doppler mode. The last image generated is "frozen" electronically and displayed as a reference for sample volume placement. The spatial region over which velocities are detected is called the "sample volume" and can be positioned as desired by the operator. The white line across the image defines the Doppler orientation while the bright dot along that line defines the sample volume location. The white arrows show that the operator has control over sample volume location, both left to right, and in depth along the transducer axis. In this way, any site within the image can be examined for the presence of flow. If the scan head or patient moves, it is easy to switch back and forth between modes in order to insure desired sample volume placement. The important diagnostic information found to date, is contained in the display of Doppler frequency, F_d, vs time. The Doppler frequencies correspond to the distribution of red blood cell velocities within the sample volume and can be displayed in a grey scale format.

Figure 2 illustrates the important features of the velocity waveform that we find both interesting and meaningful. Normally, in large peripheral arteries the velocity profile is blunt, with velocity gradients near the vessel wall, since flow must go to zero at this boundary. With the sample volume placed at mid-stream, flow is laminar and the velocity vectors are uniform. Because of the narrow range of velocities in the sample volume the Doppler waveform at this site exhibits a corresponding, narrow range of frequencies. This is shown in the velocity tracing above, with the relatively narrow band of Doppler frequencies, F_d, plotted as a function of time for two cardiac cycles. With disease present, the following observations are made. In moderate disease states the velocity vectors are neither uniform nor laminar. A wider distribution of velocities occurs within the sample volume, as reflected by the increased range of Doppler frequencies displayed in the velocity waveform. This is called spectral broadening. With greater diameter reduction, an increase in peak velocity is apparent. These increased velocities may be accompanied with vortex and eddy formations, resulting from high shear rates generated by the narrowed segment. The latter is easily recognized by increased Doppler frequencies concurrent with spectral broadening. The features of peak velocity and spectral broadening are the key features that we have found diagnostic to date.

Since disease classification is based primarily upon analysis of the velocity waveform, considerable care is taken to insure that the data are recorded properly. A block diagram of the pulsed Doppler unit is shown in Fig. 3. The audio output of the Doppler signal is useful to the operator as direct feedback for qualitative assessment of the signal. Although lesions greater than 50% diameter reduction can be detected audibly by the increased frequencies, lesser amounts of disease require frequency analysis in order to detect spectral broadening in the velocity waveform. In our system, the Doppler waveform is broken down into fundamental frequency components by Fourier analysis. Spectra of amplitude vs frequency are sent to a grey

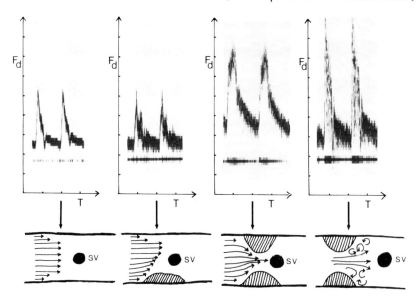

VELOCITY WAVEFORMS WITH PROPOSED MODELS(sv:sample volume)

Figure 2. Frequency analysed pulsed Doppler waveforms are shown in grey scale format along with schematic representations of the flow velocity fields in a carotid blood vessel. The sample volume is placed at centre stream locations in each case. Illustrated from left to right are: centrestream laminar, uniform flow velocities associated with the relatively blunt profile in a carotid artery; velocity gradients in centrestream are produced by minimal disease and noted by increased spectral broadening in the deceleration phase of systole; increased Doppler frequencies are seen at the site of a stenosis; distal to the stenosis increased Doppler frequencies can be seen alongwith increased spectral broadening due to post-stenotic velocity gradients and vortices.

scale recorder where the amplitudes are displayed as a function of time and frequency. This is the directional velocity waveform that is used in the assessment of disease.

The velocity waveforms are acquired from centrestream sites within the artery. In addition, the Doppler angle is monitored and kept as close to 60° as possible. This is important as a normalization factor for direct comparison of velocity waveforms acquired at other anatomical sites and in serial studies.

After recording, the velocity waveforms are analyzed and displayed in grey scale format for visual classification into one of five categories designated A to E. These categories correspond to specific internal carotid arterial states as defined by arteriography.

The A category represents the normal internal carotid. Specific features of this category include: a peak systolic frequency less than 2 KHz, a

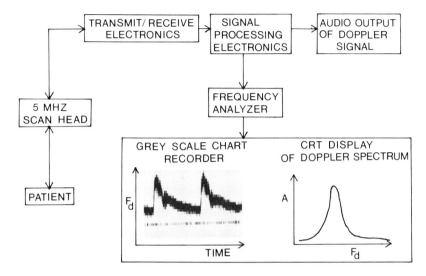

PULSED DOPPLER BLOCK DIAGRAM

Figure 3.   A block diagram is shown for the pulsed Doppler part of the duplex scanner. Following acquisition, the pulsed Doppler signal is sent to speakers for audio interpretation. However, the Doppler signal is also sent to a frequency analyser in order to appreciate subtle changes in frequency content of the Doppler signal. Both the two dimensional display of Amplitude vs Time and the three dimensional display of Doppler Frequency vs Amplitude vs Time are useful in analysis.

relatively narrow band of frequencies throughout the cardiac cycle and especially during systole, and a non-zero diastolic frequency consistent with the low distal impedance of the brain.

The B category is consistent with less than 10% diameter reduction as determined by arteriography. The difference between this, and the normal or A category is a small, but definite amount of spectral broadening noted during systole. The peak velocity and level of diastolic flow remain similar to that of the A category.

The C category designates disease in the 10–49% diameter reduction range. The outstanding feature associated with this category is increased spectral broadening which fills in the velocity waveform. Peak systolic velocities remain near the 2 kHz level.

The D category is consistent with a 50–99% diameter reduction and is recognized by increased peak velocities above 2 kHz with significant amounts of spectral broadening.

The E category is that of total occlusion and is applied when no flow velocities can be detected with the sample volume clearly positioned within the vessel.

Although our numbers are small, we have had considerable success when comparing this method with arteriography (Fell *et al.*, 1981).

Future Efforts Include

(1) Continuation of the methods presented in order to establish our accuracy.
(2) Application of ensemble averaging and computer pattern recognition techniques (Greene *et al.*, 1982) to the velocity waveforms. This objective approach will allow us to look at clinical questions related to disease progression and its natural course.
(3) Comparison of velocity waveforms along a specific artery as well as bilaterally. These efforts will aid in the understanding of why the waveforms look the way they do. There are few independent methods through which haemodynamic information can be obtained in the human carotid system.
(4) Instrument application and evaluation of new techniques. Improvements in waveform signal analysis and new devices related to flow imagining will become available and are potentially useful diagnostic methods (Eyer *et al.*, 1981; Stevenson *et al.*, 1981).

Ultrasound methods used for assessment of atherosclerotic disease will only increase in popularity and future use. The complement of pulsed Doppler to conventional imaging techniques permits important functional aspects of an arterial segment to be examined and will continue to play an important role in the clinical diagnosis and management of atherosclerotic disease.

Acknowledgements

The work outlined here is the result of a group effort of engineers, clinicians and technicians over a period of many years. The importance of a "group effort" cannot be underestimated in our experience. This work is supported by National Institutes of Health grant number HL-20898.

References

Chikos, P. M., Fischer, L., Hirsch, J. H., Harley, J. D., Thiele, B. L. and Strandness, D. E., Jr *Stroke* (in press).
Eyer, M. K., Brandestini, M. A., Phillips, D. J. and Baker, D. W. (1981). *Ultrasound Med. Biol.* **7**, 21.

Fell, G., Phillips, D. J., Chikos, P. M., Harley, J. D., Thiele, B. L. and Strandness, D. E. Jr (1981). *Circulation* **64**, 1191.

Greene, F. M., Beach, K., Strandness, D. E. Jr, Fell, G. and Phillips, D. J. (1982). A Computer Based Pattern Recognition Approach to Quantification of Carotid Arterial Disease Using Pulsed Doppler Ultrasound. *Ultrasound Med. Biol.* **8**, 161.

Phillips, D. J., Powers, J. E., Eyer, M. K., Blackshear, W. M. Jr Strandness, D. E. Jr and Baker, D. W. (1980). *Ultrasound Med. Biol.* **6**, 205.

Stevenson, G. J., Kawabori, I. and Brandestini, M. A. (1981). "Echocardiology" (Rijsterborgh, H., Ed.) pp. 399. Martinus Nijoff, The Hague.

Thiele, B. L., Young, J. V., Chikos, P. M., Hirsch, J. H. and Strandness, D. E., Jr. (1980). *Neurology* **30**, 1041.

A Non-Invasive Approach to Detect Transient Mechanical Changes Due To Acute Myocardial Ischaemia in Man: Role of M-mode and Two-dimensional Echocardiography*

A. DISTANTE[1], D. ROVAI[2],
E. PICANO[1], C. PALOMBO[1],
E. MOSCARELLI[2],
M. A. MORALES[2], F. SABINO[1],
L. LANDINI[1], C. MICHELASSI[1],
A. BENASSI[1], G. VALLI[1]
and A. L'ABBATE[1]

[1] Institute of Clinical Physiology, CNR and Institute of Patologia Medica, University of Pisa, Pisa, Italy; and [2] Associazione per la Ricerca Medica, Pisa, Italy

* This work has been partially supported by CNR, Project for Biomedical Technology, Subproject BIOI 4, Contracts n. 204121/86/81787 – 212310/86/8002395 – 104520/86/8002396 – 102060/86/8002397.

Introduction

Ichaemic heart disease was one of the earliest targets of diagnostic echography: in a pioneering study, Wild *et al.* (1957) showed the possibility to distinguish, by means of a rudimental "echoscope", areas of acute infarction from normal segment in the same excised heart. Nevertheless ischaemic heart disease remained for many years on the fringes of the main interest in diagnostic ultrasound (only 12 pages in the first edition of Feigenbaum's classical textbook, 1972).

In time, the urge to exploit a technique as enriching as echocardiography for the study of ischaemic heart disease promoted a progressive growth of interest and observations as documented by the extension of relative chapters and references in subsequent editions of Feigenbaum's (1981) textbooks (35 pages in the second edition and 44 pages in the third one, 1981). The main goal in this field has been represented by the detection of global or regional left ventricular asinergies caused by ischaemia; thus, acute and chronic infarction with relative complications entered the domain of clinical ultrasonic diagnosis. Today's "echo-frontiers" stop, however, before detection of acute transient ischaemia: such a pathological model – which is surrounded by great interest from both the physiopathological and clinical points of view – has remained until now almost neglected by clinical echocardiography and is only marginally discussed in the literature in the form of sporadic case reports (Widlansky *et al.*, 1975; Gerson *et al.*, 1979).

Experimental studies (Kerber *et al.*, 1976, 1979) have shown that echo techniques are capable of detecting beat by beat changes in cardiac mechanics caused by coronary occlusion, just a few seconds after ligation of the vessel.

Clinical studies (Maseri *et al.*, 1978; Maseri, 1980) proved that episodes of angina at rest with ST-segment elevation or pseudonormalization of a basally negative T wave (Parodi *et al.*, 1981) are caused by a sudden reduction in coronary blood supply, thus resembling the "stop flow" pattern of experimental acute ischaemia.

Thus, it appears reasonable to figure out that echocardiographic techniques might be of some use in the clinical study of angina at rest. Moving from these premises, we continuously recorded by M-mode and two-dimensional echocardiography episodes of transient myocardial ischaemia at rest, with the purpose of studying mechanical changes induced by ischaemia and also of assessing the relationships between these changes and symptomatic, electrocardiographic and haemodynamic markers of ischaemia. The present work represents, therefore, a small contribution in order to displace "a little bit farther" today's echo frontiers in coronary artery disease, in view of a possible clinical role of this technique in angina pectoris at rest.

Materials and Methods

Characteristics of the Patients

Among the population admitted to the Coronary Care Unit because of frequent episodes of angina at rest, we selected 34 patients in whom a continuous M-mode and/or B-mode (two-dimensional) echocardiogram could be recorded during an episode of myocardial ischaemia at rest (spontaneous or induced by ergonovine maleate) with ST-segment elevation or pseudonormalization of basally negative T wave.

Indirect evidence of transient primary reduction in coronary blood flow (Maseri *et al.*, 1978; Maseri, 1980) was reached in all patients by the following findings: *clinical* (anginal attacks at rest); *electrocardiographic* (transient ST-segment elevation or pseudonormalization of basally negative T wave); *radioisotopic* (transient transmural defect in 201-Thallium uptake); *angiographic* (coronary vasospasm). *Continuous haemodynamic monitoring* was also performed in four patients, showing that increase in myocardial metabolic demand was not responsible for the ischaemic event since heart rate, systolic blood pressure, left ventricular end-diastolic pressure and dP/dt did not increase before the onset of electrocardiographic ischaemic changes.

Instrumentation and Protocol of the Study

M-mode and two-dimensional echocardiographic recordings were obtained by commercially available equipments: Echocardiovisor 03 (Organon Teknika) (only M-mode tracings) and SSD 800 (Aloka) (both M-mode and B-mode). The line of view, to explore left ventricular structures according to the standard position in M-mode, was obtained either by means of a single element focused transducer (24 episodes) or by appropriate line selection from two-dimensional images as obtainable by electronic equipments (ten episodes). The latter approach permitted to verify that the same regions of left ventricle were insonated throughout the study. Tracings were obtained by means of a fibre optic or dry silver recording system at a paper speed of 2·5 or 5·0 cm/s. Echocardiograms were continuously recorded during ischaemic episodes with ST-segment elevation or pseudonormalization of basally negative T wave in one or both of the following circumstances:

(a) From the appearance of electrocardiographic changes or onset of pain during a routine echo examination or, having the instrumentation ready at the bedside, in selected patients with frequent spontaneous ischaemic attacks at rest.

(b) During the ergonovine maleate test (from 0·025 to 0·2 mg i.v.), which reproduces ischaemic changes similar to the spontaneous ones.

During echocardiographic examination the selected electrocardiographic lead was the one where ischaemic changes had been observed in previously documented episodes.

In four patients echocardiograms were recorded simultaneously to haemodynamic monitoring, undertaken for diagnostic purposes, and left ventricular pressure with its dP/dt were superimposed on echo tracings (Chierchia *et al.*, 1980).

During each study, which could last up to several minutes, the operator held the transducer as stable as possible at the acoustic window.

Data Analysis

M-mode: tracings were selected according to criteria of sharpness of signals from right and left septal endocardium and from posterior wall endocardium and epicardium. Selected recordings were analysed by a previously described semi-automatic approach which includes a digitizer (HP 9874 A) linked by a HP–IB interface to a HP 1000/45 computer, network, some peripherals, magnetic tapes and electrostatic printer-plotters (Distante *et al.*, 1980). Blocks of at least four complete cardiac cycles were sampled by graph-pen every 10–20 s during the phase of induction (transient-in) and the phase of recovery (transient-off) of myocardial ischaemia or every 1–2 min during steady states. We digitized the outline of right and left septal endocardium, of posterior wall endocardium and epicardium, the onset of R wave on ECG and, when available, left ventricular pressure and peak dP/dt of contraction and relaxation. The following parameters were obtained from each block:

(a) Excursion, end-systolic and end-diastolic thickness, systolic percentual thickening of both septal and posterior walls.
(b) End-systolic and end-diastolic left ventricular internal diameter and percentual fractional shortening.
(c) Heart rate.
(d) Left ventricular systolic and end-diastolic pressure.
(e) Peak dP/dt of contraction and relaxation.

B-mode: two-dimensional images did not undergo any computer processing; therefore evaluation of regional and global left ventricular function was expressed on a purely qualitative basis.(Distante *et al.*, 1983).

Results

In 34 patients we recorded echocardiograms during 72 episodes (34 spontaneous and 38 ergonovine induced) of transient myocardial ischaemia at rest with ST-segment elevation. Thirty-four episodes were recorded by M-mode and 38 by two-dimensional technique.

Fifteen M-mode tracings were rejected because of poor quality of printed signals; most of the rejected tracings came from studies performed by single element transducer while only one came from the studies where a line of

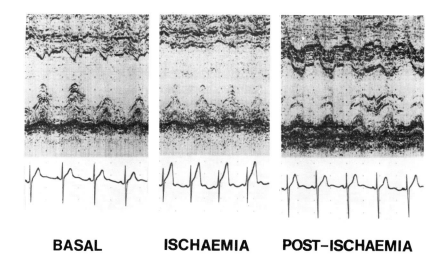

BASAL   ISCHAEMIA   POST–ISCHAEMIA

Figure 1.   Three blocks of an M-mode echocardiogram continuously recorded during a spontaneous ischaemic attack. On the left, under basal conditions (BASAL) the electrocardiogram (V_s) appears normal and left ventricular walls show normal movement and percentual systolic thickening. In the central panel, during ISCHAEMIA with ST-segment elevation (electrocardiogram on the bottom) interventricular septum shows a reduction in movement and highly reduced percentual systolic thickening and left ventricular cavity appears enlarged. On the right (POST-ISCHAEMIA) the electrocardiogram shows no ST-segment elevation; interventricular septum and posterior wall do move and do thicken more than under basal conditions with a consequent reduction in left ventricular cavity.

view had been selected from two dimensional images. By means of M-mode technique interpretable tracings were obtained and semiautomatically analysed in 19 episodes (eight spontaneous and 11 induced). Transient changes in left ventricular walls and cavity, as shown in Fig. 1, were observed in 17 episodes while in two episodes echocardiographic tracings, although good in quality, did not show any changes when compared to basal state.

Two dimensional technique allowed to detect such changes in all the studied patients (38 episodes). The results obtained are summarized as follows:

(1) Echocardiographic signs of ischaemia detectable by both M-mode and B-mode techniques: these signs occur in a well defined time sequence during the anginal episode (points a to d).
(2) Echocardiographic signs detectable by B-mode only (e).
(3) Temporal relationship with other clinical markers of ischaemia, such as electrocardiographic changes and anginal pain (f and g).
(4) Relationship between haemodynamic parameters (such as dP/dt and LV pressure) and echocardiographic indices (such as fractional shortening and left ventricular end diastolic diameter) (h, i).

Specific signs, sequence and relationship of echocardiographic changes due to myocardial ischaemia are reported below:

(a) Ischaemic wall shows, before the onset of ECG changes (in the 11 induced ischaemic attacks), an early *reduction of motion* (up to paradox in some cases) and *systolic thickening* (Fig. 2).

(b) *A diastolic thinning* of the ischaemic wall can become evident shortly before or contemporary to the onset of ECG changes.

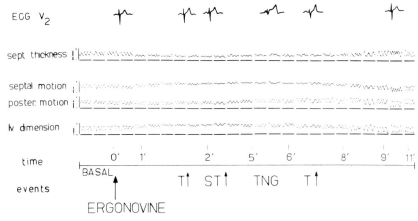

Figure 2. Computer print-out of an M-mode echocardiographic tracing, continuously recorded during an ischaemic attack induced by ergonovine maleate. On ordinate, from above to below, electrocardiogram (V₂), the interventricular septal thickness (SEPT. THICKNESS) which represents the ischaemic wall in this patient, the movement of posterior wall (POSTERIOR MOTION), left ventricular diameter (LV DIMENSION), time (TIME) and events (EVENTS). It can be observed that ECG changes follow initial echocardiographic alterations and that movement and thickness alterations of the ischaemic wall precede cardiac dilatation. In post-ischaemic phase (between 8 and 11 min), septum and posterior wall hyperkinesia, it can also be seen very likely due to nitroglycerin administration (TNG). Anginal pain was not reported by the patient in this episode.

(c) After the onset of ECG ischaemic changes, an *increase in left ventri-cular end-diastolic diameter (LVEDD)* is observed. By a two-dimensional technique, the ventricular cavity also appears globular-shaped in diastole and, most of the time, with a glass-hour shape in systole.

(d) At the resolution of the ischaemic attack, a *rebound phenomenon* is observed in some cases: that is, an increase above the basal values of wall thickness and left ventricular fractional shortening together with a decrease in LVEDD (Fig. 3).

(e) At the peak of the ischaemic phase, a phenomenon is detected in systole by B-mode only: the *"step-sign"*, that is an abrupt difference in systolic thickness between spatially adjacent zones (ischaemic and not contracting region near to normally perfused and normally con-tracting segment). As shown in Fig. 4, during ischaemia the proximal part of interventricular septum has a preserved thickening capacity, while the distal ischaemic part does not thicken at all, so that a sharp "step sign" is noted between the two zones.

(f) *Time sequence* of events shows that both surface ECG and onset of pain are late indicators of ischaemia, when compared to changes of ischaemic wall, detectable by echocardiography (Fig. 2).

(g) *Anginal pain* seems to correlate with acute cardiac dilatation, since it appeared when LVEDD was increased as compared to control value; this increase is usually observed 1–3 min after the onset of definite changes on the ischaemic wall.

(h) *Contraction and relaxation dP/dt*, already well known as very early indicators of ischaemia (Chierchia *et al.*, 1980), occur together with initial impairment of motion and thickening of the involved ischaemic wall.

(i) Increase in left ventricular end-diastolic pressure is not an early event in the ischaemic phenomenon, occurring as late as the echocardio-graphic event of ventricular dilatation.

Discussion

Our study demonstrates that M-mode technique was capable of detecting transient changes (both early and late) of left ventricular mechanics in more

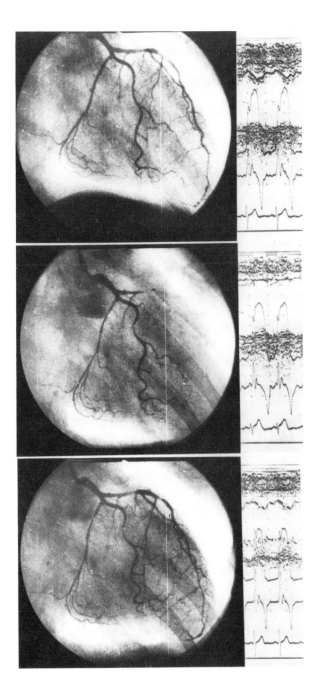

than one-half of the ischaemic episodes at rest with ST-segment elevation or pseudonormalization of basally negative T wave; on the contrary the two-dimensional technique allowed us to detect such alterations in all recorded ischaemic episodes, characterized by similar electrocardiographic changes (Distante *et al.*, 1983).

Such observations allow us to draw some conclusions:

(1) Myocardial ischaemia at rest is not preceded by an increase of any of the factors which raise myocardial oxygen consumption: left ventricular dimensions, contractility, systolic pressure, heart rate. This adds further evidence to the "proved hypothesis" that ischaemia at rest is very likely due to a reduction of coronary blood supply (Maseri, 1980).

(2) During ischaemia, besides the reduction of motion and systolic thickening, there is also a definite diastolic thinning of the involved wall; it is very likely that such a thinning is the indirect expression of a reduction in coronary blood flow. In dogs, indeed, end-diastolic wall thickness could vary up to 25% between the extremes of complete occlusion of the coronary artery on the one hand and reactive hyperaemia on the other (Gaasch and Bernard, 1977; Gaasch *et al.*, 1978).

(3) During ischaemia the onset of pain is not an early event, but rather it appears related to a certain increase in diastolic dimension (it disappears when ventricular dimensions go back toward normality) (Rovai *et al.*, 1980); such a finding appears to confirm previous experiments performed in animals in which a relation between fibre stretching and onset of painful stimuli has been postulated (Malliani and Lombardi, 1982).

(4) Some echocardiographic indices, such as wall motion and systolic thickening, do change together with well known early haemodynamic markers of ischaemia, such as dP/dt of contraction and relaxation. Moreover, left ventricular end-diastolic pressure seems to correlate with changes in left ventricular end-diastolic diameter. Therefore, it appears that a non-invasive monitoring of the ischaemic attack in the

---

Figure 3. Three blocks from a complete echocardiographic sequence of an ischaemic attack with ST elevation have been reported in order to show the rebound phenomenon of the ischaemic wall during the post-ischaemic phase. In this phase (lower panel), an increase of septal thickness and left ventricular fractional shortening above the basal values, suggesting an enhanced contractility, is well evident. Left coronary angiography obtained simultaneously to the echograms, shows a fixed stenosis on the anterior descending artery (DA) in basal conditions (upper panel). The injection of contrast during ST elevation demonstrates the full occlusion of the vessel, due to a coronary spasm at the level of a fixed stenosis (central panel). In the post-ischaemic phase (lower panel) the diameter of anterior descending artery appears diffusely increased relative to basal condition. This hyperaemic phase may provide the explanation for the "rebound phenomenon" observed by the echogram.

BASAL

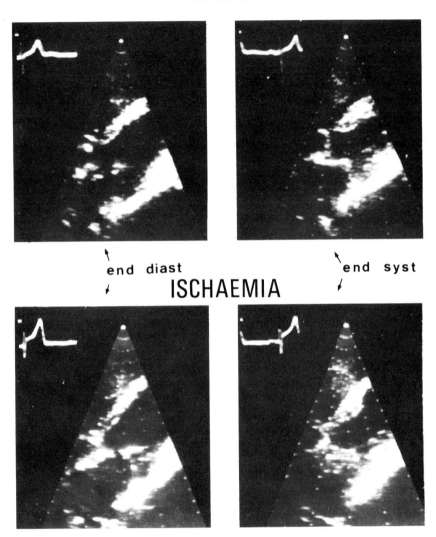

end diast   end syst

ISCHAEMIA

Figure 4.   Two-dimensional echocardiogram performed under basal conditions (BASAL) and during a spontaneous ischaemic attack with ST-segment elevation (ISCHEMIA). Basally the thickness of interventricular septum increases homogeneously throughout its length going from end-diastole (at left) to end-systole (at right), while during ST elevation the distal part of the septum does not thicken at all moving from end-diastole to end-systole. A sharp change is apparent between ischaemic and non-ischaemic area – "Step sign".

clinical setting might provide much of the information obtained – until now – only by invasive procedures.

The interest of such observations cannot, however, be confined to pathophysiology; according to our findings, echocardiography becomes a "candidate technique" for diagnostic work up of patients in whom traditional diagnostic techniques are inconclusive, particularly when (spontaneously or after provocative testing) symptomatology remains absent or atypical and electrocardiogram negative or not diagnostic.

In these situations echocardiography can indeed answer some crucial questions in the diagnosis of angina pectoris: "WHAT?" (ischaemia or not: is there any transient regional impairment in left ventricular mechanics?); "HOW?" (how great is the degree of mechanical impairment, and therefore the degree of ischaemia in the involved wall?); "WHERE?" (which wall of the left ventricle is transiently compromised?).

In conclusion, M-mode and two-dimensional echocardiography have something to offer in transient myocardial ischaemia, being not only a useful diagnostic tool, complementary to other techniques, but also helpful for a better understanding of the pathophysiological events of angina pectoris at rest in man.

Acknowledgements

We are grateful to Miss Emanuela Campani and Miss Daniela Banti for the secretarial assistance and to Mr Massimiliano Telleschi for the technical assistance.

References

Chierchia, S., Brunelli, C., Simonetti, I., Lazzari, M. and Maseri, A. (1980). *Circulation* **61**, 759.

Distante, A., Michelassi, C., Rovai, D., Benassi, A., Landini, L., Palombo, C., Pisani, P. and L'Abbate, A. (1980). *Comp. Cardiol.* IEEE Computer Society, Williamsburg, Virginia, USA, p. 219.

Distante, A., Rovai, D., Picano, E., Moscarelli, E., Morales, M. A., Palombo, C. and L'Abbate, A. (1983). *J. Am. Coll. Cardiol.* **1**, 633 (abstr.)

Feigenbaum, H. (1981). "Echocardiography", 3rd ed., p. 402. Lea and Febiger, Philadelphia.

Gaasch, W. H. and Bernard, S. A. (1977). *Circulation* **56**, 593–598.

Gaasch, W. H., Bing, O. H. L., Franklin, A., Rhodes, D., Bernard, S. A. and Weintraub, R. M. (1978). *Eur. J. Cardiol.* (suppl.) **7**, 147.

Gerson, M. C., Noble, R. J., Warm, L. S., Faris, J. N. and Morris, S. N. (1979). *Am. J. Cardiol.* **43**, 323.

Kerber, R. E., Marcus, M. L., Wilson, R., Erhardt, J. and Abbod, F. M. (1976). *Circulation* **54**, 928.

Kerber, R. E., Martins, J. B. and Marcus, M. L. (1979). *Circulation* **60**, 121.

Malliani, A. and Lombardi, F. (1982). *Am. Heart J.* **104**, 575–578.

Maseri, A. (1980). *Br. Heart J.* **43**, 648.

Maseri, A., Severi, S., De Nes, M. D., L'Abbate, A., Chierchia, S., Marzilli M., Ballestra, A. M., Parodi, O., Biagini, A. and Distante, A. (1978). *Am. J. Cardiol.* **42**, 1019.

Parodi, O., Uthurralt, N., Severi, S., Bencivelli, V., Michelassi, C., L'Abbate, A. and Maseri, A. (1981). *Circulation* **63**, 1238.

Rovai, D., Distante, A., L'Abbate, A., Palombo, C., Chierchia, S., Brunelli, C. and Maseri, A. (1980). "VIII European Congress of Cardiology", p. 71. Karger AG, Paris.

Widlansky, S., McHenry, P. L., Corya, B. C. and Phillips, J. F. (1975). *Am. Heart J.* **90**, 631.

Wild, J. J., Crawford, M. D. and Reid, J. M. (1957). *Am. Heart J.* **54**, 903.

Ultrasonic Characterization of Myocardial Tissue

J. G. MILLER

Laboratory for Ultrasonics, Department of
Physics, Washington University, St Louis,
Missouri, USA

Introduction

The long-term objective of the present research programme, which represents a collaboration between members of the Department of Physics and
members of the Cardiovascular Division under the direction of Burton E.
Sobel, MD, is the diagnostic detection and differentiation of specific types of
myocardial pathology *in vivo* non-invasively based on ultrasonic characterization of the tissue itself, as opposed to assessment of dimensions or motion.
The underlying hypothesis is that pathologic changes occurring in myocardium alter the physical properties of the tissue, and that these alterations
can be quantified with indexes based on the frequency dependences of the
ultrasonic attenuation and backscatter. Much of the work focuses on
ischaemic injury in part because of the need to detect it definitively and
quantify its progression and in part because of the wealth of information
available regarding its structural concomitants.

Background and Rationale

Ultrasound is used presently to image the heart non-invasively. However,
quantitative information defining the nature and extent of alterations in

Frontiers Cardiol. for the 80s.
0-12-220680-0

ultrasonic signals resulting from their interactions with normal and diseased tissue is not yet available. The present research is designed to obtain this information, to correlate the findings with independent biochemical criteria of tissue pathology, and to relate the ultrasonic properties of tissue to specific structural features and components.

Although myocardial scar tissue characterized by ventricular wall thinning or dyskinesis can be visualized qualitatively with conventional ultrasonic techniques, changes within the tissue itself have not been quantified (Kerber et al., 1975; Corya et al., 1976; Rasmussen et al., 1978). A number of techniques potentially useful in characterizing acoustic properties of tissue have been considered including impediography, scattering, and spectral analysis (Lele and Namery, 1972, 1974; Namery and Lele, 1972; Jones, 1972; Chivers et al., 1973; Waag and Lerner, 1973; Lizzi et al., 1976; Franklin et al., 1977). Lele and his colleagues addressed the question of whether the frequency dependence of ultrasonic attenuation might be a useful parameter for characterizing physical properties of myocardium associated with infarction (Lele and Namery, 1972, 1974; Namery and Lele, 1972). Our experimental approach employs the frequency dependence of attenuation and backscatter and has permitted characterization and differentiation of several disparate types of myocardial injury from normal in vitro and in vivo including: early ischaemic injury, completed infarction and adriamycin-induced cardiomyopathy (Mimbs et al., 1977, 1979).

Quantitative Tissue Characterization

Initial experiments in our laboratory were designed to test the hypothesis that changes in the physical properties of tissue which accompany myocardial infarction could be quantitatively detected in vitro with the use of an ultrasonic index based on the attenuation of transmitted ultrasound (as opposed to the more clinically applicable but analytically more complex reflected ultrasound). Although a method based on transmitted ultrasound does not lend itself well to clinical applications for the study of the heart, these experiments were designed as a first step to determine in the most direct fashion whether an index based on attenuation of ultrasound would be potentially capable of characterization of cardiac tissue. Myocardial injury was studied ultrasonically in two series of experiments, in investigations of animals subject to ischaemia of recent onset (minutes to hours after ligation of a major coronary artery) or remote myocardial infarction (weeks after ligation). Indexes based on ultrasonic measurements were compared with independent biochemical indexes of regional tissue injury such as creatine kinase (CK) depletion and hydroxyproline accumulation.

Our initial studies were designed to determine whether altered attenuation of transmitted ultrasound in zones of completed infarction quantitatively reflected ischaemic injury. Accordingly, we analyzed 44 regions of myocardium from 16 dogs 4–10 weeks after acute coronary artery occlusion. Attenuation of ultrasound was assessed by transmitting a broadband pulse through the tissue *in vitro* and gating the appropriate pulse into a spectrum analyser for Fourier transform analysis (frequency range 2–10 MHz). An ultrasonic index of attenuation was derived from the slope of the best fit line relating attenuation and frequency obtained from the Fourier transform. Myocardial creatine kinase content was assayed in all regions subjected to ultrasonic analysis. The extent of injury represented a range from none to severe (0–90% CK depletion). The ultrasonic index in each region correlated closely with regional CK depletion ($r = 0·80$). Thus, altered ultrasonic attenuation provides a quantitative index of regional tissue damage which could, in principle, be measured *in vivo* with the use of reflected ultrasound. Results of these studies were published in a manuscript form (Mimbs *et al.*, 1977).

A subsequent study (Mimbs *et al.*, 1979) was designed to determine whether quantitative alterations in ultrasonic attenuation were associated with changes occurring early after the onset of ischaemia, in contrast to completed, healed infarction. Specifically 517 regions of myocardium from 41 dogs were studied *in vitro* at five intervals after coronary occlusion: 15 min, 1 h, 6 h, 24 h, 3 days and 6 weeks. Quantitative indexes of ultrasonic attenuation were determined from the measured frequency dependence of the ultrasonic attenuation coefficient characterizing each myocardial region over the range 2–10 MHz. Independent definition of regions of ischaemic injury was provided by measurement of either creatine kinase depletion or colloidal carbon dye distribution. Results indicated that ischaemic myocardial regions characterized 15 min – 24 h after coronary occlusion demonstrated ultrasonic attenuation significantly decreased from that in non-ischaemic regions ($P < 0·05$). In contrast ultrasonic attenuation was significantly increased in zones of ischaemia or infarction characterized at 3 days and 6 weeks after coronary occlusion. Thus, decreased attenuation is an early manifestation of myocardial ischaemia in contrast to the increased attenuation typical of scar resulting from remote myocardial infarction.

Studies of tissue histopathology suggested the possible dependence of the altered ultrasonic properties observed on two factors, among others, namely water content and collagen content (Fields and Dunn, 1973; O'Brien, 1976). Clearly, regions of infarction exhibit increased collagen content, and oedema and swelling of mitochondria are significant early changes in myocardium rendered ischaemic (Blumgert *et al.*, 1940). Experiments conducted in our laboratory delineated quantitative relationships between ultrasonic attenuation and collagen content in hearts studied 2–11 weeks following coronary artery occlusion (O'Donnell *et al.*, 1979) and between ultrasonic properties and water content in isolated perfused heart experiments (Mimbs *et al.*, 1981).

To determine (O'Donnell *et al.*, 1979) whether increases in the ultrasonic attenuation of scar resulting from remote infarction might be attributable to increased collagen concentration, measurements were performed in hearts from 18 dogs studied at one of three intervals after coronary occlusion: 38 sites from six hearts at two weeks, 37 sites from six hearts at four weeks, and 35 sites from six hearts at six weeks. Ultrasonic analysis was performed on freshly excised myocardium within 5–45 min after the death of the animal by transmitting a broadband pulse (2–11 MHz) through the tissue. Ultrasonic indexes based on the attenuation coefficient measured as a function of frequency were determined. After ultrasonic analysis was completed, collagen content was determined in the same regions by assay of hydroxy-proline. Increases in slope of the attenuation correlated with increased regional collagen concentration in all three groups studied, with correlation coefficients $r = 0.90$ in hearts studied at six weeks, $r = 0.77$ and $r = 0.73$ in those studied four and six weeks after occlusion, respectively. Thus, collagen appears to be the principal determinant of increased attenuation in regions of scar resulting from infarct.

Because of anatomical constraints imposed by the position of the heart in the thorax, implementation of ultrasonic tissue characterization in the clinical setting requires the use of reflected rather than transmitted ultrasound. Consequently, we performed experiments with reflected ultrasound to determine quantitative values of the backscatter coefficient as a function of frequency. Backscatter is the energy redirected towards the transmitting transducer as the result of interactions with tissues. This parameter was assessed in normal and ischaemic myocardium of open-chest dogs, a preparation which avoided difficulties associated with propagating ultrasound through the intervening chest wall. Results indicated that backscatter can be used to detect acute myocardial ischaemia *in vivo*, with increased backscatter coefficient demonstrable as early as one hour after coronary ligation and with a 400% increase in backscatter over control as early as six hours after ligation (O'Donnell *et al.*, 1979; Mimbs *et al.*, 1981). These results suggest that methods of ultrasonic tissue characterization may permit early, clinical differentiation of ischaemic from normal myocardium.

In additional studies (Mimbs *et al.*, 1981) we have demonstrated that fibrotic regions of rabbit myocardium exposed to Adriamycin for 10–18 weeks exhibited significant increases in backscatter coefficient. Moderate, but significant increases in the parameter were present in myopathic but less fibrotic regions of myocardium. These findings correlated closely with local deposition of collagen. Thus, quantitative ultrasonic tissue characterization permits differentiation of normal from cardiomyopathic tissue.

In order to apply these observations in intact, closed-chest animals, and ultimately to patients, one salient experimental difficulty must be addressed – compensation for the variable amount of attenuation suffered by an ultrasonic signal as it propagates a round trip path through the intervening chest wall. Thus, an approach is required to estimate attenuation from reflected ultrasonic signals to provide a quantitative compensation for intervening tissue. Accurate estimates of attenuation will, of course, also provide the data needed for myocardial tissue characterization based on the same criteria which we have already shown to be capable of differentiating normal from ischaemic and scarred myocardium with transmitted ultrasound. Although several technically challenging obstacles remain, preliminary data from our laboratory indicates that quantitative tissue characterization can be carried out through the closed chests of dogs, thus suggesting that myocardial tissue characterization in patients may be feasible with appropriate extension of the present techniques.

References

Blumgert, H. R., Gilliginn, D. R. and Schlesinger, M. D. (1940). *Trans. Assoc. Am. Physicians* **55**, 313.
Chivers, R. C., Hill, C. R. and Nicholas, D. (1973). "Proceedings 2nd World Congress on Ultrasonics in Medicine", p. 300. Excerpta Medica, Rotterdam.
Corya, B. D., Rasmussen, S., Feigenbaum, H., Black, M. J. and Knoebel, S. B. (1976). *Am. J. Cardiol.* **37**, 129.
Fields, S. and Dunn, F. (1973). *J. acoust. Soc. Am.* **54**, 809.
Franklin, T. D. Jr, Sanghvi, N. T. and Fry, F. J. (1977). *In* "Ultrasound in Medicine", Vol. 3A (Ed., D. White). Plenum Press, New York.
Jones, J. (1972). "Proceedings of the 25th Annual Conference on Engineering in Medicine and Biology", **14**, 139.
Kerber, R. E., Marcus, M. L., Ehrhardt, J., Wilson, R. and Abboud, F. M. (1975). *Circulation* **52**, 1097.
Lele, P. P. and Namery, J. (1972). *In* "Proceedings of 25th Annual Conference on Engineering in Medicine and Biology", **14**, 135.
Lele, P. P. and Namery, J. (1974). *In* "Proceedings of San Diego Biomedical Symposium", **13**, 121.
Lizzi, F., Katz, L. Stilouis, L. and Coleman, D. J. (1976). *Ultrasonics* **13**, 77.
Mimbs, J. W., Yuhas, D. E., Miller, J. G., Weiss, A. N. and Sobel, B. E. (1977). *Circ. Res.* **41**, 192.
Mimbs, J. W., O'Donnell, M., Miller, J. G. and Sobel, B. E. (1979). *Am. J. Physiol.* **236**, H340.
Mimbs, J. W., Bauwens, D., Cohen, R. D., O'Donnell, M., Miller, J. G. and Sobel, B. E. (1981a). *Circ. Res.* **49**, 89.
Mimbs, J. W., O'Donnell, M., Miller, J. G. and Sobel, B. E. (1981b). *Am. J. Cardiol.* **47**, 1056.
Namery, J. and Lele, P. P. (1972). "IEEE 1972 Ultrasonics Symposium Proceedings", **72**, CHO 708–8, SU:491.
O'Brien, W. D. (1976). *In* "Acoustical Holography", Vol. 7, (Ed. L. Kessler). Plenum Press, New York.
O'Donnell, M., Mimbs, J. W. and Miller, J. G. (1979a). *J. acoust. Soc. Am.* **65**, 512.
O'Donnell, M., Bauwens, D., Mimbs, J. W. and Miller, J. G. (1979b). "Proceedings of IEEE Ultrasonics Symposium", **79**, CH 1482–9: 175.
Rasmussen, S., Corya, B. C., Feigenbaum, H. and Knoebel, S. B. (1978). *Circulation* **57**, 230.
Waag, R. C. and Lerner, R. M. (1973). "Proceedings of 1973 IEEE Ultrasonics Symposium", p. 63.

External Measurement of Myocardial Metabolism in Patients: Progress Using Positron Tomography

A. P. SELWYN

Royal Postgraduate Medical School, University of London, Cardiovascular Research Unit, MRC Cyclotron Unit, Hammersmith Hospital, London, UK

Introduction

In the past our knowledge of cardiac disorders was based mainly on history, examination and pathology. More recently the non-invasive techniques and catheterization have provided more insight into diagnosis and management. Nevertheless, a rational approach to treatment requires an understanding of the pathophysiological mechanisms of heart disease and this means that we need to measure disturbances of regional myocardial perfusion and metabolism in patients with coronary and other forms of heart disease. Positron emission transaxial tomography (PETT) is an attempt to accurately measure the physiological events in the myocardium. This summary presents progress in this field.

Frontiers Cardiol. for the 80s.
0-12-220680-0

Methods and Principles

PETT utilizes a ring of detectors positioned around the patient to encircle a plane of view that transects the heart. If opposing detectors are designed to register the coincidence photons from positron annihilation then multiple projections can be recorded and back projected in a computer. In this way the true distribution of positron emitting tracers can be measured in real space within the field of view. Calibration with known activity, correction for tissue attenuation, a linear response and stable sensitivity allows the method to recover the true concentration of tracer if the object is > 3 cm^3.

A variety of tracers emit positrons and some of these are listed below.

Nuclide	Source	$T_{1/2}$	Potential Application
^{82}Rb	Generator	78 s	Regional myocardial uptake of cations – detection of ischaemia
^{13}NH^{4+}	Cyclotron	13 min	Regional myocardial uptake of ammonia – detection of ischaemia
^{11}C labelled acetate palmitate	Cyclotron	20 min	Estimates of myocardial
^{18}F-deoxyglucose	Cyclotron	110 min	substrate metabolism
^{68}Ga	Generator	68 min	Microsphere – blood flow cell labelling
^{15}O as CO$_2$		123 s	Tissue water and calculation
^{11}CO		20 min	of perfusion

The above list is not complete but it does demonstrate that the tracers and molecules are short-lived and physiological.

Progress and Problems to Date

Tracers

The development of suitable compounds requires complex radiochemistry and long-term planning. The sources for ^{82}Sr – ^{82}Rb are limited, an on-line cyclotron is required for ^{13}N, ^{15}O and ^{11}C and the ^{68}Ge – ^{68}Ga generator and microsphere labelling are not yet perfected. These are just a few of the problems. In addition, the dose to the patient is a constant problem using positron emitting isotopes.

External Detectors

The commercially available instruments only record one plane through the heart and the limited sensitivity means that transient events in patients are difficult to record. Spatial resolution is limited by the instrument, statistics, heart movement and respiration. The dimensions of the left ventricular wall are significantly smaller than the dimensions required for resolution and measurement of the true concentration. The systematic loss of counts due to this effect has to be considered.

Physiological Measurements

If an available tracer can safely provide tomograms of the myocardium the investigators must then determine the physiological parameters that dominate the signals obtained.

(1) ^{82}Rb can be used to measure the regional myocardial (RM) uptake of the cation which does not measure flow alone, but can detect acute transient ischaemia.

(2) ^{11}C-acetate and palmitate can provide elimination rates that are related to RM oxygen consumption. The relationship to flow and effects of intermediate and alternative metabolic pathways must still be determined.

(3) ^{18}F-deoxyglucose can be used to measure the uptake of this analogue in tomography of the myocardium. Lump constants related to flux rates of "hot" and "cold" glucose are unknown and so are the effects of permeability and the metabolism governing uptake of this analogue. These must be determined before the RM utilization of glucose can be measured.

(4) $C^{15}O_2$ by inhalation will provide a measure of the extravascular concentration of short-lived water at equilibrium. The further calculation of perfusion requires investigations regarding the accuracy of measuring the myocardial and arterial concentrations.

All the physiological substrates used as tracers require an independent measure of flow to substantiate any changes in metabolic state. Elimination rates of ^{11}C-acetate can be measured in patients and experiments have shown that these measurements are not significantly changed by changes in flow. The external detection of the myocardial handling of these substrates will never provide detailed biochemical resolution of events in the myocardium. Therefore, it is necessary to understand the effects of different physiological states on the kinetics of the tracer before any clinical application.

Discussion and Progress to Date

PETT represents at present the most accurate way to quantify tracer concentrations in different regions of the myocardium in patients.

The clinical work has shown that absolute decreases in the RM uptake of cations occur in transient ischaemia. These ischaemic events can be prolonged for much longer than the ECG and symptoms would suggest. Ischaemic myocardium can be positively identified using ^{11}C-acetate and ^{18}F-deoxyglucose. Some of the problems have been outlined in this summary. However, the technical, physiological and clinical achievements do suggest that quantitation can be obtained in patients and these are beginning to measure different aspects of RM perfusion and metabolism. Because this may help to understand the mechanisms causing a variety of cardiac disorders this approach seems promising.

The evidence so far suggests that PETT should be used for the following purposes:

(1) *Improved diagnosis* by correlation with and improved understanding of the commonly available clinical tools (e.g. electrocardiogram).
(2) *Improved understanding of pathophysiological mechanisms* that cause myocardial ischaemia and heart muscle failure.
(3) *Initial and objective assessment of the effects of treatments* for transient ischaemia in coronary disease and metabolic derangement in heart muscle failure.

Acknowledgements

The author wishes to acknowledge the support of the British Heart Foundation.

References

Selwyn, A. P., Allan, R. M., L'Abbate, A., Horlock, P., Camici, P., Clark, J., O'Brien, H. and Grant, P. M. (1982). *Am. J. Cardiol.* **50**, 112–121.
Weis, E. S., Siegal, B. A., Sobel, B. *et al.* (1978). *In* "Principles of Cardiovascular Nuclear Medicine" (Eds, Holman, B. D., Sonnenblick, E. H. and Lesch, M.). Grune and Stratton, London.

Technology Assessment in Cardiology

L. DONATO

Institute of Patologia Medica, University of
Pisa, and Institute of Clinical Physiology, CNR,
Pisa, Italy

Technology Assessment in Cardiology

According to the definition of the National Health Care and Technology Centre of NIH, technology assessment is described as "a form of research, analysis and evaluation that attempts to examine the various impacts of a particular technology on the individual and society in terms of safety, efficacy, effectiveness, and cost-effectiveness, and its social, economic and ethical implications, and to identify those areas requiring further research, demonstration or evaluation".

Under the term "technologies" are currently included all kinds of procedures, drugs, devices or equipment used in the delivery of health services for prevention, diagnosis, treatment of illness and rehabilitation.

Over the last ten years the issue of technological assessment has become a very hot one, and a territory of conflict between the medical profession (claiming that progress cannot be denied to the patient, and advocating clinical judgement as the only ethically acceptable decisional tool for the use of a new technology) and health care specialists and administrators stressing the need for more systematic and possibly objective assessment of the actual value of new technological developments.

The real and practical problem facing the health care system in presence of continuously rising costs and continuous development of new technologies, is how to prevent their uncontrolled introduction into practice, without obstructing diffusion of new and possibly advantageous innovation.

Cardiology has been one of the areas of medicine in which new technologies have been introduced at a faster rate over the last few decades, and are likely to continue to be so in the next decade, as has been shown during this conference. Proposed innovations have ranged from screening methods, preventive interventions, early diagnostic approaches, quantitation and visualization of disease states, treatment of acute phase or chronic illness, replacement of defective structures, artificial organs and rehabilitation procedures.

Usually it is relatively easier to establish the technical performance of a technology and its safety than to draw conclusions on its clinical value and cost-effectiveness. As an example it is relatively easy to establish whether a venous graft implant is adequate to restore flow in an occluded coronary vessel, and to assess the risk of the operation, but it is much more complex to establish the actual value of the procedure to the patient.

In the assessment of the clinical value of a technology a very large number of variables come into play. They include:

– the kind of technology (drug, physical method, device, equipment, laboratory procedure, etc.; invasive, non-invasive, automated, manual, etc.);
– the purpose of use (preventive, diagnostic, used for treatment, rehabilitation, etc.);
– the class of subjects for which its use is proposed (healthy individuals, subjects at risk, acutely ill patients, chronically ill subjects, etc.; young or old, male or female);
– characteristics and expertise of the provider (self administration, general physician, specialist office, out-patient department, hospital ward, operating theatre, etc.);
– expected consequences of the intervention in terms of decision or effect;
– time lag between application of the technology and the expected consequences;
– side- and/or undesirable effects;
– availability of alternative approaches.

The above list could be indefinitely extended if it had to cover all possible combinations in which the practical application of a technology may take place: no wonder the problem of assessing the clinical value is so complex. As a matter of fact, no satisfactory nor systematic definition of means and ways to this critical aspect of technological assessment is yet available.

We shall attempt here to develop a few considerations on this topic; they do not pretend to establish guidelines, but simply to attract the attention of the physician on a critical area.

First of all an attempt should be made to *separate the technical performance and safety aspects* from those of the clinical relevance: in most instances the main element in performance is not the technology itself but the provider and the population to which it is applied. This is well known in the clinical chemistry laboratory, and it has led to the development of inter- and intra-laboratories quality control in terms of precision and accuracy, sensitivity and specificity, predictive value of positive or negative results. Very limited efforts are currently made to extend this approach to functional diagnosis, monitoring and imaging techniques. Examples from this conference concern inter-observer variability in the examination of the ocular fundus (Ghione and Donato, this volume, p. 35), and the sensitivity in detecting ischaemic episodes in the CCU (Biagini *et al.*, this volume, p. 61). They should be extended to the variety of procedures used in diagnostic cardiology.

Assessment of technical performance and safety of therapeutic technology in a specific environment should also become a regular procedure both at a medical and surgical level: in general, more critical attention should be given and more detailed reporting should be made available, on the dependence on the provider's ability, and resources of the resulting performance and on the safety of applying a certain technology in a given environment. A good example is represented by the prediction of mortality at operation in coronary surgery.

Assuming that technical performance and safety could be covered, we are back to the problem of assessing the clinical value of a diagnostic or therapeutic procedure. The main difficulty is that only very few technological developments are "critical" in the sense that their successful application will produce a clear-cut, non-ambiguous, and important effect on the therapeutic decision or on the course of the illness.

The visualization of a narrowed calcific mitral ring by echocardiography may be critical in order to decide whether a patient should be operated or not; the application of a cardiac pacemaker may be critical in order to restore an adequate heart rate in a patient with A–V block; the detection of an increased CK level after chest pain with ambiguous ECG may be critical for the diagnosis of myocardial infarction. In all these cases there is *a clear connection between the use of a given technology and the production of an effect of critical "clinical" importance.*

In most instances the clinical relevance of the technology is much less obvious: most often a specific and critical consequence cannot be identified because of lack of adequate knowledge of the disease pathophysiology and consequently *lack of identification of a specific decisional or therapeutic role of the technology.* From this conference it has come out, for instance, that systematic renin assay in arterial hypertension seems to be of limited value In these latter cases of therapeutic technologies lacking immediate and obvious clinical relevance of the produced effect, *assessment of their clinical value requires the definition of a rigid protocol.* Such a protocol may take two forms. The first is in fact a kind of *long-term appraisal of the performance of a therapeutic technology in selected groups of patients*: criteria for patients selection, classification, functional, anatomical and pathological assessment, standardization of procedure, scheduling and content of their follow-up, are the essential components of such studies. Examples from this conference are the protocols for surgical intervention in patients with arrhythmias by Dr Bentall (p. 215), that for pediatric cardiac surgery by Dr Chalant (p. 209), and that for heart transplantation by Dr English (p. 203). If carefully conducted for a sufficiently long time these studies will permit a retrospective analysis in which it will be possible to relate the outcome of the technological intervention with the conditions at entry in the study, and consequently to set up some *predictory schemes for better selection of patients* for that particular technological application.

One of the risks of such studies may be that of missing a positive result because of inappropriate selection of patients: a typical case is that reported by Dr Gattinoni (p. 235) in which a first trial on Extra–Corporeal Membrane Oxygenation in patients with Adult Respiratory Distress Syndrome gave poor results in comparison with standard treatment partly because inappropriate criteria for selection of patients, while lowering criteria for patient admission and modification of the protocol reversed the judgement on the clinical value of the method.

The second approach is that of the so-called *clinical controlled trials*, in which patients are randomized between different forms of treatment which are then tested one against the other. This approach can be very productive, provided the end-points are very clearly identified, and the characterization of the patients is adequate. The practical value of these studies, however, depends heavily on the size of the population required to give statistical significance to the difference between the two forms of treatment, the extent of the difference, the duration of the study, the nosographic homogeneity of the subjects entered in the study (which in turn is a function of the knowledge of the pathophysiology of the disease), the possible multiplicity of effects of the tested treatment, and the evolution of knowledge on the disease and its treatment during the study.

For instance, assessment of the actual clinical value of multi-annual studies of coronary artery bypass surgery requires taking into account the evolution in pharmacological treatment which has occurred during the years of the study, and the evolution in the conception of angina with identification of subgroups with primary or secondary angina.

Finally great care should always be taken in extrapolating the results of a population trial to the individual patients. One should always remember, for instance, that *the same level of mortality for two different forms of treatment in the same disease, might not mean that the two treatments are equivalent*: it could be that the subjects who would have died if submitted to the first treatment have survived when exposed to the second treatment, which in turn has not prevented the death of an equal number of subjects which would have survived if submitted to the first treatment. This would express the actual inhomogeneity of the apparently homogenous group of patients which has been submitted to the trial and it stresses the need on the one hand for adequate characterization of the patients entering a trial, and on the other for careful extrapolation of the results of trials to daily practice.

Are we then facing a hopeless situation? Certainly not, although a very complex one. But these difficulties should stimulate the intelligence and the responsibility of the physicians for better design of protocols and better interpretation of the data. They should also discourage too rapid incorporation of new technologies in everyday practice, before reasonable and objective evidence of their value has been produced by studies of adequate size and design.

Index